ALLE · ZEIT · WACH · 1842

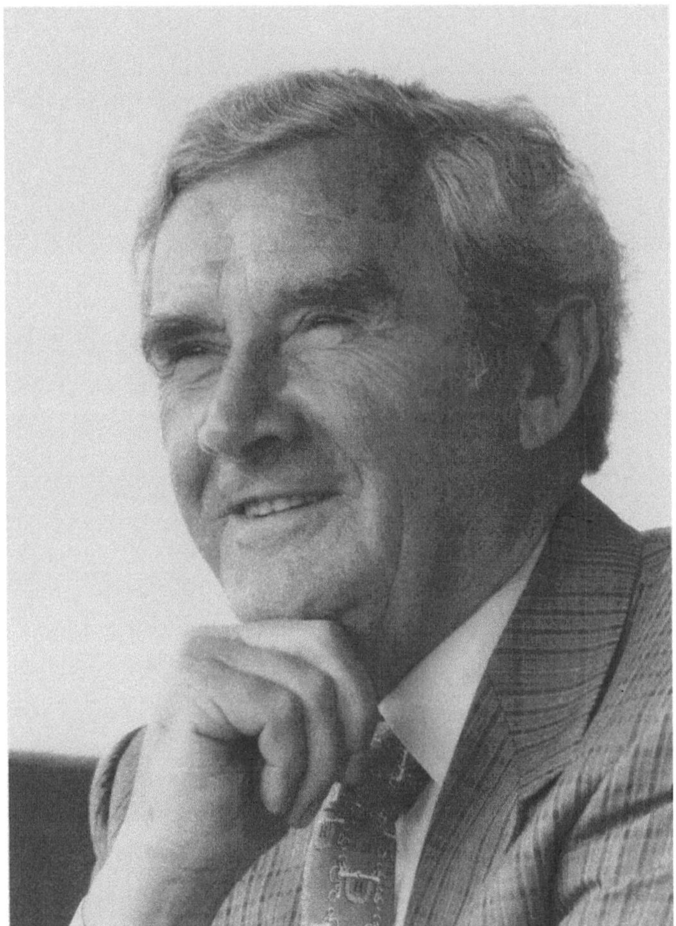

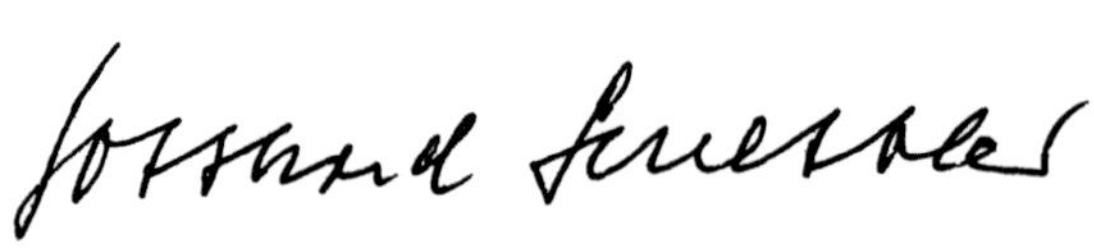

G. Schlierf H. Mörl (Eds.)

Expanding Horizons in Atherosclerosis Research

To Gotthard Schettler on his 70th Birthday

With 89 Figures and 75 Tables

Springer-Verlag
Berlin Heidelberg New York
London Paris Tokyo

Prof. Dr. Günter Schlierf
Klinisches Institut für Herzinfarktforschung,
Medizinische Universitätsklinik
Bergheimer Straße 58, 6900 Heidelberg, FRG

Prof. Dr. Hubert Mörl
Innere Abteilung am Diakonissenkrankenhaus
Mannheim, Speyerer Straße 91-93, 6800 Mannheim 1, FRG

Cover picture: Exposed foam cells after 3 months of hypercholesterolemia. A lipid-laden macrophage can be seen in what is interpreted as egress from the artery wall in a monkey that had been on the diet for 3 months. Note the numerous lamellipodia at the luminal aspects of the cell that suggest that its direction of motion may be into the arterial lumen. Bar = 10 u.

Source: Agostino Fagiotto, Russell Ross, Laurence Harker: Studies of hypercholesterolemia in the nonhuman primate. Arteriosclerosis 4: 323-340, 1984

ISBN-13: 978-3-642-71755-0 e-ISBN-13: 978-3-642-71753-6
DOI: 10.1007/978-3-642-71753-6

Library of Congress Cataloging-in-Publication Data. Expanding horizons in atherosclerosis research. Includes bibliographies. 1. Atherosclerosis-Congresses. 2. Schettler, Gotthard. I. Schettler, Gotthard. II. Schlierf, Günter. III. Mörl, Hubert. (DNLM: 1. Arteriosclerosis. WG 550 E96) RC692.E97 1987 616.1'36 87-4287

Softcover reprint of the hardcover 1st edition 1987

Preface

On 29 February 1964, a group of European scientists met in Paris to discuss a subject of common interest, namely atherosclerosis research, with particular reference to international communication and collaboration. After a second meeting on 15 May 1964, they founded the European Atherosclerosis Group which was to comprise individuals engaged in the various disciplines of atherosclerosis research in Eastern and Western Europe. Since then this group has initiated multidisciplinary discussion and scientific collaboration across Europe, in accordance with the objects and aims written in its statutes:

1. To hold colloquia and symposia dealing with research in the field of atherosclerosis and allied sciences
2. To encourage meetings and exchanges between scientists in the group engaged in the investigation of atherosclerosis
3. To encourage collaborative work between national and international centers engaged in atherosclerosis research
4. To encourage the publication of reviews, etc., on atherosclerosis research which may be considered of value
5. To promote research fellowships, particularly for younger research workers, for studies within the field of atherosclerosis and allied sciences
6. To accept dues, endowments, grants, funds, and bequests to be used for the above purposes

The European Atherosclerosis Group has helped to bring together what was separated during the second world war and the postwar period in Europe and to reestablish ties with the leading American teams. One or two meetings per year in member and nonmember countries have dealt with subjects of acute interest at the time, and the list of topics now gives a historical view of research frontiers as they have been seen during the last three decades.

The European Atherosclerosis Group was also instrumental in promoting first the International Symposia on Atherosclerosis and later the International Atherosclerosis Society, which by now has more than 4000 members in some 24 countries all over the world.

Gotthard Schettler was the group's first chairman and has steered it for 10 years. His wide range of interests in the field of atherosclerosis research, his integrating power, and his sincere interest in the people who are behind scientific achievements, meant that he continued to support the group's activities when the chairmanship moved to his scientist friends Lars Carlson, Jean Louis Beaumont, and Rodolfo Paoletti.

It is in honour of and as a tribute to Professor Schettler that, with hardly any exceptions, the members have contributed to this volume. With great mourning we regret that the contribution of Esko Nikkilä "Lowering of LDL or raising HDL: which is more important?" could not be delivered because of the death in a traffic accident of this eminent scientist and founding member of the European Atherosclerosis Group. From pathogenesis and morphology to risk factors, therapy and prevention, this monograph gives an integrated and up-to-date review of a topic which has not only stimulated fascinating research, as evidenced by the Nobel prize-winning work of Goldstein and Brown, but is of the greatest impact on health policy in affluent countries.

With their contributions, all the members of the group and his friends within the scientific community express their best wishes on the occasion of the 70th birthday of Prof. Dr. Dr. h. c. mult. Gotthard Schettler.

Many happy returns!

Heidelberg, April 1987

Günter Schlierf
Hubert Mörl

European Atherosclerosis Group Meetings

No.	Date	Place	Chairman	Title of meeting
1	29 February 1964	Paris	J. Cottet	Business only
2	18 May 1964	Milan	S. Garattini	Business only
3	7 November 1964	Milan	S. Garattini	Plasma lipids and atherosclerosis
4	28 May 1965	Heidelberg	G. Schettler	International Symposium on Pathophysiological and clinical aspects of lipid metabolism
5	15 September 1965	Milan	R. Paoletti	International Symposium on Drugs affecting lipid metabolism
6	8 January 1966	Basle	A. Studer	The Duguid hypothesis
7	29 May 1966	Athens	C. J. Miras	International Symposium on Recent advances in atherosclerosis
8	6 January 1967	Milan	S. Garattini	Drugs affecting FFA metabolism
9	27 September 1967	Leiden	F. Böttcher	Metabolic and transport processes in the arterial wall
10	28 March 1968	Munich	N. Zöllner	Experimental nutrition and vascular disease
11	10 September 1968	Milan	R. Paoletti	International Symposium on Drugs affecting lipid metabolism
11 A	13 December 1968	London	G. S. Boyd	Triglycerides
12	16 June 1969	Frankfurt	G. Schettler	Platelets and fibrin deposition
13	1 November 1969	Chicago	R. Wissler	International Symposium on atherosclerosis
14	19 October 1970	Lindau	G. Schettler	International Symposium on Fundamental data on reactions of vascular tissue in man
15	29 October 1970	Paris	J. L. Beaumont	Les lipoprotéines du sang et de la paroi artérielle
16	25 April 1971	Brussels	H. Peeters/ H. Vastesaeger	Risk factors in coronary heart disease
17	7 September 1971	Philadelphia	W. Holmes	Drugs affecting lipid metabolism
18	14 April 1972	Oberursel	G. Schettler	Lipid metabolism, obesity and diabetes mellitus: impact upon atherosclerosis
19	11 October 1972	Munich	N. Zöllner	Symposium on Xanthoma formation and other tissue reactions to hyperlipidemia
20	13 April 1973	Rome	P. Ricci/R. Paoletti	Plasma lipids and lipoproteins
21	27 October 1973	Berlin	G. Schettler	IIIrd International Symposium on Atherosclerosis
23	29 May 1974	Stockholm	L. A. Carlson	Tissue utilization of lipids

24	8 September 1974	Milan	R. Paoletti	Vth Symposium on Drugs affecting lipid metabolism
25	21 May 1975	Venice	P. Avogaro	Genetic versus environmental factors in atherosclerosis
26	2 September 1975	London, Ontario	D. Haust	International Workshop Conference on atherosclerosis
27	27 May 1976	Athens	C. J. Miras	Lipid clinics, screening and early detection of disease
28	26 August 1976	Tokyo	Y. Goto	IVth International Symposium on Atherosclerosis
29	6 May 1977	Brügge	H. Peeters	Comparative aspects of lipoproteins
30	10 November 1977	Milan	R. Paoletti	International Conference on Atherosclerosis
31	10 May 1978	Paris	J. L. Beaumont	Evaluation of advances in the methods in use for atherosclerosis Research
32	28 September 1978	Capri	M. Mancini	Nutrition and other environmental factors as related to atherosclerosis
33	17 May 1979	Dresden	M. Hanefeld	Interrelation of physical activity, lipid metabolism and atherosclerosis
34	8 November 1979	Houston	A. M. Gotto Jr.	Vth International Symposium on Atherosclerosis
35	30 May 1980	Milan	R. Paoletti	VIIth International Symposium on Drugs affecting lipid metabolism
36	24 September 1980	Cambridge	A. N. Howard	Animal models in atherosclerosis research
37	25 May 1981	Padua	G. Crepaldi	Atherosclerotic brain disease
38	2 October 1981	Lugano	G. Noseda	Lipoproteins and coronary atherosclerosis
39	15 June 1982	Berlin	G. Schettler/ G. Schlierf	VIth International Symposium on atherosclerosis
40	7 October 1982	Paris	J. L. de Gennes	Latent dyslipoproteinemia
41	3 June 1983	Stockholm	L. A. Carlson/ A. G. Olsson	Treatment of hyperlipoproteinemia
42 a	28 July 1983	Philadelphia	D. Kritchevsky	VIIIth International Symposium on Drugs affecting lipid metabolism
42 b	9 September 1983	Athens	C. J. Miras	Atherosclerosis in developing countries
43	5 March 1984	Munich	N. Zöllner	Genetics of vascular disease
44	5 October 1984	Perugia	L. Ventura/ G. Crepaldi	Extracoronary atherosclerosis
45	14 March 1985	Montreux	D. Pometta	Dyslipoproteinemias, diabetes and atherosclerosis
46	6 October 1985	Melbourne	P. Nestel	VIIth International Symposium on atherosclerosis
47	18 June 1986	Naples	M. Mancini	Biochemical evaluation of the coronary patient

Table of Contents

Pathogenesis and Morphology

Pathogenesis of Atherosclerosis: - Current Status
M. Daria Haust 3

The Extracellular Matrix of the Vessel Wall, Its Role and Modification During the Atherosclerotic Process
L. Robert 13

Changing Views of the Morphology of Atherosclerosis
G. A. Gresham 23

Atherosclerosis as a Recurrent Cycle of Inflammation and Repair
C. W. M. Adams 27

Non-Arterial Deposition of Lipids and Lipoproteins: Significance in Relation to Atherogenesis
K. W. Walton 39

On the Role of Lipoprotein Antibody Immuno Complexes in Atherogenesis
A. N. Klimov 52

Role of Different Agents Affecting Endothelial Cells in the Process of Atherosclerosis - In Vitro Examinations
H. Jellinek, E. Csonka, A. Somogyi, and E. Takács 59

On the Delayed Experimental Pathologic Involvement of Cerebral Arteries in Hypercholesterolemic Monkeys, Rabbits and Spontaneously Hypertensive Rats
G. Weber, L. Resi, and P. Tanganelli 70

Enzyme-Acylalcohol-Alcohol Interactions in the Arterial Wall
J. Patelski, T. Szwajca, and K. Świdzińska 76

The Effect of Balloon De-Endothelialization on Arterial Enzymes and Metabolic Intermediates in Rabbits
T. Zemplenyi, D. W. Crawford, D. F. Tidwell, and M. A. Cole . 82

Epidemiology, Risk Factors

Coronary Heart Disease Epidemiology – Perspectives
F. H. Epstein 89

Obesity and Cardiovascular Disease
P. Björntorp 96

Lipoproteins and Apolipoproteins in the Prediction of Coronary Artery Disease
G. Assmann 102

Prevalence of Hyperlipidaemia in British Compared with North American Men
G. R. Thompson, D. Robinson, S. L. Allaway, E. A. Bevan, and C. D. Ritchie 114

Low-Density Lipoprotein: Its Metabolic Determinants and Its Role in Coronary Heart Disease
B. Lewis 122

Plasma Levels of Lipoproteins and Apolipoproteins in Octo- and Nonagenarians
P. Avogaro, G. Bittolo-Bon, G. Cazzolato, A. Bottecchia, and R. Brugiolo 126

Cholesteryl Ester Transfer, Lipoproteins, Hypertriglyceridemia, and Atherosclerosis
S. Eisenberg 132

Importance of Hypertriglyceridemia as an Independent Risk Factor: Investigations with Familial Combined Hyperlipidemia and Familial Hypertriglyceridemia
M. Hanefeld 140

The Plasma Lipoproteins in Hypertriglyceridemia as Risk Factors for Atherosclerosis
G. Crepaldi and E. Manzato 147

Myocardial Infarction in Women on Oral Contraceptives: Risk Factors and Mechanism
V. Beaumont and J. L. Beaumont 153

Combined Oral Contraceptives: From Risk to Benefit?
L. W. Hessel 161

Bile Acids, Lipoproteins, and Atherosclerosis
B. Angelin 165

Metabolic Abnormalities in Cerebral and Peripheral Arteriosclerosis
R. Fellin and G. Valerio 173

Elastase-Type Enzymes and Their Relation to Blood Lipids and Atherosclerosis
M. Bihari-Varga and L. Keller 180

DNA Polymorphisms for the Genetic Analysis of Atherosclerosis
D. J. Galton 187

Lipoproteins

Chylomicron Catabolism and Uptake by the Liver
E. Windler and H. Greten 197

Lipoprotein Lipase, Synthesis and Regulation
O. Stein, Y. Stein, G. Friedmann, and T. Chajek-Shaul 204

Structural and Clinical Aspects of the Plasma Phospholipid Subclasses
V. Blaton and D. Hollez 213

Irregular Working Hours and Lipid Levels in Men
G. de Backer, M. Kornitzer, M. Dramaix, H. Peeters, and F. Kittel 217

Identification and Computer Modeling of Functional Domains in Plasma Apolipoproteins
M. Rosseneu, H. de Loof, R. Brasseur, and J. M. Ruysschaert . 225

New Perspectives in Human Apolipoprotein B Metabolism
J. Shepherd and C. J. Packard 236

Fish Eye Disease: Implications for the Understanding of Cardiovascular Disease and Plasma Lipoprotein Metabolism
L. A. Carlson and L. Holmquist 242

Diabetes

Vascular Growth Factors and Atherogenesis in Diabetes Mellitus
T. Koschinsky and F. A. Gries 251

Cholesterol Biosynthesis in Diabetes Mellitus
E. Andersén and K. Hellström 260

Effects of Diet Fat Composition on Serum Lipids and Lipoproteins in Patients with Insulin-Dependent Diabetes Mellitus
J. Boberg, L. Abrahamsson, C. Berne, I.-B. Gustafsson, and T. Pollare 264

Platelets and Thrombosis

β_2-Glycoprotein-I (Apolipoprotein H): Possible Role in Platelet Activation and Coagulation
J. Nimpf and G. M. Kostner 273

Diet, Lipoproteins and Atherosclerosis

Changes in Diet, Serum Cholesterol, and Mortality from Coronary Heart Disease in Spain
R. Carmena 283

Modified Fat Diets and Serum Lipoproteins
P. Schwandt and P. Weisweiler 286

Essential Fatty Acids, Marine Oils, Olive Oil and Coronary Heart Disease
M. F. Oliver 293

What Are the Alpha-Linolenic Acid Supplies to Be Recommended to the Normal Adult?
B. Jacotot 299

Animal and Vegetable Protein Effects in Experimental Atherosclerosis
D. Kritchevsky 304

Food Proteins and Atherosclerosis
G. Debry 309

Cholesterol-Lowering and High-Density Lipoprotein-Raising Properties of Lecithinated Soy Proteins in Type II Hyperlipidemic Patients
G. Noseda, C. R. Sirtori, and G. C. Descovich 317

Prevention and Therapy

From Theory to Practice: Community-Based Studies on the Prevention of Coronary Heart Disease
P. Puska 323

Regression of Atherosclerosis in Man
A. G. Olsson 329

Plasma Exchange and Its Development in the Treatment of Familial Hypercholesterolemia
M. Mancini, A. Postiglione, and A. Gnasso 338

The HELP System: A Novel Technique for the Extracorporeal Treatment of Familial Hypercholesterolemia
V. W. Armstrong and D. Seidel 345

Plasma Exchange for Severe Forms of Familial Hypercholesterolemia: 10 Years' (23 Patient Years') Experience
N. Zöllner, C. Keller, and G. Wolfram 352

List of Contributors

L. Abrahamsson
Department of Geriatrics, University of Uppsala, Box 641, 751 27 Uppsala, Sweden

C. W. M. Adams
Department of Pathology, Guy's Hospital Medical School (UMDS), St. Thomas's Street, London SE1 9RT, Great Britain

S. L. Allaway
MRC Lipid Metabolism Unit, Hammersmith Hospital, Ducane Road, London W12 OHS, Great Britain

E. Andersén
3rd Department of Medicine, Södersjukhuset, Sachsska barnsjukhuset, Box 38100, 10064 Stockholm, Sweden

B. Angelin
Department of Medicine, Huddinge University Hospital, 14186 Huddinge, Sweden

V. W. Armstrong
Abteilung für Klinische Chemie, Georg-August-Universität Göttingen, Medizinische Klinik und Poliklinik, Robert-Koch-Straße 40, 3400 Göttingen, Federal Republic of Germany

G. Assmann
Institut für Klinische Chemie und Laboratoriumsmedizin, Westfälische Wilhelms-Universität, Albert-Schweitzer-Str. 33, 4400 Münster, Federal Republic of Germany

P. Avogaro
Ospedale Regionale, Divisione Medica II a, 30100 Venezia, Italy

G. de Baker
Department of Hygiene and Social Medicine, University Hospital, De Pintelaan 185, 9000 Gent, Belgium

J. L. Beaumont
Unité de Recherches sur les Dyslipidémies et l'Athérosclérose, INSERM (U 32), Hôpital Henri Mondor, 51, avenue du Maréchal de Lattre de Tassigny, 94010 Créteil Cedex, France

V. Beaumont
Unité de Recherches sur les Dyslipidémies et l'Athérosclérose, INSERM (U 32), Hôpital Henri Mondor, 51, avenue du Maréchal de Lattre de Tassigny, 94010 Créteil Cedex, France

C. Berne
Department of Geriatrics, University of Uppsala, Box 641, 751 27 Uppsala, Sweden

E. A. Bevan
MRC Lipid Metabolism Unit, Hammersmith Hopital, Ducane Road, London W12 OHS, Great Britain

M. Bihari-Varga
2nd Department of Pathology, Semmelweis Medical University, Biochemica Division Ullöi ut 93, 1091 Budapest, Hungary

G. Bittolo-Bon
Ospedale Regionale, Divisione Medica II a, 30100 Venezia, Italy

P. Björntorp
Department of Medicine I, Sahlgrenska sjukhuset, 413 45 Göteborg, Sweden

V. Blaton
Department of Clinical Chemistry, A. Z. St.-Jan van het O. C. M. W., Ruddershove 10, 8000 Brugge, Belgium

J. Boberg
Département de médecine, Division de diabétologie, Hôpital cantonal universitaire de Genève, 1211 Genève 4, Switzerland

A. Bottecchia
Ospedale Regionale, Divisione Medica II a, 30100 Venezia, Italy

R. Brasseur
Laboratoire d' Epidémiologie et de Médicine Sociale, ESP, ULB, 1180 Bruxelles, Belgium

R. Brugiolo
Ospedale Regionale, Divisione Medica II a, 30100 Venezia, Italy

L. A. Carlson
Karolinska Institutet, Konung Gustaf V: s forskningsinstitut, Box 600 04, 10401 Stockholm, Sweden

R. Carmena
Facultad de Medicina, Universidad de Valencia, Av. Blasco Ibañez, 17, 46010 Valencia, Spain

G. Cazzolato
Ospedale Regionale Divisione Medica II a, 30100 Venezia, Italy

T. Chajek-Shaul
Lipid Research Laboratory, Department of Medicine B, Hadassah University Hospital, POB 12000, Jerusalem 91120, Israel

M. A. Cole
School of Medicine, University of Southern California, Los Angeles County USC Medical Center, Los Angeles, CA 90033, USA

D. W. Crawford
School of Medicine, University of Southern California, Los Angeles County USC Medical Center, Los Angeles, CA 90033, USA

G. Crepaldi
Istituto di Medicina Interna, Università di Padova, Policlinico,
Via Giustiniani 2, 35128 Padova, Italy

E. Csonka
2nd Department of Pathology, Semmelweis Medical University, Ullöi ùt 93,
P.O. Box 41, 1450 Budapest, Hungary

G. Debry
Centre de Nutrition Humaine, Université de Nancy, INSERM U 59,
40, rue Lionnois, 54000 Nancy, France

G. C. Descovich
Clinica Medica II, Università di Bologna, Via Masarenti 9, Policlinico S. Orsale,
40138 Bologna, Italy

M. Dramaix
Laboratoire d' Epidémiologie et de Médecine Sociale, ESP, ULB,
1180 Bruxelles, Belgium

S. Eisenberg
Department of Internal Medicine B, Hadassah University Hospital, POB 12000,
Jerusalem i1-91-120, Israel

F. H. Epstein
Institut für Sozial- und Präventivmedizin der Universität Zürich,
Sumatrastraße 30, 8006 Zürich, Switzerland

R. Fellin
Istituto di Medicina Interna, Università di Padova, Policlinico,
Via Giustiniani 2, 35128 Padova, Italy

G. Friedmann
Lipid Research Laboratory, Department of Medicine B, Hadassah University
Hospital, P.O. Box 1172, Jerusalem 91120, Israel

D. J. Galton
Department of Medicine, St. Bartholomew's Hospital, West Smithfield,
London E.C. 1., Great Britain

A. Gnasso
II. Clinica Medica, Nuovo Policlinico, Via Sergio Pansini 5, 80131 Naples, Italy

G. A. Gresham
Department of Morbid Anatomy and Histopathology, The John Bonnett
Clinical Laboratory, Addenbrooke's Hospital, Hills Road, Cambridge CB2 2QQ,
Great Britain

H. Greten
Universitäts-Krankenhaus Hamburg-Eppendorf, Martinistraße 52,
2000 Hamburg 20, Federal Republic of Germany

F. A. Gries
Diabetes-Forschungsinstitut der Universität Düsseldorf, Klinische Abteilung,
Auf'm Hennekamp 65, 4000 Düsseldorf, Federal Republic of Germany

I.-B. Gustafsson
Department of Geriatrics, University of Uppsala, Box 641, 75127 Uppsala, Sweden

M. Hanefeld
Medizinische Akademie "Carl Gustaf Carus", Medizinische Klinik, Fetscherstraße 74, 8019 Dresden, German Republic

M. D. Haust
Department of Pathology, Health Sciences Centre, The University of Western Ontario, Ontario, Canada N6A 5C1

K. Hellström
3rd Department of Medicine, Södersjukhuset, 10064 Stockholm, Sweden

L. W. Hessel
TNO Gaubius Instituut, Herenstraat 5 d, 2313 AD Leiden, The Netherlands

D. Hollez
Department of Clinical Chemistry, Pharmaceutical Institute, KU Leuven, Van Evenstraat 4, 3000 Leuven, Belgium

L. Holmquist
Karolinska Institutet, Konung Gustaf V: s forskningsinstitut, Box 60004, 104 01 Stockholm, Sweden

B. Jacotot
Unité de Recherches sur les Dyslipidémies et l'Athérosclérose, INSERM (U32), Hôpital Henri Mondor, 51, avenue du Maréchal de Lattre de Tassigny, 94010 Créteil Cedex, France

H. Jellinek
2nd Department of Pathology, Semmelweis Medical University, Űllöi út 93, P.O. Box 41, 1450 Budapest, Hungary

C. Keller
Medizinische Poliklinik der Universität, Pettenkoferstraße 8 a, 8000 München 20, Federal Republic of Germany

L. Keller
1st Department of Medicine, István Hospital, 1091 Budapest, Hungary

F. Kittel
Laboratoire d'Epidémiologie et de Médecine Sociale, ESP, ULB, 1180 Bruxelles, Belgium

A. N. Klimov
Institute of Experimental Medicine, Academy of Medical Science, Kirovsky Prospekt 69/71, Leningrad 22, USSR

M. Kornitzer
Laboratoire d'Epidémiologie et de Médecine Sociale, ESP, ULB, 1180 Bruxelles, Belgium

T. Koschinsky
Diabetes-Forschungsinstitut an der Universität Düsseldorf, Klinische Abteilung, Auf'm Hennekamp 65, 4000 Düsseldorf 1, Federal Republic of Germany

G. M. Kostner
Institut für Medizinische Biochemie, Universität Graz, 8010 Graz, Austria

D. Kritchevsky
The Wistar Institute of Anatomy and Biology, 36th Street at Spruce, Philadelphia, PA 19104-4268, USA

B. Lewis
Department of Chemical Pathology and Metabolic Disorders, St. Thomas's Hospital Medical School, London SE1 7EH, Great Britain

H. de Loof
Department of Clinical Biochemistry, AZ Sint-Jan, 8000 Brugge, Belgium

M. Mancini
II. Clinica Medica, Nuovo Policlinico, Via Sergio Pansini 5, 80131 Naples, Italy

E. Manzato
Istituto di Medicina Interna, Università di Padova, Policlinico, Via Giustiniani, 2, 35128 Padova, Italy

J. Nimpf
Institut für Medizinische Biochemie, Universität Graz, 8010 Graz, Austria

G. Noseda
Internal Medicine, Ospedale Beata Vergine, 6850 Mendrisio, Switzerland

M. F. Oliver
Cardiovascular Research Unit, Hugh Robson Building, George Square, Edinburgh EH8 9XF, Great Britain

A. G. Olsson
Linköping University, Medical School, Department of Internal Medicine, 581 85 Linköping, Sweden

C. J. Packard
University Department of Pathological Biochemistry, Royal Infirmary, Glasgow G4 OSF, Great Britain

J. Patelski
Department of General Chemistry, Medical Academy, ul. Grunwaldzka 6, 60-780 Poznań, Poland

H. Peeters
Institute for Medical Biology, Alsembergsesteenweg 196, 1180 Bruxelles, Belgium

T. Pollare
Department of Geriatrics, University of Uppsala, Box 641, 751 27 Uppsala, Sweden

A. Postiglione
II. Clinica Medica, Nuovo Policlinico, Via Sergio Pansini 5, 80131 Naples, Italy

P. Puska
National Public Health Institute, Department of Epidemiology, Mannerheimintie 166, 00280 Helsinki, Finland

L. Resi
Istituto Anatomia e Istologia, Patologica, Via Della Scotte, Università, 53100 Siena, Italy

C. D. Ritchie
MRC Lipoprotein Team, Hammersmith Hospital, Ducane Road, London W12 OHS, Great Britain

L. Robert
Laboratoire de Biochimie du Tissu Conjonctif (UACNRS 580), Faculté de Médecine, 8, rue du Général-Sarrail, 94010 Créteil Cedex, France

D. Robinson
MRC Lipoprotein Team, Hammersmith Hospital, Ducane Road, London W12 OHS, Great Britain

M. Rosseneu
Department of Clinical Biochemistry, A. Z. St.-Jan van het O. C. M. W., Ruddershove 10, 8000 Brugge, Belgium

J. M. Ruysschaert
Laboratory of Macromolecules at Interfaces, ULB, 1050 Bruxelles, Belgium

P. Schwandt
Medizinische Klinik II, Klinikum Grosshadern, Marchioninistraße 15, 8000 München 70, Federal Republic of Germany

D. Seidel
Abteilung Klinische Chemie und Zentrallabor der Universitätsklinik Göttingen, Robert-Koch-Straße 40, 3400 Göttingen, Federal Republic of Germany

J. Shepherd
Department of Pathological Biochemistry, Royal Infirmary, University of Glasgow, 84 Castle Street, Glasgow G4 OSF, Great Britain

C. R. Sirtori
Cattedra di Chemioterapia, Centro E Grosse Paoletti, Università di Milano, Via A. del Sarto 21, 20129 Milano, Italy

A. Somogyi
2nd Department of Pathology, Semmelweis Medical University, Ullöi ùt 93, P. O. Box 41, 1450 Budapest, Hungary

O. Stein
Department of Experimental Medicine and Cancer Research, The Hebrew University, Hadassah Medical School, POB 1172, Jerusalem 91010, Israel

Y. Stein
Lipid Research Laboratory, Department of Internal Medicine B, Hadassah University Hospital, POB 12000, Jerusalem 91120, Israel

K. Świdzińska
Department of General Chemistry, Medical Academy, ul. Swiecickiego 6, 60-781 Poznań, Poland

T. Szwajca
Department of General Chemistry, Medical Academy, ul. Swiecickiego 6,
60-781 Poznań, Poland

E. Takács
2nd Department of Pathology, Semmelweis Medical University, Ullöi ùt 93,
P. O. Box 41, 1450 Budapest, Hungary

P. Tanganelli
Istituto Anatomia e Istologia, Patologica, Via Delle Scotte, Università,
53100 Siena, Italy

G. R. Thompson
MRC Lipoprotein Team, Hammersmith Hospital, Ducane Road,
London W12 0HS, Great Britain

D. F. Tidwell
School of Medicine, University of Southern California, Los Angeles County
USC Medical Center, Los Angeles, CA 90033, USA

G. Valerio
Istituto di Medicina Interna, Università di Padova, Policlinico,
Via Giustiniani, 2, 35128 Padova, Italy

K. W. Walton
Queen Elizabeth Hospital, Medical Centre, Edgbaston, Birmingham B15 2TH,
Great Britain

G. Weber
Istituto Anatomia e Istologia, Patologica, Via Delle Scotte, 6, Università di Siena,
53100 Siena, Italy

P. Weisweiler
Medizinische Klinik II, Klinikum Grosshadern, Marchioninistraße 15,
8000 München 70, Federal Republic of Germany

E. Windler
Universitäts-Krankenhaus Hamburg-Eppendorf, Martinistraße 52,
2000 Hamburg 20, Federal Republic of Germany

G. Wolfram
Medizinische Poliklinik der Universität, Pettenkoferstraße 8 a,
8000 München 20, Federal Republic of Germany

T. Zemplenyi
LAC/USC Medical Center, Department of Medicine, Rm. 7900,
1200 N. State Street, Los Angeles, CA 90033, USA

N. Zöllner
Medizinische Poliklinik der Universität, Pettenkoferstraße 8 a,
8000 München 20, Federal Republic of Germany

Pathogenesis and Morphology

Pathogenesis of Atherosclerosis: - Current Status*

M. Daria Haust

Introduction

Atherosclerosis has been recognized as a complex multifaceted arteriopathy which is characterized by three forms of focal intimal lesions of inception, each with the potential to develop into the clinically important atherosclerotic plaques [23, 30, 31]. The latter in turn may become complicated lesions when processes of ulceration, thrombosis, hemorrhage and calcification ensue alone or combination [33, 34].

It is of interest to note that until recent times, theories intended to explain the pathogenesis of atherosclerosis were largely concerned with one or the other aspect of this arteriopathy, ignoring the multitude of other features. Each of the theories had its own followers who promoted one concept only to the exclusion of the other proposed pathogenetic mechanisms. It is perhaps no coincidence that in an era stretching from the fifth to the seventh decade of this century no single gathering of scientists in this field was designed to review and reconcile these various (and numerous) hypotheses, as if avoiding the "confrontation of theories".

It is largely to the credit of the organizers of the symposium held at the 68th Annual Meeting of the American Association of Pathologists and Bacteriologists in Montreal, 7-9 March 1971 [71], that the various theories were reviewed in an accomodating rather than confronting manner, and what emerged was largely a reaffirmation of the validity of the unifying concept of the pathogenesis of atherosclerosis as proposed some two years earlier [22].

The Problems of, and the Valid Elements in the Older Theories

It became apparent in assessing the older theories of the pathogenesis of atherosclerosis that in many instances it was difficult to ascertain to which aspect or phase of the disease reference was being made. For example, it was not clear whether a given theory proposed the pathogenesis of early lesions (all forms?, only one form?), mechanisms involved in their progression, or both; whether it referred to the pathogenesis of complicated lesions (vide supra), or of those largely responsible for the "precipitation" of clinical manifestations, i.e., the illness itself. It had been largely overlooked that several different mechanisms could be accountable, for example, for lipid accumulation in the arterial wall, and that there could be several

* Supported by grant-in-aid T.3-11 from the Heart and Stroke Foundation of Ontario, London, Ontario, Canada.

mechanisms (but not necessarily the same ones) promoting the cellular proliferation or fibrosis.

Over a period of at least a decade and a half immediately prior to 1969 (vide infra), it emerged that although none of the theories could explain or account for all features of the disease, some measure of truth was contained in almost each theory proposed for the pathogenesis of atherosclerosis, and that most of the hypotheses were not exclusive, but rather complementary to each other. This concept was slow in developing because of the usual tendency to ascribe one cause and one mechanism to one tissue reaction and one disease. Overlooked was the fact that many diseases of man may be caused by diverse etiological factors and/or by different pathways, and conversely, that a given etiological element may elicit various tissue reactions in different hosts. It has been learnt that the same principle applies to atherosclerosis.

The recently developed concept in atherosclerosis recognized, perhaps for the first time, that several of the theories proposed as pathogenetic mechanisms may account for some segments in the successive (sequential) order, or in the continuous spectrum of the disease from the inception, development and progression of lesions to the atherosclerotic plaque, its complications, and finally the clinical manifestations. Although it has been recognized of late that certain mechanisms may be operational at almost all levels of atherosclerosis, others may be involved only in one or a few aspects of the disease.

Of the older theories proposed, three may be singled out as those "furnishing a basic component" that is largely valid in today's generally accepted unifying concept of the pathogenesis of atherosclerosis (vide infra). Thus, the oldest of these, von Rokitansky's thesis [61] on the role of encrustation of blood constituents upon the arterial wall (thrombogenic theory), may explain the inception of one of the early lesions (microthrombi), the mechanism of growth of the already established lesion by the process of episodic mural thrombosis (with subsequent organization), and some complications (occlusive thrombosis). This theory was revided in the forties [11, 12] and expanded later by Canadian investigators [27, 37, 41, 54, 56, 57] taking into account the more recent knowledge of the mechanism of thrombosis, and experimentation.

The lipid theory, firmly established by Anitschkow [1] (originally implicating hypercholesterolemia, but since "refined" considerably with respect to the nature of lipids involved [8, 16–18, 50, 58, 64] is applicable to the pathogenesis of other early lesions, i.e., the fatty dots and streaks, to the interrelation between blood lipids, coagulation mechanisms, and some risk factors (smoking, stress), and to certain other parameters of atherosclerosis [65, 66].

The third of these theories, the permeability of perfusion theory modified by Doerr [9, 10], explains the inception of the last form of the early lesions, i.e., the focal gelatinous elevation (resulting from insudation of plasma constituents into the intima) [23]; the same process may also account for the growth of an already established atherosclerotic plaque [30, 31, 34].

Each of the three theories explains (at least) one of the main tissue changes that are observed in the early phases of atherosclerotic lesions: focal intima edema, lipid accumulation, and (micro-) thrombosis. Other formerly proposed theories (aging, intimal hemorrhages and several others) may also be "accomodated" at other points of the spectrum of atherosclerosis, but even if pertinent, these processes would seem to have only a minor role.

Injury and Repair - The Unifying Concept of Pathogenesis

It was suggested in several publications written in the early forties by pathologists that the tissue changes (in the main their focal nature) observed in atherosclerosis resemble tissue reactions to injury. Rössle [62] in particular elaborated on this subject in the context of his thesis that atherosclerosis represents a form of serous inflammation manifesting itself by the early lesion of gelatinous elevation. However, Rössle and the other authors referring to the possible injuries to the arterial wall that may culminate in atherosclerosis, concerned themselves with one or other segment of the disease or one type of lesion, leaving other aspects unexplained.

It was not until 1969 that, on the occasion of the Second International Symposium on Atherosclerosis in Chicago, an all-embracing concept of "injury and repair" as a unifying pathogenetic mechanism operating in atherosclerosis was presented for the first time [22] and was reinforced and broadened shortly thereafter [24, 26, 43]. In developing this concept a concerted effort was made to take into consideration in the most general terms, all the factors known or proposed to play a major or minor role in atherogenesis (see also [5, 19, 47, 49, 51, 69, 70]).

In the broadest terms the concept of injury and repair (as the pathogenetic mechanisms operating in atherosclerosis) takes into account that factors injurious to the arterial wall and specifically to the intima may be derived from three main sources, i.e., from the blood (its constituents or elements in transit) (vide supra), hemodynamics (of the circulation), [6, 15], and the arterial wall itself.

Injurious factors (see Fig. 1) "originating" from the arterial lumen (i.e., either from the blood or from hemodynamics) may injure the endothelium [28] (functionally and/or structurally) and affect its selective permeability and abolish its active control mechanism of filtration. Indiscriminate influx of blood constituents into the intima will ensue and be reflected in the appearance of one form of the early atherosclerotic lesions, i.e., the grey gelatinous elevation (focal intimal edema). Other factors derived from the lumen may not affect the functional integrity of the endothelium, but "acting" upon the subendothelial intima may cause injury to its constituents (cells and/or interstitial components). Thus, involved (subendothelial) intima may not only manifest that injury in a form of another early leasion, i.e., the fatty dot or streak, but may in turn affect the overlying endothelium, with consequent altered permeability as outlined above.

The functionally changed endothelium (whether the change be primary or secondary; vide supra) may become the site of microthrombus deposition (the third form of the early lesion). However, microthrombi may represent a primary phenomenon, i.e., when factors in the blood or in circulation promote their deposition on apparently unaltered endothelium.

Elements representing "injury" may originate from within the arterial wall itself [22, 24]. These may be divided into at least two distinct groups: factors that represent inherent genetic (mis)information and thus aberrations of the "make-up" of the

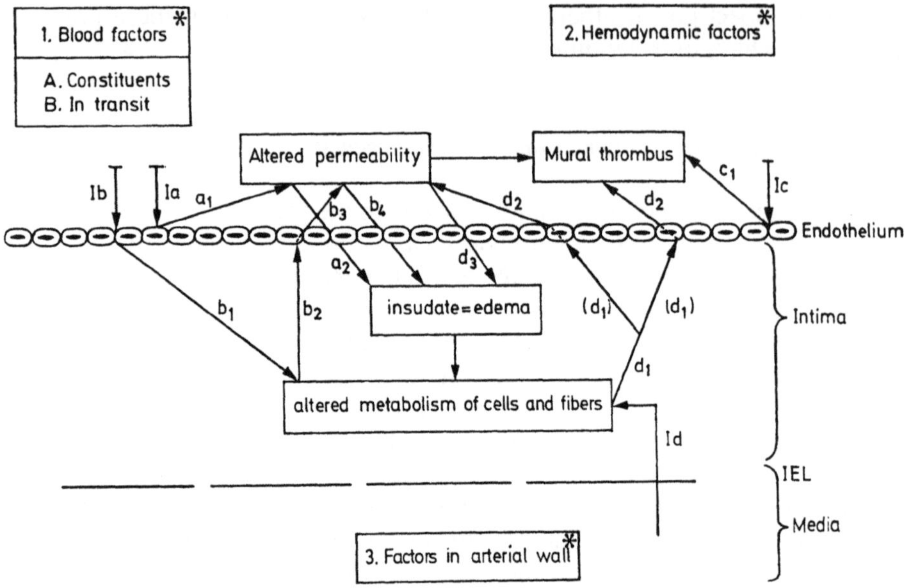

Fig. 1. Schematic representation of "injury and repair" in the pathogenesis of atherosclerosis. Injurious factors derived from the lumen (either from blood or from hemodynamics of circulation) *(Ia)* may act upon endothelium whose selective permeability may be altered (a_1) resulting in insudation of blood constituents into the intima (a_2). This insudate in turn may affect the metabolism of the intimal cells and fibers aggravating the local conditions. Other injurious elements derived from the lumen (either from blood or from hemodynamics of circulation) *(Ib)* may "pass" through the endothelium without affecting it, but instead alter the metabolism of intimal cells and/or connective tissues (b_1). This in turn will ultimately affect the integrity of endothelial cells (b_2), followed by altered permeability (b_3) and insudation (b_4). Some injurious factors originating from the lumen *(Ic)* may promote the precipation of mural (micro-)thrombi (c_1). Factors derived from the wall itself *(Id)*, and relating to an altered metabolism of the mural cells and connective tissues, will influence the endothelial integrity via the latter (d_1); mural thrombosis and/or altered permeability (d_2) and insudation (d_3) may thus ensue. *Ia–Id*, injurious factors; initiating and promoting factors; *IEL*, internal elastic lamina. (Reprinted with permission from [22])

arterial wall (e.g., in inborn errors of metabolism) [24, 39], and those that may relate to the deviation from normal vascular and neural supply, or vasospasm [7]; the entire area relevant to the group of injurious factors "residing" (directly or indirectly) in the arterial wall itself has received little attention to date.

Experimentally, many factors have been shown to be injurious to arterial endothelium, intima, or both, producing lesions that in some aspects resemble those of human atherosclerosis. These include chemical, metabolic, physical, and biological forms of injury (see [22, 70]).

The repair process that follows injuries to the arterial intima is important in determining the outcome and the nature of the lesions. The most remarkable feature of this repair process is the central role played by the intimal smooth muscle cells (SMCs), a feature that is a hallmark ot this arteriopathy [13, 35]. The SMCs proliferate to replace those that become necrotic in the initial phases of the process; they "organize" in an avascular mode the plasma proteins that either entered the intimal substance or were deposited upon its surface as thrombi [44, 55], and elaborate all the connective tissue elements similar to those of the intima [31, 42]. Since the original observations on the role of SMCs in the repair of intimal damage in atherosclerosis [40, 45, 46], these cells have proved to be extremely versatile. By virtue of their contractile properties they add to the "pliability" of the atherosclerotic plaque, they synthesize the components of the basal lamina (laminin, "minor" collagens, fibronectin, and proteoglycans), collagen fibrils (types I and III; see [35]), microfibrils [20], units of elastic tissue, and glycosaminoglycans (of the extracellular matrix; see [34, 35]), and secrete formed precursors of an arterial elastase [68]. They have the ability to migrate and by proliferating provide new lines of SMCs. It was recently established that in atherosclerotic lesions the SMCs give rise to so-called "myohistiocytes" [32, 38]. The latter have an appearance of cells with some features of SMCs and in certain other characteristics resemble histiocytes. They are capable of phagocytosis, a property not inherent in their progenitors - SMCs. The intimal SMCs also possess receptors for low-density lipoproteins (LDL) and the complement of enzymes that regulate intracellular cholesterol metabolism. By accumulating intracellular fat droplets they become (myogenic) foam cells [2, 14, 21, 25, 29, 36]. The numerous pinocytotic vesicles and Porter pits at the plasma membranes enable the uptake by SMCs of various substances, including proteins, from the extracellular space. These serve as building blocks for the intracellular synthesis of the many (vide supra) secretory products for "export." Thus, all phases of the intimal reactions to injury are governed by the SMCs.

The repair that follows injury is basically intended as a healing process. Usually, however, this process proceeds beyond the actual needs for replacement of tissues lost, and in this sense the initially well "intentioned" repair process contributes to the progression of the lesion to a prominent and clinically important atherosclerotic plaque [22, 24]. It may be stated on the basis of the nature of the repair tissue that the injuries sustained by the arterial wall are not severe, but rather subtle. It is probable that the arterial intima (including the endothelium) may be susceptible to injurious factors that are of a relatively low intensity and which in other tissues represent stimuli within the physiological range.

Whereas some injurious elements may be involved in the initiation, others may be largely responsible for the progression of atherosclerotic lesions. Certain forms of injury may be involved at several levels of the disease. For example, plasma lipoproteins have assumed an important role in atherosclerosis because they were shown to influence the process at almost every step. High concentrations of certain plasma lipoproteins, or the absolute or relative low levels of others probably create an abnormal milieu (injury) for arterial endothelium [28] with consequent influx of plasma into the intima and/or thrombosis; high concentration of these lipoproteins in plasma will be reflected in their high content in the intimal lesion and all the known consequences. Certain plasma lipoproteins are known to promote thrombosis either by altering the fibrinolytic system or by influencing the function of platelets. Some plasma lipids were shown to promote SMC proliferation or to influence the composition and thus properties of the intimal connective tissues. Of particular importance is the recently recognized fact that it is not so much the level of plasma lipoproteins as their composition (both with respect to the nature of the apoproteins and of the fatty acids) that plays a dominant role in this process (see references on lipoproteins in the section on the older theories). Similarly, support can be given to the belief that the two other risk factors for atherosclerosis, i.e., hypertension and the (presumably) "active principles" in cigarette smoke, exert their deleterious influences at several levels of the spectrum of the atherosclerotic process [6, 7, 15].

Comments and Conclusions

Since the concept of injury and repair was formulated in 1969 [22, 24, 26, 43] as the all-embracing pathogenetic mechanism of atherosclerosis, at least three additional pathogenetic theories were proposed in the seventies: the so-called monoclonal, the clonal-senescence and the immunological theories. The last of these was not an entirely new thesis, as in the past several investigators drew attention to data indicating that many aspects of atherosclerosis have features characteristic of immunological reactions [63]. However, it was not until 1979 that Klimov and his colleagues provided a very comprehensive account supporting and clearly formulating the immunological theory of atherogenesis [48].

The so-called monoclonal theory as proposed by Benditt and Benditt [4] was based on the observation that in some black women who were heterozygous for the X-linked enzyme glucose-6-phosphate dehydorgenase (G6PD), the normal intima contained both, cells with the A- and the B-isoenzyme of G6PD, but the atherosclerotic plaques consisted of cells with either only one or other isoenzyme. This was interpreted as indicator that each lesion contained a clone of cellular elements derived from only one smooth muscle cell, and represented a benign neoplasm originating from a cell transformed by viruses or chemical agents [3, 4]. Pearson and colleagues extended these studies to fatty dots and streaks [59, 60]. It is irrelevant to this discussion whether the lesions are monoclonal or monotypical in nature, as subsequently proposed by Thomas and his colleagues [67].

The clonal-senescence theory relates to aging, - a phenomenon that throughout the decades of this century has been proposed on and off as being the basis of the atherosclerotic process. However, as formulated in the seventies by Martin and his colleagues [52, 53], the thesis took into consideration a more basic approach (cellular elements and genetic information) than was ever the case in the past, and herein lies its attraction. In short, the thesis proposes that normally the replication of the arterial SMC stem cells is regulated by a feedback mechanism via "chalones" secreted by the SMCs. This regulatory mechanism, inhibiting the replication of the SMC stem cells beyond physiological needs (of replacement), fails with age (and in atherosclerosis). Although the effect of this process is not important in the arterial media, because this layer contains large numbers of both the stem cells and (pre)existing SMCs, the decreased diffusion of chalones in (to) the intima results in an unchecked focal replication of the intimal SMCs giving rise to the (fibrous) atherosclerotic plaques.

Attractive as all the above three theories are (as was the case with the many theses prior to 1969), they again either address themselves to only one narrow aspect (i.e., the proliferative aspect of the entire atherosclerotic process; ([monoclonal] proliferation of SMCs, failure of replication-control of SMCs), or propose an immunological basis that in the majority of instances cannot be proven to prevail in atherosclerosis.

On the other hand, each of these newly proposed theories may be easily "embraced" by, or accommodated within the concept of "injury and repair" of atherogenesis. Thus, the proliveration of the SMCs (whereas not always necessarily monoclonal or even monotypical) may in fact represent a repair in response to injurious factors such as viruses and chemicals (proposed in the monoclonal theory), or represent a failed control of SMC-s-replication with aging, i. e., a factor relating to the arterial wall itself as a source of "injury". Similarly, immunological processes may also represent some forms of injury either to the endothelium and/or to the entire intima, and the theory as proposed by Klimov and his colleagues may also be "fitted" into the broad concept of injury and repair as the pathogenesis of atherosclerosis.

It may be anticipated that with advancing knowledge many other important aspects of atherosclerosis will be uncovered and found to play a role in the mechanisms operating in the inception, progression and complications of this disease. There is reason to believe that all of these (anticipated factors) could be easily accommodated in the sequence of events that fall either into the phase of injury or of repair in the overall pathogenesis of atherosclerosis.

Acknowledgements. The author wishes to thank Mr Roger Dewar for this technical assistance and Paula Fenner for efficient typing of the manuscript.

References

1. Anitschkow NN (1967) A history of experimentation on arterial atheroscerosis in animals. In: Blumenthal HT (ed) Cowdry's arteriosclerosis, 2nd edn. Thomas, Springfield, pp 21-44
2. Balis JU, Haust MU, More RH (1964) Electron microscopic studies in human atherosclerosis. Cellular elements in aortic fatty streaks. Exp Mol Pathol 3: 511-525
3. Benditt EP (1977) Implications of the monoclonal character of human arterosclerotic plaques. Am J Pathol 86: 693-702
4. Benditt EP, Benditt JM (1973) Evidence for a monoclonal origin of human atheroscerotic plaques. Proc Natl Acad Sci USA 70: 1753-1756
5. Björkerud SU (1979) Mechanisms of atherosclerosis. In: Ioachim HL (ed) Pathobiology annual, vol 9. Raven Press, New York, pp 277-301
6. Bomberger RA, Zarins CK, Taylor KE, Clagov S (1980) Effect of hypotension on atherogenesis and aortic wall composition. J Surg Res 28: 402-409
7. Boyd GW (1978) Stress and disease: the missing link. A vasospastic theory. II. The nature of degenerative arterial disease. Med Hypotheses 4: 420-430
8. Brown MS, Goldstein JL, Fredrickson DS (1983) Familial type 3 hyperlipoproteinemia (dysbetalipoproteinemia). In: Stanbury JB, Wyngaarden JB, Fredrickson DS, Goldstein JL, Brown MS (eds) The metabolic basis of inherited diseases, 5th edn. McGraw-Hill, New York, pp 655-671
9. Doerr W (1963) Perfusionstheorie der Arteriosklerose. In: Bargmann W, Doerr W (eds) Zwanglose Abhandlungen aus dem Gebiet der Normalen und Pathologischen Anatomie, vol 13. Thieme, Stuttgart
10. Doerr W (1970) Arterioslcerose. In: Doerr W (ed) Allgemeine Pathologie der Organe des Kreislaufes. Springer, Berlin Heidelberg New York, p 568
11. Duguid JB (1946) Thrombosis as a factor in the pathogenesis of coronary atherosclerosis. J Pathol Bacteriol 58: 207-212
12. Duguid JB (1949) Pathogenesis of arterosclerosis. Lancet 2: 925-927
13. Geer JC, Haust MD (1972) Smooth muscle cells in atherosclerosis. Monographs on atherosclerosis, vol 2. Karger, Basel

14. Geer JC, McGill HC, Strong JP (1961) The fine structure of human atherosclerotic lesions. Am J Pathol 38: 263-287
15. Glagov S (1972) Hemodynamic risk factors: mechanical stress, mural architecture, medial nutrition and the vulnerability of arteries to atherosclerosis. In: Wissler RW, Geer JC (eds) The pathogenesis of atherosclerosis. Williams and Wilkins, Baltimore, pp 164-199
16. Goldstein JL, Brown MS (1983) Familial hypercholesterolemia. In: Stanbury JB, Wyngaarden JB, Fredrickson DS, Goldstein JL, Brown MS (eds) The metabolic basis of inherited diseases, 5th edn. McGraw-Hill, New York, pp 672-712
17. Goldstein JL, Kita T, Brown MS (1983) Defective lipoprotein receptors and atherosclerosis. Lessons from an animal counterpart of familial hypercholesterolemia. New Engl J Med 309: 288-296
18. Grundy SM (1984) Pathogenesis of hypertriglyceridemia in man. In: Carlson LA, Olsson AG (eds) Treatment of hyperlipoproteinemia. Raven Press, New York, pp 21-34
19. Hauss WH, Mey J, Grünwald J (1981) Modernes Konzept über den Mechanismus der Pathogenese der Arteriosklerose. In: Breddin K (ed) Thrombose und Atherogenese. Witzstrock, Köln, pp 3-16
20. Haust MD (1965) Fine fibrils of extracellular space (microfibrils). Their structure and role in connective tissue organization. Am J Pathol 47: 1113-1137
21. Haust MD (1968) Electron microscopic and immunohistochemical studies of fatty streaks in human aorta. In: Miras CJ, Howard AN, Paoletti R (eds) Progress in biochemical pharmacology,.vol 4. Karger, Basel, pp 429-437
22. Haust MD (1970) Injury and repair in the pathogenesis of atherosclerotic lesions. In: Jones RJ (ed) Atherosclerosis; proceedings of the second international symposium. Springer, New York Heidelberg Berlin, pp 12-20
23. Haust MD (1971 a) The morphogenesis and fate of potential and early atherosclerotic lesions in man. Human Pathol 2: 1-29
24. Haust MD (1971 b) Arteriosclerosis. In: Brunson JG, Gall EA (eds) Concepts of diesease. A textbook of human pathology. Macmillan, New York, pp 451-487
25. Haust MD (1972) Regressive and progressive changes of intimal smooth muscle cells in atherosclerosis. Ver Dtsch Ges Inn Med 78: 1124-1138
26. Haust MD (1974) Reaction patterns of intimal mesenchyme to injury, and repair in atherosclerosis. Adv Exp Med Biol 43: 35-57
27. Haust MD (1977 a) Thrombosis in the inception and progression of coronary atherosclerotic lesion. In: Schettler G, Horsch A, Mörl H, Orth H, Weizel A (eds) Der Herzinfarkt. Schattauer, Stuttgart, pp 120-135
28. Haust MD (1977 b) Arterial endothelium and its potentials. Adv Exp Med Biol 82: 34-51
29. Haust MD (1977 c) Myogenic foam cells in explants of fatty dots and streaks from rabbit aorta. Morphological studies. Atherosclerosis 26: 441-464
30. Haust MD (1978 a) Light and electron microscopy of human atherosclerotic lesions. Adv Exp Med Biol 104: 33-59
31. Haust MD (1978 b) Zur Morphologie der Arteriosklerose. Internist (Berlin) 19: 621-626
32. Haust MD (1980) The nature of bi- and trinuclear cells in atherosclerotic lesions in man. Ultrastructural studies of aortic fatty dots and streaks. Atherosclerosis 36: 365-377
33. Haust MD (1981) The natural history of atherosclerotic lesions. In: Moore S (ed) Vascular injury and atherosclerosis. Dekker, New York, pp 1-23
34. Haust MD (1983 a) Atherosclerosis-lesions and sequelae. In: Silver MD (ed) Cardiovascular pathology, vol 1. Churchill Livingstone, New York, pp 191-315
35. Haust MD (1983 b) Atherosclerosis and smooth muscle cells. In: Stephens NL (ed) Biochemistry of smooth muscle, vol 2, no 6576. CRC Press, Boca Raton, pp 189-250
36. Haust MD (1983 c) The derivation and fate of foam cells in atherosclerosis. G Arterioscler 1 [Suppl 1]: 55-81
37. Haust MD (1985) Thrombosis and atherosclerosis - some unresolved problems. Ann NY Acad Sci 454: 154-161
38. Haust MD (1986) Myohistiocytes and ciliated smooth muscle cells in human atherosclerotic lesions. In: Fidge NH, Nestel PJ (eds) Atherosclerosis VII. Excerpta Medica, Amsterdam, pp 377-380
39. Haust MD (1987) Arterial involvement in genetic diseases. Am J Cardiovasc Pathol, in press

40. Haust MD, More RH (1958) New functional aspects of smooth muscle cells. Fed Proc 17: 440
41. Haust MD, More RH (1960) The thrombotic basis of arteriosclerosis. Heart Bull 9: 90-92
42. Haust MD, More RH (1963) Significance of the smooth muscle cell in atherogenesis. In: Jones RJ (ed) Evolution of the atherosclerotic plaque. University of Chicago Press, Chicago, pp 51-63
43. Haust MD, More RH (1972) Development of modern theories on the pathogenesis of atherosclerosis. In: Wissler RW, Geer JC (eds) The pathogenesis of atherosclerosis. Williams and Wilkins, Baltimore, pp 1-19
44. Haust MD, More RH, Movat HZ (1959) The mechanisms of fibrosis in arteriosclerosis. Am J Pathol 35: 265-273
45. Haust MD, More RH, Movat HZ (1960) The role of smooth muscle cells in the fibrogenesis of arteriosclerosis. Am J Pathol 37: 377-389
46. Haust MD, Movat HZ, More RH (1957) Organization by smooth muscle cells. Am J Pathol 33: 626
47. Kinlough-Rathbone RL, Mustard JF (1981) Atherosclerosis, - current concepts. Am J Surg 141: 638-643
48. Klimov AN, Zubzhitsky YN, Nagornev VA (1979) Immunochemical aspects of atherosclerosis. In: Paoletti R, Gotto AM (eds) Atherosclerosis reviews, vol 4. Raven Press, New York, pp 119-156
49. Kottke BA, Subbiah MTR (1978) Pathogenesis of atherosclerosis. Concepts based on animal models. Mayo Clin Proc 53: 35-48
50. Lippel K, Tyroler H, Eder H, Gotto A, Vahouny G (1981) Relationship of hypertriglyceridemia to atherosclerosis. Arteriosclerosis 1: 406-417
51. Mahley RW (1983) Development of accelerated atherosclerosis. Concepts derived from cell biology and animal model studies. Arch Pathol Lab Med 107: 393-399
52. Martin GM, Ogburn C, Sprague C (1975) Senescence and vascular disease. In: Cristafalo VJ, Roberts J, Adelman RC (eds) Exploration in aging. Plenum Press, New York, pp 163-193
53. Martin GM, Sprague CA (1973) Life histories of hyperplastoid cell lines from aorta and skin. Exp Mol Pathol 18: 125-141
54. Moore S (1973) Thromboatherosclerosis in normolipemic rabbits. A result of continued endothelial damage. Lab Invest 29: 478-487
55. More RH, Haust MD (1961) Atherogenesis and plasma constituents. Am J Pathol 38: 527-535
56. More RH, Movat HZ, Haust MD (1957) Role of mural fibrin thrombi of the aorta in genesis of arteriosclerotic plaques. Report of two cases. AMA Arch Pathol 63: 612-620
57. Mustard JF (1976) The Gordon Neilson Lecture. Function of blood platelets and their role in thrombosis. Trans Am Clin Climatol Assoc 87: 104-127
58. Nikkilä EA (1983) Familial lipoprotein lipase deficiency and related disorders of chylomicron metabolism. In: Stanbury JB, Wyngaarden JB, Fredrickson DS, Goldstein JL, Brown MS (eds) The metabolic basis of inherited diseases, 5th edn. McGraw-Hill, New York, pp 622-642
59. Pearson TA, Kramer EC, Solez K, Heptinstall RH (1977) The human atherosclerotic plague. Am J Pathol 86: 657-664
60. Pearson TA, Wang A, Solez K, Heptinstall RH (1975) Clonal characteristics of fibrous plagues and fatty streaks from human aortas. Am J Pathol 81: 379-388
61. Rokitansky K (1852) A manual of pathological anatomy, vol 4. Sydenham Society, London, pp 261-273
62. Rössle R (1944) Über die serösen Entzündungen der Organe. Virchows Arch Path Anat 311: 252-284
63. Scebat L, Renais J, Groult N (1967) Pouvoir immunogène et pathogène de la paroi artérielle. Rev Atheroscler (Paris) 9: 50-61
64. Schaefer EJ, Levy RI (1985) Pathogenesis and management of lipoprotein disorders. New Engl J Med 312: 1300-1310
65. Schettler G (1983) Atherosclerosis. The major problem in man. In: Schettler G, Gotto AM, Middelhoff G, Habenicht AJR, Jurutka KR (eds) Atherosclerosis VI, Springer, Berlin Heidelberg New York, pp 3-11
66. Schettler G, Gross R (1985) (eds) Arteriosklerose-Grundlagen, Diagnostik, Therapie. Deutscher Ärzte-Verlag, Köln
67. Thomas WA, Reiner JM, Florentin RA, Janakidevi K, Lee KJ (1977) Arterial smooth muscle

cells in atherogenesis: birth, deaths and clonal phenomena. In: Schettler G, Goto Y, Hata Y, Klose G (eds) Atherosclerosis IV. Springer, Berlin Heidelberg New York, pp 16-23
68. Trillo A, Haust MD (1975) The granulovasicular bodies of the arterial wall. Lab Invest 32: 105-110
69. Wissler RW (1974) Atherosclerosis - its pathogenesis in perspective. Adv Cardiol 13: 10-31
70. Wissler RH (1980) Principles of the pathogenesis of atherosclerosis. In: Braunwald E (ed) Heart disease: a textbook of cardiovascular medicine. Saunders, Philadelphia, pp 1221-1245
71. Wissler RW, Geer JC (1972) (eds) The pathogenesis of atherosclerosis. Williams and Wilkins, Baltimore

The Extracellular Matrix of the Vessel Wall, Its Role and Modification During the Atherosclerotic Process

L. Robert

Introduction

It is a special pleasure and honour to contribute to this volume dedicated to Prof. Gerhard Schettler for his 70th birthday. Since I entered this field in 1964 I have often had the opportunity of meeting Professor Schettler, listening to his lectures and presenting my results under his presidency. I have especially appreciated his wide interest in every aspect of experimental medicine and biology related to the still wide-open field of atherosclerosis research. In this respect, he certainly deserves to belong to the highly prestigious family of great German physicians who have contributed so much to our understanding of human diseases.

As far as my own field is concerned it was in the foreground of the early histopathological studies on atherosclerosis because of the relatively specific staining methods devised by pathologists since the end of the nineteenth century. Fragmentation of elastic lamellae, increase of collagen, especially in the fibrous plaques, early increase of protoeoglycans ("acid mucopolysaccharides") were all described in the early part of this century. The detailed knowledge of the extracellular matrix of the vessel wall had however to await the advent of the modern era of molecular and cellular biology of extracellular matrix (EM). It has only become clear in the last decades that most cells of the organism secrete an EM of a specific composition which represents its "ecological niche". The constituents of EM remain in close contact with the cells through specific receptors and anchoring molecules such as fibronectins, elastonectin and others. This is especially true for the vessel wall which is rich in EM components.

Figure 1 shows part of a rabbit aorta with the smooth muscle cells (SMC) embedded in the extracellular matrix they synthesise. The understanding of the biology and pathology of the vessel wall is therefore largely dependent on the precise knowledge of its extracellular matrix. The following section gives a short summary of the macromolecular composition of the EM of vessel walls and of its pathological modifications especially in atherosclerosis.

Composition of the Extracellular Matrix of the Vessel Wall

The macromolecular composition of the EM of the vessel wall reflects the state of phenotypic differentiation of its cellular components. These belong essentially to three different cell types: endothelial cells, smooth muscle cells and fibroblasts. All three cell types contribute to the biosynthesis and secretion of EM macromolecules.

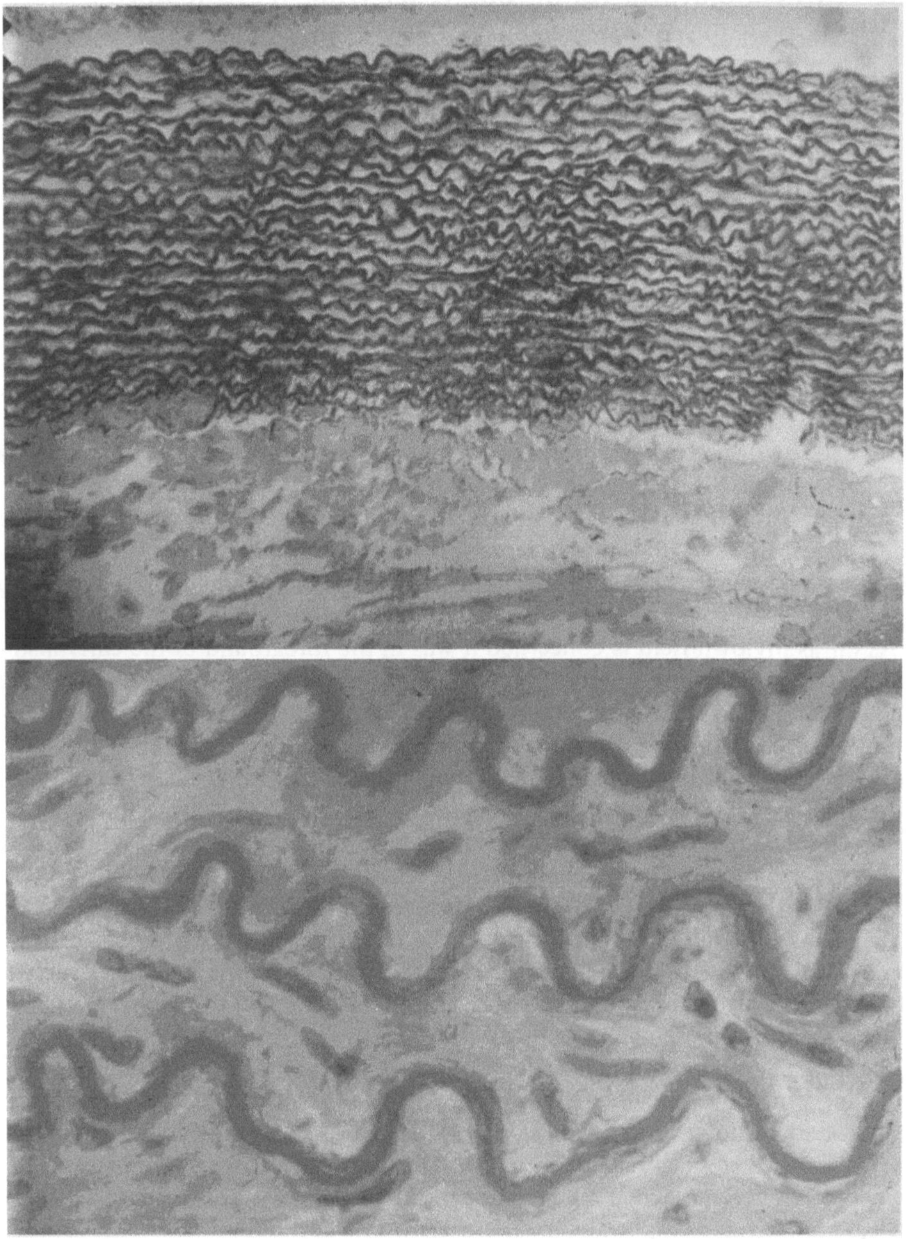

Fig. 1. Smooth muscle cells in the normal rabbit aorta. They are surrounded by the extracellular matrix they synthesise and are anchored in the matrix by specific anchorage proteins (fibronectin, elastonectin, anchorines). *Above:* Low magnification of a rabbit aorta showing the elastic fibres (acid-orcein straining ×210). *Below:* Higher magnification showing the smooth muscle cells between the elastic fibres (phosphotungstic acid 1% eosine aque 1%, haematoxylin staining ×1200. (Photo by G. Godeau)

Table 1. Extracellular matrix macromolecules synthesized by the different cells of the vessel wall

Cell type	Collagens	Elastin	Proteoglycans	Structural glycoproteins
Endothelial cells	Type III, IV, VI	±	HS	FN, VW, TSp, N, Lam
Smooth muscle cells	Type I, III, V, VI	+ + +	DS, CS, HA	FN, EN, and others less well-characterised [32]
Fibroblasts	Type I, III	±	CS, DS, HA	FN, EN and others

Proteoglycans: HS, heparan sulphate proteoglycan; DS, dermatan sulphate proteoglycan; CS, chondroitin sulphate proteoglycan; HA, hyaluronate.
Structural glycoproteins: FN, fibronectin; VW, von Willebrandt factor; TSp, thrombospondine; N, nidogen; Lam, laminin; EN, elastonectin.

EM components belong to four major families (see Table 1): (a) the collagens; (b) elastin; (c) proteoglycans; and (d) structural glycoproteins. Table 1 shows the selective expression of some macromolecules of these four families by the above three cell types during their differentiation.

Cell differentiation with respect to EM biosynthesis as well as the phenotype of mesenchymal cells can be defined by this selection of some of the EM macromolecules which will be synthesized by the differentiating cells. This selection process implies a quantitative and a qualitative aspect; the qualitative aspect concerns the selection of the genes coding for the EM macromolecules which will be expressed. The quantitative aspect concerns the amplification and/or repression of the expression of these genes in order to increase or to decrease their biosynthetic products. The interplay of these two processes will then result in the production of a specific matrix corresponding structurally and functionnally to the requirements of that part of the vascular tree to which the cells belong. The EM synthesized by the cells mentioned above will therefore differ according to the anatomical localization of the vascular structure. For example, the matrix components synthesized by the endothelial cells are different in capillaries and in the intima of the major elastic arteries. Another example is the changing ratio of elastin to collagen in the different parts of the aorta: this ratio is about 2 to 1 in the thoracic aorta, which is especially rich in elastin, and 1 to 2 in the abdominal aorta which contains more collagen than elastin.

The composition of the EM changes with age qualitatively and quantitatively [1, 2]. As shown recently using conjunctival biopsies, the ratio of collagen type III to chollagen type I increases with age [3]. The progressive rigidification of elastic arteries such as the aorta appears to be the result of the fragmentation of elastic lamellae and a relative increase of collagen (increase of the collagen/elastin ratio) [4]. Other modifications were also described, such as the exponential decrease of EM biosynthesis as a function of age of rabbit aorta SMCs in organ culture [5]. The electron microscopic studies of Kern et al. clearly showed that the width of capillary basement membranes increases with age in non-diabetics as well as in diabetics; the diabetic curve starts at a higher level than the normal and ramains above it at all ages (for a review, see [1, 2]). According to the recent studies of Labat-Robert et al. [6, 7], these modifications appear to depend on an increased biosynthesis of fibronectin.

All the modifications mentioned above (and others) result in a continuously changing vascular wall with increasing rigidity and modified permeability and filtration capacity. These continuous and progressive modifications, which we prefer to designate as *arteriosclerosis,* often underly the focal, localized modifications of the vessel wall which lead to the development of the *atherosclerotic* plaque.

Pathological Modifications

Although this distinction between a generalized arteriosclerosis and a more localised atheromatosis may appear to be more of a didactic and semantic nature than a realistic one, we believe that it does correspond to two distinct processes which can be concomitant but of a different nature. This distinction rests today on firm cell-biological grounds. The formation of the atherosclerotic plaque requires radical modifications of the behaviour of the SMCs of the media. These modifications can be schematically separated in several successive steps (Table 2). The modification of the behaviour of SMCs participating in the formation of the plaque may well be designated as proposed by the Campbells [8] as "phenotypic modulation". This designation is based on a relatively sudden modification of SMCs in culture after several passages [8, 9]. In the arterial wall, the sequence of events must be different because the cells are firmly anchored in their extracellular matrix. Therefore in vivo the first steps of this change of phenotype from a sessile and contractile state to a mobile, dividing and biosynthetically activated one *must start with the detachment of the cells from the surrounding matrix*. Recent experiments carried out in our laboratory with Hornebeck and Tixier showed that SMCs synthesise a specific adhesive protein which mediates their interaction with elastin. We proposed its designation as *elastonectin* [10]. The synthesis of elastonectin is induced by the presence of elastin in its fibrous or peptide form. But SMCs also express an elastase-type of protease [11].

Table 2. Modifications of the phenotypic behaviour of smooth muscle cells of the media during the development of the atherosclerotic plaque. Consecutive steps involved in this process and possible mechanisms

Process	Possible mechanism
1. Detachment from the surrounding matrix and loss of contractility	Elastase-type proteases of SMC membrane and from migrating cells
2. Mitoses	Growth factor (PDGF and others), viral genome integration, oncogene activation
3. Migration towards the intima	Chemotactic factors - PDGF, elastin peptides
4. Oversynthesis of extracellular matrix macromolecules and fibrous plaque formation	PDGF, elastin peptides, other hormonal or growth factors
5. Lipid deposition	Intracellular: LDL receptors, etc. Extracellular: matrix-lipid interactions [22, 23]

The synthesis of this enzyme increases with age in vivo [12] and in vitro [13]. We proposed that this enzyme is involved in the detachment of the SMCs from their surrounding matrix. It was also shown by Senior et al. [14] that elastin degradation products are chemotactic for mesenchymal cells and monocytes. SMCs will therefore migrate towards the site of degradation of elastin. We could show recently that this migration depends on the elastase-type enzyme of migrating cells: its inhibition abolishes migration [15]. The experiments also showed that elastin degradation products induced an increased synthesis of the elastase-type enzymes in leucocytes [15]. We have, therefore, all the elements of a vicious circle. There remains the problem of the nature of the primary trigger of these events.

This is an old problem in atherogenesis. Platelets, growth factor, lipoproteins and more recently, inflammatory and immune factors as well as viruses and activation of oncogens have been proposed as playing this role. Figure 2 shows these (hypothetical) mechanisms schematically. Immunization with elastin can induce arteriosclerotic lesions (with no addition of lipid to the diet) [16, 17] and anti-elastin antibodies have been detected in a large number of human sera [18, 19]. There is also increasing evidence for the oncogen-type activation of cell division in the arteriosclerotic plaques.

Whatever the triggering mechanism, the migrating and dividing SMCs will eventually reach the lumen of the vessel. The increased synthesis of EM macromolecules will result in the construction of the fibrous plaque (Fig. 3). Matrix elements also play in important role in the retention of lipoproteins. A dermatan sulphate proteoglycans isolated from porcine aorta was shown to form insoluble complexes with low-density lipoprotein (LDL) [20].

It appears, therefore, that the modified cell behaviour (phenotypic modulation)

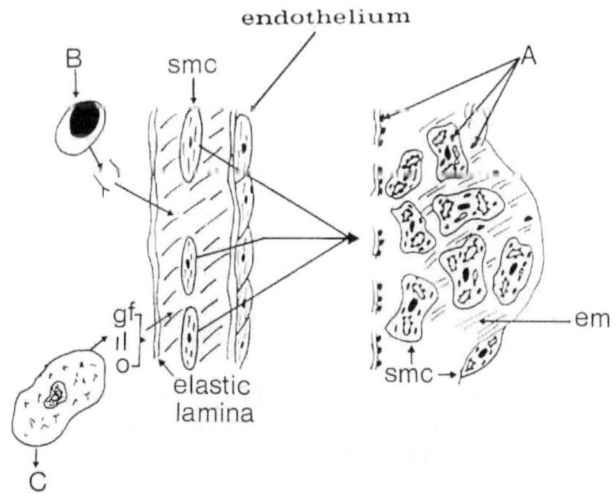

Fig. 2. Schematic representations of the (theoretical) mechanisms involved in the genesis of the atherosclerotic plaque. *Left:* Section of a normal media; *A,* lipid deposition; *B,* inflammatory and immune mechanisms; *C,* triggering of cell division by oncogene activation [viruses, "mutational" events, oncogenes *(o),* growth factors *(gf),* interleukins *(il)*]. *Right:* The fibrous atherosclerotic plaque. These mechanisms result in the phenotypic modulation of the smooth muscle cells which then divide, degrade the surrounding matrix, migrate to the intima, oversynthesise extracellular matrix *(em)* and build up the atherosclerotic plaque (see also Table 2)

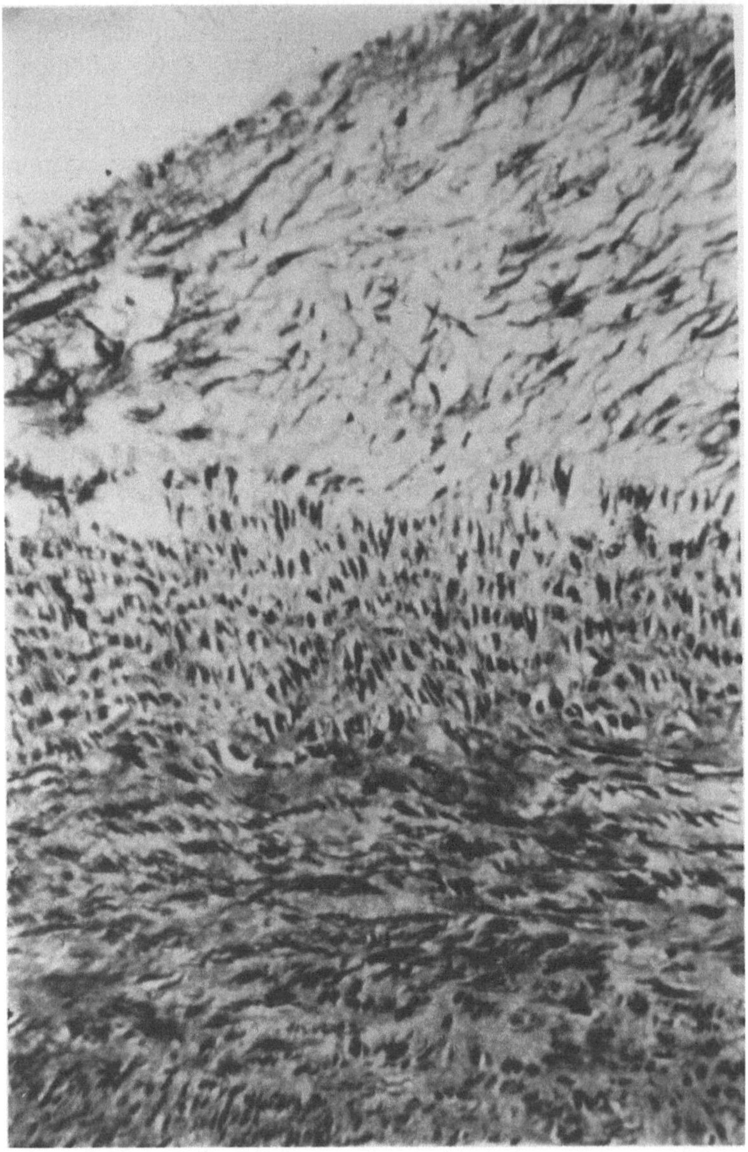

Fig. 3. A typical atherosclerotic plaque of a rabbit aorta fed with a lipid-rich diet (1% cholesterol and 5% primrose oil). The modification of the orientation and matrix surroundings of the cells can be clearly seen. (From [31])

also involves far-reaching changes in cell-matrix interactions and matrix biosynthesis. This is particularly well-reflected by the changing composition of the EM components of the atherosclerotic plaque.

Recent studies by Labat-Robert et al. [21] showed the presence of increased amounts of fibronectin colocalising with type III collagen in fresh plaques of

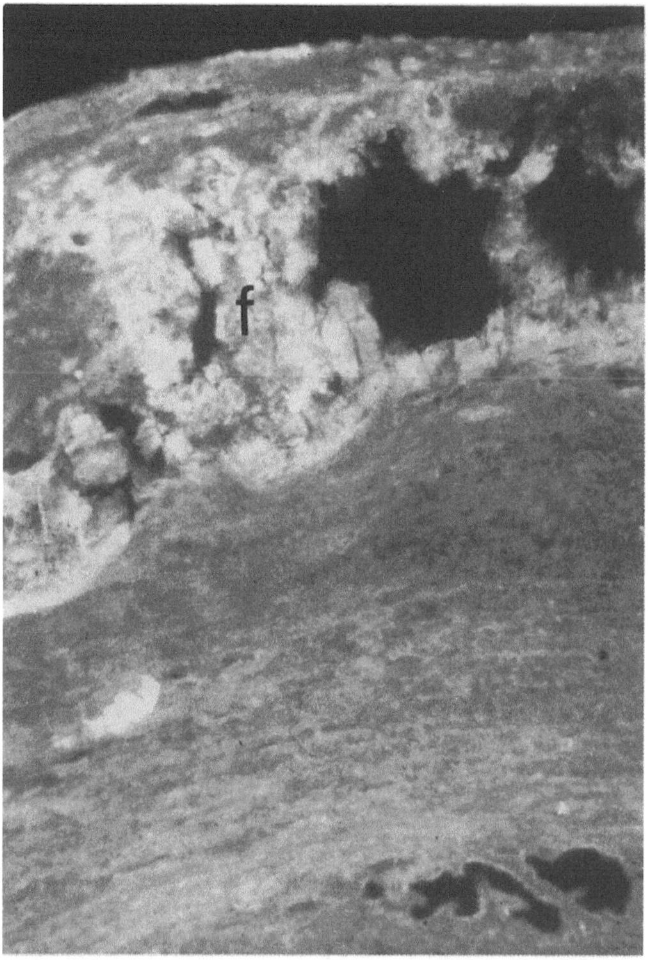

Fig. 4. Massive deposition of fibronectin (*f*) colocalising with collagen type III in fresh human atherosclerotic plaque. (From [21])

human aorta (Fig. 4). In later stages, as well as in the aging arterial intima, collagen type I appears to increase (Fig. 5). Lipid retention was also shown to occur in EM macromolecules. We have already mentioned the role of a particular family of proteoglycans. This corresponds to early histochemical observations (for review see [21 a]) concerning the early rise in plaque areas of "acid mucopolysaccharides". We demonstrated with Beaumont and Jacotot's team the role of other EM components in lipid deposition. Elastic fibres and also structural glycoproteins play a crucial role in this respect [22, 23]. Lipid deposition (especially of free fatty acids and of cholesterol esters) in elastic fibres accelerates their degradation, preceded by the loss of their rheological properties [24].

The modifications of the vessel wall described above apply to elastic arteries which develop atherosclerotic modifications. The smaller vessels and the capillaries

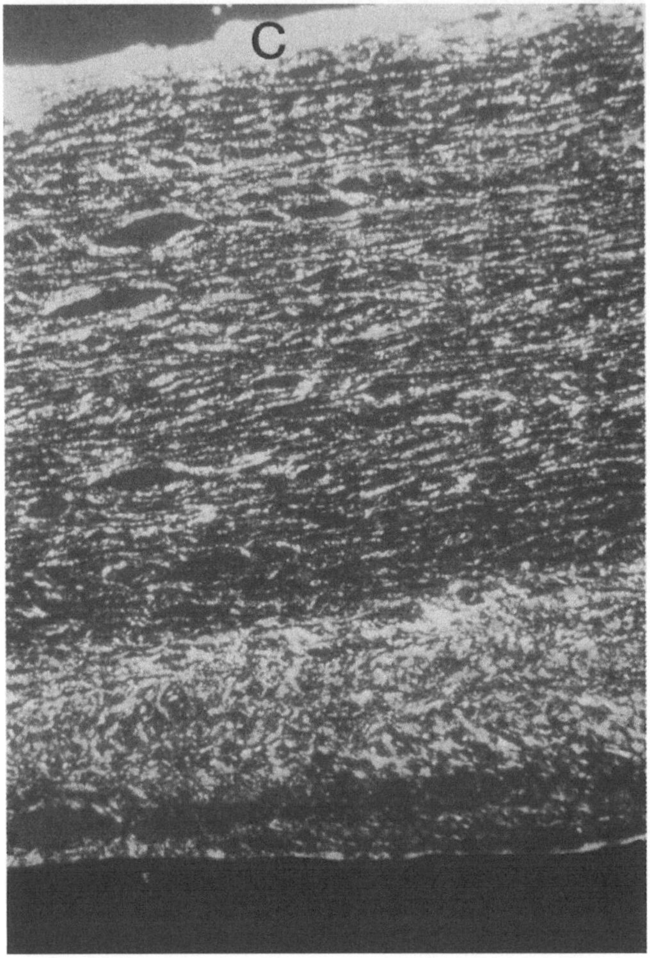

Fig. 5. Deposition of collagen type I *(C)* on the intima of aging human aorta as shown by picro Syrius red staining on a plaque-free area. (From [21])

also change with age and in pathological conditions. The width of capillary basement membranes increases linearly with age [1, 2, 25]. The slope of this age-dependent increase is about the same as the one obtained for diabetic capillaries according to the measurements of Kern et al. [26]. Diabetics, however, start at a higher value. The same holds for the collagen type III/I ratio which is also increased in diabetic tissues (skin, conjunctiva) as compared with age-matched controls [27, 28].

There is, however, a continuous increase with age of the collagen III/I ratio in non-diabetics, as also shown by Kern's studies in our laboratory [3]. Lipid deposition also affects all tissues during aging (arcus senilis) and especially in atherosclerosis-prone individuals (hyperlipaemia) as was shown experimentally by Beaumont's team [29]. We presented evidence for lipid deposition in brain capillary wall basement membranes in cholesterol-fed rabbits [30] with consecutive changes in the biology of the capillary wall. These modifications were prevented by calcitonin treatment.

Discussion and Conclusions

The above description of the composition and age-dependent modifications of extracellular matrix clearly shows the importance of cell-matrix interactions in the biology of the vessel wall. The pathological modifications are also accompanied and possibly triggered by the modifications of cell-matrix interaction. The development of the atherosclerotic plaque involves far-reaching modifications of the composition of the extracellular matrix of the vessel wall. We tried to separate the continuous age-dependent modifications of the extracellular matrix *(arteriosclerosis)* from the local modifications accompanying the development of the atherosclerotic plaque. We also emphasized the importance of age-dependent modifications of the microvascular wall and the acceleration of this process in diabetes.

These modifications affect the increased and perturbed permeability properties of microvessels. Although lipids and lipoproteins play an important role in these processes, they are not the only factors in the development of the atherosclerotic disease. Cell and matrix biology and cell-matrix interactions play an important role in this respect.

References

1. Robert L, Robert B (1973) Aging of connective tissues-skin. In: Robert L (ed) Frontiers of matrix biology, vol 1. Karger, Basel
2. Robert L, Labat-Robert J, Hornebeck W (1987) Aging and atherosclerosis. Atheroscler Rev 14 (in print)
3. Kern P, Sebert B, Robert L (1986) Increased type III/type I collagen ratios in diabetic human conjunctival biopsies. Clin Physiol Biochem 4 (2): 113-119
4. Robert L, Robert AM (1980) Elastin, elastase and arteriosclerosis. In: Robert AM, Robert L (eds) Frontiers of matrix biology, vol 8. Karger, Basel, pp 130-173
5. Moczar M, Ouzilou J, Courtois Y, Robert L (1976) Age dependence of the biosynthesis of intercellular matrix macromolecules of rabbit aorta in organ culture and cell culture. Gerontology 22: 461-472
6. Labat-Robert J, Leutenegger M, Llopis G, Ricard Y, Derouette JC (1984) Plasma and tissue fibronectin in diabetes. Clin Physiol Biochem 2: 39-48
7. Labat-Robert J, Phan Thanh L, Robert L (1985) Modification of plasma and tissue fibronectin in diabetes. In: Reddi AH (ed) Extracellular matrix: structure and function, vol 25. Liss, New York, pp 421-426
8. Campbell JH, Campbell GR (1986) The smooth muscle cell. CRC Press, Boca Raton, (in press)
9. Campbell GR, Chamley-Campbell JH (1981) The cellular pathology of atherosclerosis. Pathology 13: 423-440
10. Hornebeck W, Tixier JM, Robert L (1986) Inducible adhesion of mesenchymal cells to elastic fibers: elastonectin. Proc Natl Acad Sci USA 83: 5517-5520
11. Hornebeck W, Brechemier D, Bourdillon MC, Robert L (1981) Isolation and partial characterization of an elastase-like protease from rat aorta smooth muscle cells. Possible role in the regulation of elastin biosynthesis. Connect Tissue Res 8: 245-249
12. Hornebeck W, Derouette JC, Roland J, Chatelet F, Bouissou H, Robert L (1976) Corrélation entre l'âge, l'artériosclérose et l'activité élastinolytique de la paroi aortique humaine. C R Seances Acad Sci 282: 2003-2006

13. Hornebeck W, Brechemier D, Soleilhac JM, Bourdillon MC, Robert L (1985) Studies on rat aorta smooth muscle cells' elastase activity. In: Reddi AH (ed) Extracellular matrix: structure and function, vol 25. Liss, New York, pp 269-282
14. Senior RM, Griffin GL, Mecham RP (1982) Chemotactic responses of fibroblasts to tropoelastin and elastinderived peptides. J Clin Invest 70: 614-618
15. Hornebeck W, Soleilhac JM, Tixier JM, Moczar E, Robert L (1987) Inhibition by elastase inhibitors of the formyl Met Leu Phe-induced chemotaxis of rat polymorphonuclear leukocytes. Cell Biochem Function (in press)
16. Robert AM, Grosgogeat Y, Reverdy V, Robert B, Robert L (1971) Lésions artérielles produites chez le lapin par immunisation avec l'élastine et les glycoprotéines de structure de l'aorte. Etudes biochimiques et morphologiques. Atherosclerosis 13: 427-449
17. Jacob MP, Hornebeck W, Lafuma C, Bernaudin JF, Robert L, Godeau G (1984) Ultrastructural and biochemical modifications of rabbit arteries induced by immunization with soluble elastin peptides. Exp Mol Pathol 41: 171-190
18. Stein F, Pezess MP, Robert L, Poullain N (1965) Antielastin antibodies in normal and pathological human sera. Nature 207: 312-313
19. Horsch AK, Brechemier D, Robert L, Horsch S (1977) Anti-elastin Antikörper bei der Thrombangiitis obliterans. Verh Dtsch Ges Inn Med 83: 1757-1762
20. Wegrowski J, Moczar M, Robert L (1986) Proteoglycans from pig aorta. Comparative study of their interactions with lipoproteins. Biochem J 235: 823-831
21. Labat-Robert J, Szendroi M, Godeau G, Robert L (1985) Comparative distribution patterns of type I and III collagens and fibronectin in human arteriosclerotic aorta. Pathol Biol 33: 261-265
21 a. Adams CWM (1967) Vascular Histochemistry. Lloyd-Luke, London
22. Jacotot B, Beaumont JL, Monnier G, Szigeti M, Robert B, Robert L (1973) Role of elastic tissue in cholesterol deposition in the arterial wall. Nutr Metab 15: 46-58
23. Claire M, Jacotot B, Robert L (1976) Characterization of lipids associated with macromolecules of the intercellular matrix of human aorta. Connect Tissue Res 4: 61-71
24. Robert AM, Robert L (eds) (1980) Biology and pathology of elastic tissues. Karger, Basel (Frontiers of matrix biology, vol 8)
25. Robert L (1980) Mécanismes cellulaires et moléculaires du vieillissement. Masson, Paris
26. Kern P, Regnault F, Robert L (1976) Biochemical and ultrastructural study of human diabetic conjunctiva. Biomedecine 24: 32-38
27. Robert AM, Boniface R, Robert L (1979) Biochemistry and pathology of basement membranes. Role in diabetes. Karger, Basel (Frontiers of matrix biology, vol 7)
28. Kern P, Moczar M, Robert L (1979) Biosynthesis of skin collagens in normal and diabetic mice. Biochem J 182: 337-345
29. Beaumont JL, Grosgogeat Y, Richard JL, Claude JR (1963) La teneur en cholestérol de l'aorte et d'autres organes chez le lapin nourri avec du cholestérol. J Atheroscler Res 3: 210-221
30. Robert AM, Miskulin M, Godeau G, Tixer JP, Milhaud G (1982) Action of calcitonine on the atherosclerotic modifications of brain microvessels induced in rabbits by cholesterol feeding. Exp Mol Pathol 37: 67-73
31. Robert L, Chaudiere J, Jacotot B (1984) Interaction between lipids and the intercellular matrix of the arterial wall: its role in the evolution of atherosclerotic lesions. In: Malinow MR, Blaton VH (eds) Regression of atherosclerotic lesions. Experimental studies and observations in humans. NATO ASI Life Sciences 79: 145-173
32. Moczar M, Lafuma C (1986) Structural glycoproteins from aorta and lung. In: Robert L (ed) Frontiers of matrix biology, vol 11. Karger, Basel, pp 42-57

Changing Views of the Morphology of Atherosclerosis

G. A. Gresham

What is atherosclerosis? This is a question which was easily answered in the days when Schettler was a student. He would have been told of a degenerative disease characterized by lipid, thrombus, calcium and so on which blocked arteries and led to ischaemic damage.

Were he to ask his numerous friends and colleagues in Europe, America and the Far East the same question today he would get many different answers. Over the past 50 years research into atherosclerosis has expanded rapidly. Chemists, immunologists, histopathologists, haematologists and many others have persued there own special interests. Each discipline has concentrated on its own theme often to the exclusion of others.

The main change in approach in more recent times has been to direct attention to the early stages in the development of the atherosclerotic lesion. In the past the advanced complicated lesion was regarded as the prototype of the disease but this lesion is the result of the complex interaction of many factors and its study no longer occupies attention.

The central question about human coronary atherosclerosis remains unanswered. The question is why man is so peculiarly affected and killed by this disease in sharp contrast to most other animals. The answer must lie in the nature of the human arterial wall and the reaction of its various components to noxious stimuli of one sort or another.

Research into atherogenesis has persued several lines of thought. A common method for the clinician is to identify known risk factors such as smoking, hypertension, diabetes mellitus and hyperlipidaemia and then attempt to modify these factors in order to see if the effects of atherosclerosis are reduced. The end points in such investigations are death and clinical evidence of myocardial infarction or ischaemia. Such end points do not necessarily indicate the extent of coronary disease because other factors such as vascular spasm may be modified by altering risk factors.

Research by the epidemiologist often involves the identification of the risk of ischaemic heart disease in different communities. Significant differences exist in the incidence of ischaemic heart disease in different countries. For example the mortality incidence is high in Scotland and low in France. Differences in incidence such as these are only partly explicable by involving the presence of known risk factors. But the differences are not fully explained, which suggests that hitherto unrecognized provoking factors for atherogenesis exist.

Clinical and epidemiological research has been accompanied by experimental studies in a wide variety of animals. The early studies of Anitschkow used the rabbit and this animal model held sway for many years of this century. The rabbit is exquisitely sensitive to the atherogenic effects of dietary cholesterol. A few weeks of feeding as little as 1% cholesterol in the diet can lead to large intimal accumulations of foamy macrophages on the intimal surface. Later, if the dietary regime is continued, the lesions become capped with fibrous tissue. Because of its rapid response to cholesterol feeding, the rabbit has been regarded by many as atypical and not a suitable model for atherogenic studies. However, it still provides a suitable model for the study of certain aspects of atherogenesis. Attempts to produce regression of experimentally induced lesions in this animal have been successful but only occur with those lesions that are not encased with fibrous tissue. The Watanabe rabbit provides another interesting facet of study. It has a genetically determined deficiency of cell receptors for low-density lipoproteins (LDL) and develops severe atherosclerosis. Models with genetically determined risk factors implanted in their constituion are not common but have proved very useful. The white Cerneau pigeon develops severe atherosclerosis spontaneously and is valuable for studies of reversion of lesions. Animals with spontaneous hypertension such as the turkey and strains of rat can be used to demonstrate the potent effects of hypertension as an atherogenic agent.

No animal model is fully acceptable as being equivalent to man himself for the study of atherogenesis. However non-human primates have been much used and a variety of provoking factors have been applied to produce lesions that resemble human atherosclerotic disease. Most of the lesions that have been produced are of the fatty streak or fibromuscular types. The effects of dietary lipid, hypertension, allergens, smoking have all been studied. Some primates seem to be more susceptible to atherogenic regimes than others. Some, like the marmoset monkey, are resistant and this may be related to the high levels of high-density lipoproteins (HDL) in the plasma of these animals.

Over the years, experiments in animals have contributed a good deal to the understanding of the factors that provoke atherogenesis, those that modify or ameliorate it and those that may cause it to disappear. None of them have solved the precise problem of the early steps in atherogenesis. It seems most likely that some factor or factors acting at the plasma endothelial cell interface are likely to be important in this regard. For this reason work in recent times has emphasized the need to study the cells that might interact at this plasma endothelial interface.

Some years ago the blood monocyte transformed to a macrophage was considered to be a likely candidate for study. Interest in this cell waned, only to be revived in the past few years. The role of the macrophage as a scavenger has been accepted for years and the notion that these cells become the lipid-laden foam cells of atherosclerosis was generally accepted. However the macrophage has other properties that make it a likely candidate for an atherogenic role. For example it possesses powerful hydrolytic enzymes such as elastases that are capable of damaging the arterial wall. It produces mitogenic growth factors that may cause cell proliferation and contribute to the bulk of the atherosclerotic lesion. The macrophage is concerned in cholesterol esterification and in lipoprotein catabolism and the presence of oxidised lipid within the cell can render it powerfully histotoxic by virtue of this ability to produce injury to cell membranes.

Cholesterol feeding causes macrophages to adhere to the endothelial surface and in time the endothelium is damaged by the presence of these cells. Macrophages and platelets then adhere to the exposed collagen and smooth muscle cell proliferation ensues from the mitogenic action of growth factors produced by both of these cell types. It appears then that blood cells which are usually extraneous to the vessel wall are capable of initiating atherosclerosis. This supports a modified view of the thrombogenic hypothesis which postulated the role of thrombus incorporation as an atherogenic factor.

Endothelial cells themselves may also play an important part in the process. These cells are damaged by a variety of factors that have been postulated as atherogenic. In hypertension a number of amines may be circulating in the blood and these can have a direct effect on endothelial cells or on endothelial cell junctions rendering the endothelial sheet more permeable to plasma constituents. Substances such as angiotensin II, epinephrine and tyramine have such effects. Once the sheet of cells develops leaks then all the constituents of the plasma can gain entry to the vessel wall. Some are harmless but others such as LDL can create damage giving rise to death and subsequent proliferation of smooth muscle in the arterial media. Some authors have claimed that smooth muscle proliferation can be induced without endothelial damage: for example, by the administration of vitamin D to the rat. This causes medial damage and calcification followed by cell proliferation. However, the suggestion that changes of endothelial permeability do not occur in such experiments is not convincing.

Endothelium has many other potentially protective and contributary roles in atherogenesis. The cells produce prostacyclin and antithrombotic substances which are advantageous. They are also capable of producing collagen and elastin which may be contributary to intimal thickening.

Blood platelets have often been suspected of having an atherogenic role. The argument against this is based on the view that endothelial damage must occur before platelets can interact with the vessel wall. So that whilst platelets may contribute to intimal thickening they do not primarily initiate it.

The blood platelet is richly endowed with potential atherogens such as mitogenic growth factors. They play an important role in the accelerated version of atherosclerosis that occurs in the arteries of transplanted organs such as heart, liver and kidney. This relentless arterial occlusion is a common frustrating cause of organ failure in allograft recipients. The fact that it can be ameliorated by anti-platelet drugs such as dipyridamole and sulphinpyrazone lends support to the role of the blood platelet in atherogenesis.

In recent years most attention has been paid to the smooth muscle cell and its behaviour in the atherosclerotic process. It can assume various forms such as contractile or secretory, and its growth can be affected by a variety of mitogens derived from cells such as platelets and monocytes. It seems that LDL which has entered the vessel wall can have a profound effect upon these cells. LDL enters the vessel wall following a change in endothelial permeability, which may be brought about in a number of ways. Within the media, LDL becomes anchored to glycosaminoglycans which envelop the lamellar units of the vessel wall and from this point of vantage they stimulate smooth muscle cell growth.

The secretory phase of smooth muscle cell function is associated with the production of collagen and elastin and for this and other reasons the smooth muscle cell has been regarded as the central figure in the atherosclerotic process. These cells proliferate in the media and in the intima and a variety of stimuli induce this reaction. In many respects they are similar to the myofibroblasts of granulation tissue concerned in collagen and scar formation.

Atherosclerosis can be regarded as a basic inflammatory reaction in the vessel wall and because of the muscular structure of the artery it is the muscle cells that have a dominant role. The result is thickening of the wall of the artery leading to relative hypoxia in the expanded inner media. These hypoxic conditions promote lipid accumulation which forms the main occlusive component of atheroma.

An acceptable modern hypothesis of atherogenesis is that injury occurs to the endothelium but the precise nature of this injury is yet to be determined. Following this cellular proliferation occurs, a repair reaction, which further compromises the vessel wall leading to a chain of secondary events such as lipid accumulation. The nature of the initial damage to the arterial wall, be it single or multiple, is the question that many of us in atherosclerosis research seek to answer.

Atherosclerosis as a Recurrent Cycle of Inflammation and Repair

C. W. M. Adams

In the last century, Virchow first drew attention to the inflammatory aspect of atherosclerosis, and pointed to endarteritis as a factor in the multifactorial pathogenesis of the disease [37]. This observation has been largely ignored, mainly because most doctors regard inflammation as having only a microbiological connotation. Even though it has been suggested that herpes or other viruses may play a part in atherogenesis [18], there are many other types of inflammation apart from those caused by microbial agents. Trauma induced inflammatory changes that parallel those seen in atherosclerosis, such as fibrinous exudation in tenosynovitis and the reparative aspects of a peptic ulcer (namely epi- or endothelial, macrophage and fibroblastic activity). Immune reactions result in an inflammatory response marked mainly by lymphocytoid and plasmocytoid infiltration and by macrophage activation or arming. Some of these responses are seen in advanced atherosclerosis. Acute inflammation also causes foci of necrosis, either as a result of the cytotoxic nature of the inflammatory agent (e.g. the carbuncle caused by staphylococcal toxins) or compression of the local blood supply by inflammatory oedema. Necrosis is an important feature of atherosclerosis with clinical manifestations. Indeed, the arterial wall at various sites and at different ages shows all these manifestations of subacute or chronic inflammation, and inflammatory events often alternate with repair processes in a recurrent cycle producing "geological layers" in the lesion [27].

In discussing inflammation in atherogensesis, it is appropriate first to consider what roles physical and humoral agents play in the disease. Increased endothelial permeability may in part be a response to the haemodynamic trauma of blood flow, as in the turbulent areas at the orifices of branch arteries [39]. Increased shear is accompanied by an immediately increased influx and thickening of the arterial wall [10, 16]. Hypertension, as well as increasing the amplitude of the pulse wave, may be accompanied by the formation of vasoactive compounds, promoting increased vascular permeability [31]. Other simple injuries may result in endothelial damage with resulting endothelial proliferation. Newly formed endothelial cells are particularly permeable [15] and will permit increased influx into the arterial wall. Hypercholesterolaemia itself seems to act as a chemical injurious agent promoting endothelial damage and proliferation, with resulting increased permeability to Evans blue or its isomer [5, 9, 39].

Another humoral aspect of inflammation is the formation of fibrin, which is a defence mechanism to limit and contain the contents of the inflammatory exudate and other agents that have penetrated the extravascular space. Indeed, fibrinogen, inter alia, enters the arterial wall in large quantity in the process termed insudation or, in more extreme form, plasmatic vasculosis, including fibrinoid necrosis [24].

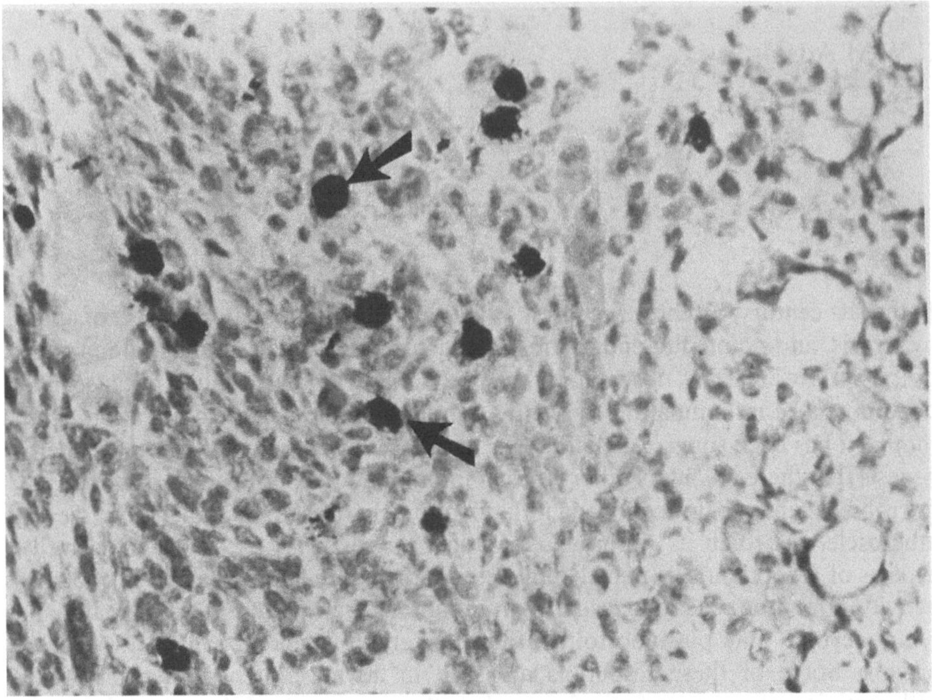

Fig. 1. Macrophages *(arrows)* on surface of aortic endothelium. *Hautchen en face* preparation. Cytochrome oxidase, × 170

Fibrin forms a fine fibrous network within tissues which, as well as entrapping bacteria, may reduce the flow of metabolites across the arterial wall. Indeed, Lendrum [24] suggested that the fenestrations in elastic fibres may be blocked by fibrin and, thus, efflux across the arterial wall is impeded.

Complement or part of the complement cascade seems to be involved in the formation of the atherosclerotic plaque [36]. Apart from chemotaxis of macrophages (see below), there is at present not much concrete evidence about the role of vasoactive peptides (such as kinins), leukotrienes (prostacyclin B) and lymphokines (including interleukins) in the development of atherosclerosis. However, other prostaglandins do control certain functions of the arterial wall. Thus, prostacyclins C, D and E promote smooth muscle relaxation and vasodilation, whereas thromboxanes promote thrombus formation. The relation of these events to smoking and their effect on permeability [40] remain to be clarified. Clearly, this area constitutes a growing point and is part of the widening horizon of atherosclerosis research.

The margination of macrophages, their adherence to arterial endothelium (Fig. 1) and their entry into the subendothelial tissues (Fig. 2; [28]) parallels the margination and diapedesis of polymorphonuclear leucocytes in acute inflammation. It is not clear what vasoactive agents stimulate the entry of macrophages into the arterial wall, but it has been suggested that locally formed interleukin I and leukotriene B4 may initiate and maintain the chemotaxis of macrophages [35]. Once inside the arterial wall, macrophages appear to be mainly concerned with phagocytosing lipid

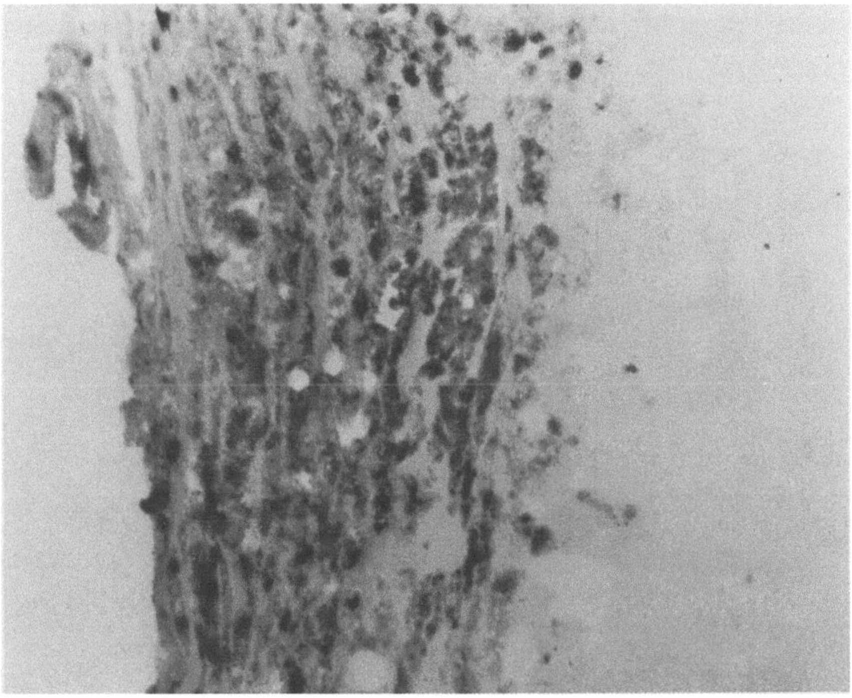

Fig. 2. Macrophages in superficial fatty-streak lesion of human atherosclerotic aorta. Non-specific esterase, × 170

material. Perhaps it is the presence of free lipid, possibly opsonized by fibronectin, that in part determines macrophage entry into the arterial intima. Nevertheless, in severely hypercholesterolaemic animals such as the cholesterol-fed-rabbit, the monocyte precursor of the macrophage actually carries lipid from the blood into the arterial intima [22]. Such extreme examples of hypercholesterolaemia are analogous to that seen in homozygous familial hypercholesterolaemia and similar conditions in man, where lipid storage within macrophages is a feature [4, 30]. However, such an explanation is clearly not tenable with the usual ranges of serum cholesterol, and macrophage entry into the arterial wall must be seen as an inflammatory response to remove debris in preparation for repair by organization. If this is so, then the early fatty-streak lesion in the tunica intima represents a reparative or phagocytic response by the macrophage to foci of lipid deposited in the subendothelium, rather than a specific invasive focus of blood monocytes. The end stage of atherosclerosis, where thrombosis and ulceration have occurred, is accompanied by vascularization from the intima [17, 20]. Endothelial proliferation and formation of new capillaries precedes monocyte entry into an organizing inflammatory (granulating) lesion. Such vascularization of the arterial wall allows macrophages to enter deeply into the plaque, and here they pallisade around cholesterol crystals or even coalesce to form giant cells in the central necrotic gruel (Fig. 3).

As well as the traumatic inflammatory and reparative mechanisms outlined above, the human coronary arterial wall may show evidence of lymphocytic infiltra-

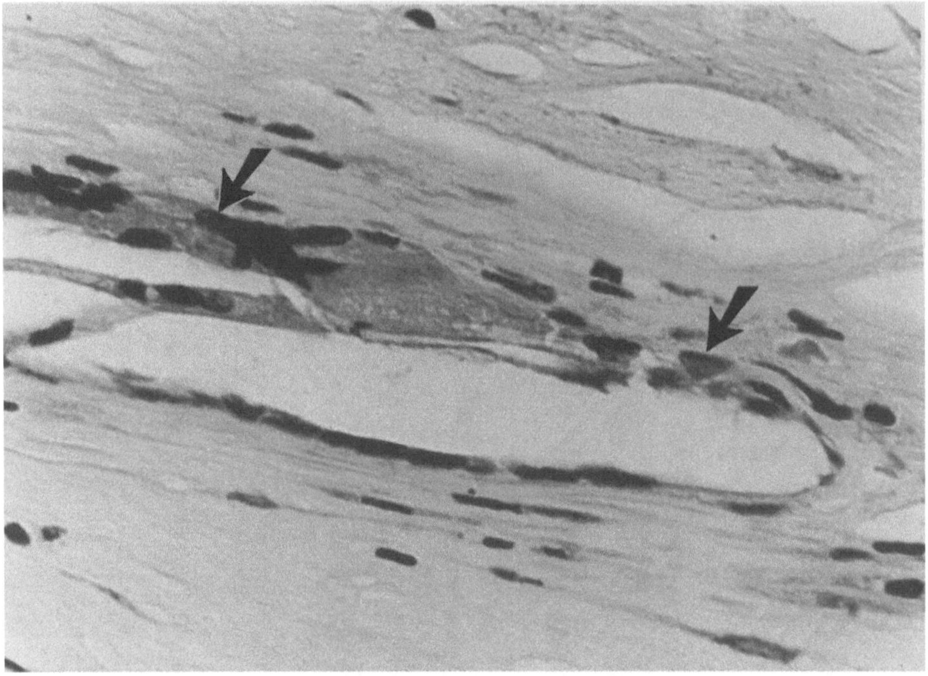

Fig. 3. Macrophages *(arrows)* pallisading around a cholesterol cleft in human atherosclerotic aorta, ×220

tion in the adventitia [29] and, in addition, macrophage infiltration of the smooth muscle fibres in the media [2, 21]. These inflammatory infiltrates, together with some damage to the tunica media, are seen in the coronary arteries of about 3% of subjects over 70 years in age, and could well be the expression of a local immune disorder.

For many years, Hauss and his colleagues [19] have been concerned with the reactions of the mesenchyme in atherosclerosis. These mesenchymal responses include the formation of matrices, such as collagen and elastin, and the ground substance. The main synthetic cell in the arterial wall is the smooth muscle cell (SMC), which is capable of synthesizing glycosaminoglycan, contractile protein, collagen and elastin [33]. This is in effect saying that the SMC can synthesize the full range of extracellular matrices and intracellular filaments and, in addition, retains its potential for contractility [8]. In addition to its synthetic, mesenchyme and contractile roles, the SMC also seems to subserve the function of an inflammatory cell. It proliferates and secretes in response to injury and trauma (Fig. 4) and is also capable of marked endocytosis or even phagocytic activity. Whether the removal of lipoprotein by SMC represents true scavenger uptake is not clear, but certainly the cell can be regarded as analogous to an inflammatory cell and has an active reparative function in the process of organization.

The early stages of atherosclerosis are not accompanied by ischaemic changes, but advanced lesions frequently develop a necrotic gruel-like core (Fig. 5). This

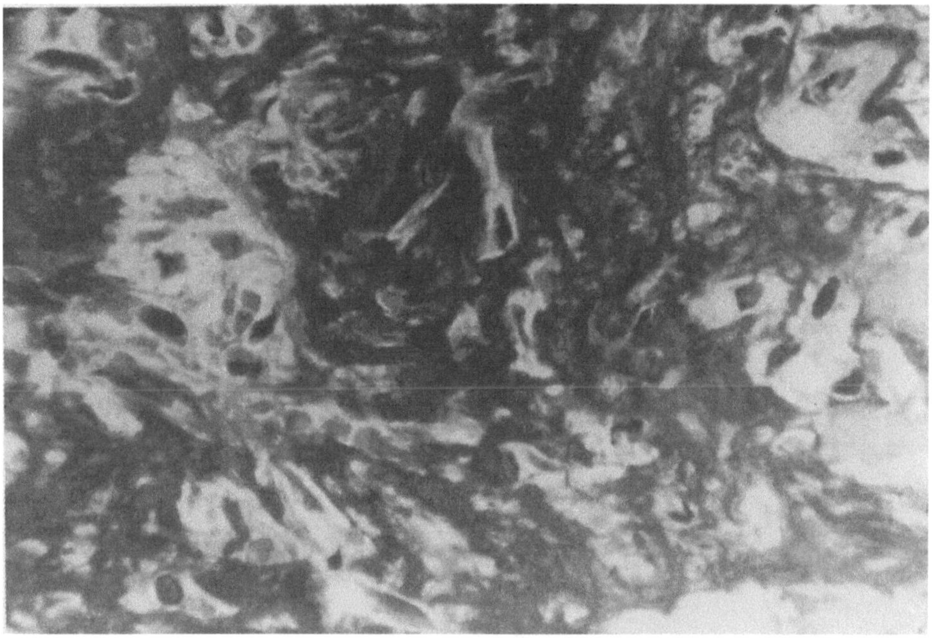

Fig. 4. Proliferating smooth muscle in intima. Intimo-medial junction at right. Elastic-trichrome-MSB, ×350

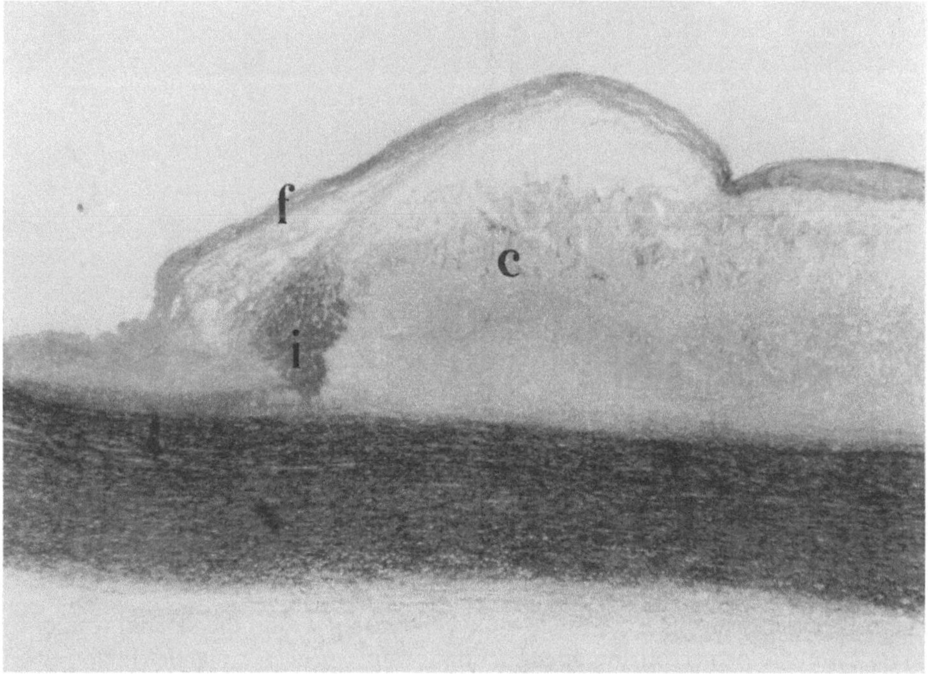

Fig. 5. Necrotic atheromatous core of dome-shaped human aortic atherosclerotic plaque. *c*, Cholesterol clefts; *f*, fibrous cap; *i*, insudation of fibrin. Elastic-trichrome-MSB, ×20

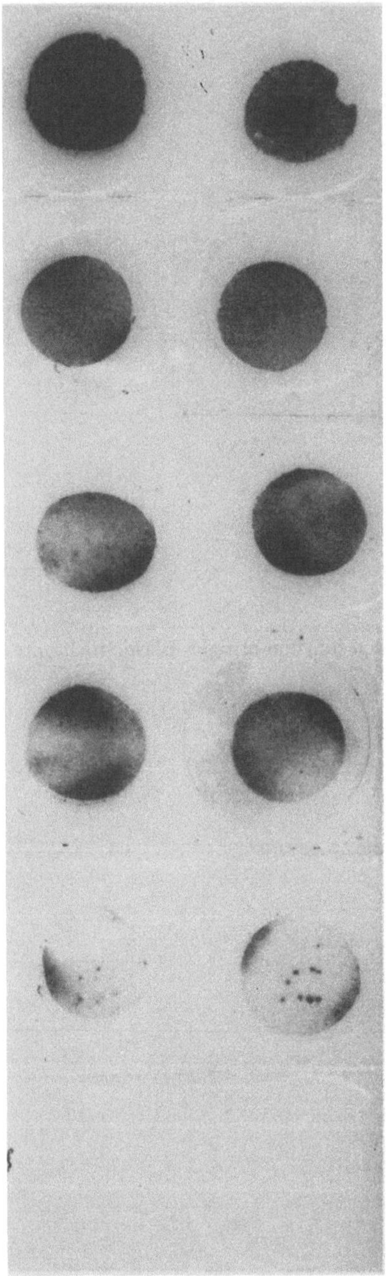

Fig. 6. Effect of oxysterols on culture wells of human fibroblasts. From *left* to *right*: cholestane-3,5,6-triol, 35-hydroxycholesterol, cholesterol oxidized in UV light, dibromo-purified cholesterol, cholesterol-5,6-epoxide, control. Toluidine blue, ×1

necrosis possibly results from the low oxygen tension within the arterial wall or to some cytotoxic or necrotizing agent acting locally, such as a platelet factor or an oxysterol formed by oxidation of the surfaces of cholesterol crystals (Fig. 6; see [7, 26]). In addition, the obstructive action of layers of collagen, water-repellant lipid and calcium salts impedes perfusion into the deeper intima and promotes further

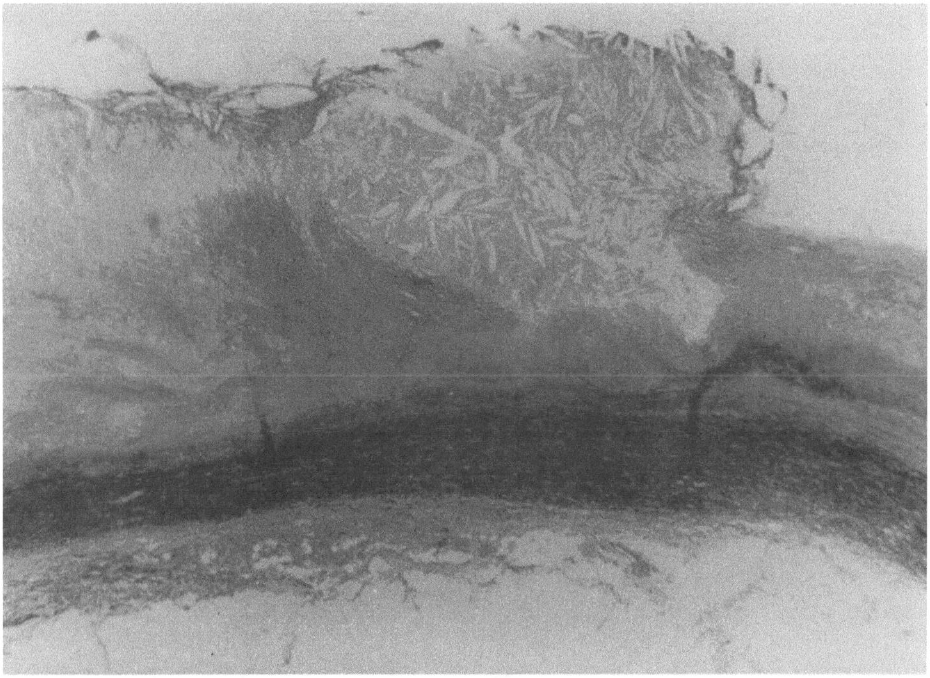

Fig. 7. Ruptured human atherosclerotic plaque. Compare with Fig. 5. Elastic-trichrome-MSB, ×20

hypoxia. However, it remains uncertain what the precise cause is of the necrosis of the centre of the advanced atherosclerotic lesion.

Local ischaemia and necrosis in the atherosclerotic intima induces ulceration of the surface (Figs. 5, 7) and this, in turn, provides a nidus for thrombus formation, perhaps partly as a result of exposure of collagen in the underlying intima [23]. Ulceration of a substantial area of an atherosclerotic plaque is commonly seen in the aorta, but cracks or fissures are the more usual manifestations of necrosis in the coronary arteries (Fig. 8; [11]). However, sizeable areas of coronary atherosclerosis sometimes undergo ulceration, and the extruded atheromatous material causes coronary embolization. This process seems to be the pathological explanation for crescendo or unstable angina [14]. The integrity of the cap of fibrous tissue over an atherosclerotic plaque is clearly a most important factor in preventing local thrombosis and distant embolism. The mural thrombus that forms over such denuded ulcerated areas introduces a risk of embolism, but the platelet-derived growth factors (PDGF and endothelial growth factor [34, 35]) that it contains are powerful factors in promoting connective tissue and endothelial growth to repair the defect. The mural thrombus can, in a way, be regarded as an immediate but risky defence mechanism, a rubber patch to prevent the immediate discharge of the atheromatous gruel in the floor of the "ulcer" into the circulation. Subsequently, the patch becomes organized to form a new and safe retaining fibrous cap over the lesion which, to pursue the analogy, is akin to the torn tyre being repaired by vulcanization.

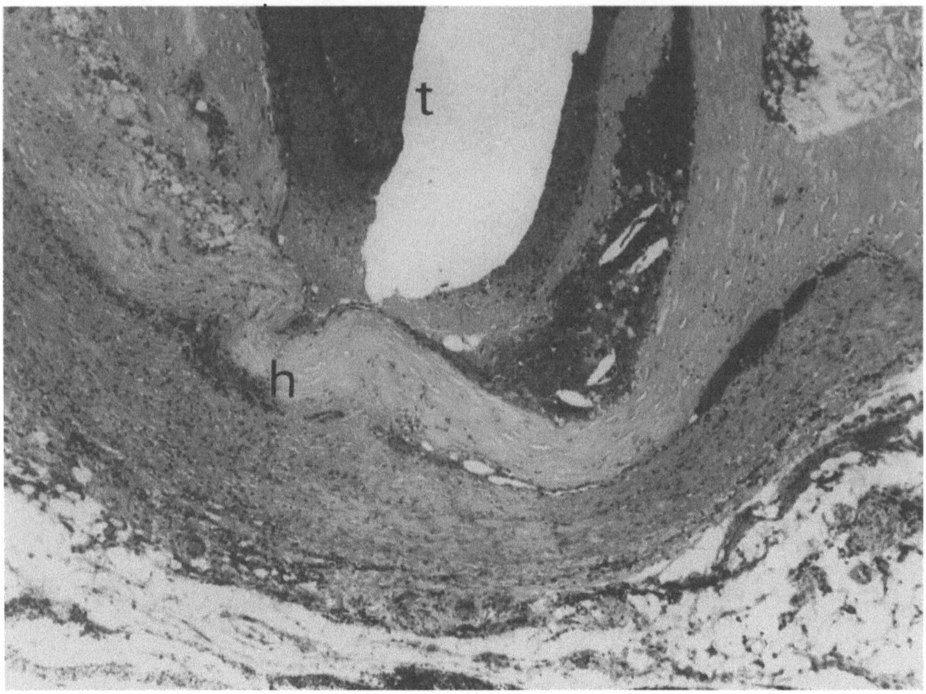

Fig. 8. Crack in atherosclerotic plaque of human coronary artery. *t*, Thrombus; *h*, intimal haemorrhage. Elastic-trichrome-MSB, ×4

In addition to the organizing activity resulting from repair of an ulcer or thrombus, certain lipids (notably cholesterol, its saturated and *trans* esters, certain oxysterols and some free fatty acids) promote inflammation (Fig. 9), necrosis and fibrotic repair [3, 7]. These reactions may be an important factor in promoting fibrosis around the lipid deposits within the plaque. Additionally, deposits of fibrin or fibrin degradation products promote fibrosis and repair by organization [13]. Clearly, fibrosis as a healing mechanism over an atherosclerotic plaque is in general beneficial, but fibrosis in the depths of the lesion can only be seen as adding to the thickness of the lesion and in further obstructing the flow of oxygen and metabolites into and out of the wall. Indeed, Osborn [27] pointed to the importance of "geological layering" of alternating or recurrent thrombotic and healing events during the "incubation period" of clinical coronary disease.

Fibrotic repair with type I collagen and consequent replacement of type III structural collagen sometimes results in scar formation and contractures. These may impair function, such as in pyloric stenosis complicating gastric ulcer and in hydrocephalus following acute or chronic meningitis. It has previously been mooted that scarring or contracture of collagen in the atherosclerotic artery may result in arterial stenosis. However, such fibrotic stenosis does not seem to occur in practice, possibly because the kinetic engery of blood flow is continually promoting vascular dilation and lengthening of the collagen fibre.

With advancing age the arterial wall undergoes dilatation, both in a radial and in

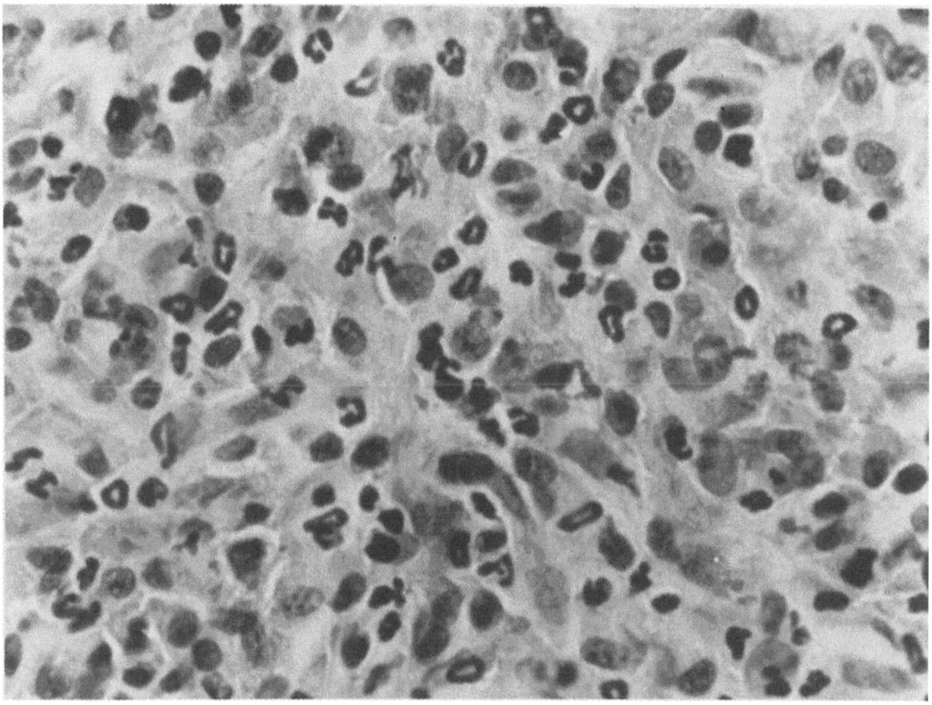

Fig. 9. Inflammatory response to 25-hydroxycholesterol. Note abundant polymorphonuclear leucocytes and macrophages. Subcutaneous implant at 7 days, H & E, ×480. (From *Atherosclerosis* with permission)

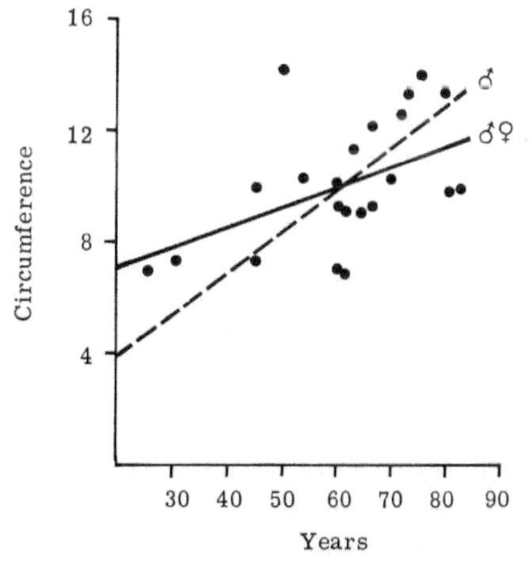

Fig. 10. External circumference of human coronary arterial wall with advancing age (sum of circumferences at six sites in coronary arterial tree, using formaldehyde perfusion at 108 mmHg). (From *Atherosclerosis* with permission)

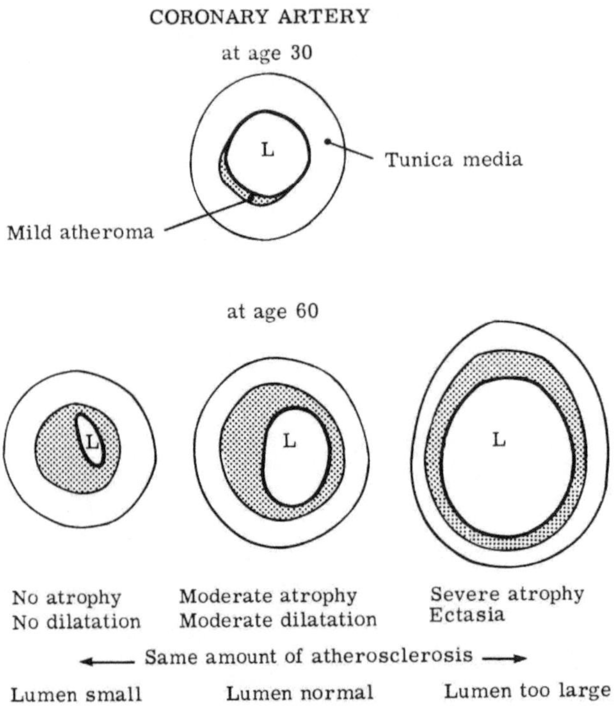

Fig. 11. Effect of different degrees of mural dilatation on coronary lumen. The *middle lower* diagram shows dilatation matching inward encroachment by atherosclerosis, whereas the *right lower* diagram shows the enlarged lumen in ectasia. (From *Atherosclerosis* with permission)

a longitudinal direction. This dilatation has been measured in the coronary artery (Fig. 10; [32, 38 and others]), aorta [25] and renal arteries (L. Denmark and C. W. M. Adams, unpublished observations). Duguid [12] first drew attention to the general process of arterial dilatation with advancing age and, clearly, this would tend to offset the stenosing effect of atherosclerosis (Fig. 11; [38]). M. F. Oliver has suggested that the expectation of such dilatation, together with reasonable efforts to prevent further increase in atherosclerosis, constitute an effective clinical policy for the management of established atherosclerotic disease. However, in some instances arterial dilatation is excessive and forms local ectatic enlargements or even aneurysms. Ectasia [6] is a dangerous condition because it alters local haemodynamics, particularly reducing flow rate and promoting wave-reflection and local turbulence. The resulting poor perfusion through these drain-pipe arteries carries a very real risk of thrombosis [1].

The development of coronary ectasia as outlined above could result from senile atrophy of connective tissues, the direct pressure effects of atherosclerotic fibro-fatty or calcified lesions or from medial damage induced by an immune reaction, as evidenced by the lymphocytic and macrophage infiltration described above. A current study [21] suggests that loss of medial smooth muscle fibres (as an index of coronary ectasia) correlates best with the degree of atherosclerosis, rather than with age and immune damage to the media. However, this is not to deny that age-dependent atrophy is not a more important causal mechanism for simple dilatation without thinning of the media.

This brief discussion underlines the importance of the reparative role of connective tissues (including their proliferation and degeneration) in the progression and unfolding of the atherosclerotic process. The lipid contant of a human atherosclerotic lesion occasionally forms mor than one-half the total area seen in histological sections, but it more usually occupies one-quarter to one-third of the lesion, sometimes even less than this. Thus, in most instances the connective tissues are the predominant constituents of the plaque. Certainly, changes in these matrices seem to be the major factors determining and regulating the onset of clinical arterial disease (namely, cracking of the human coronary intima, plaque ulceration, thrombosis and organization thereof, atrophic aneurysm, dissecting aneurysm, and atrophy or hypertrophy of the arterial tunica intima and media).

As emphasized in this essay, the bulk mass of the human coronary atherosclerotic lesion does not arise as a sudden monophasic event. Rather, it is built up by recurrent inflammatory events, including periods of platelet deposition and increased permeability to fibrinogen and plasma lipoproteins, followed by a stage of repair.

References

1. Adams CWM (1987) Disordered structure and function in the atherosclerotic artery. In: Olssen AG (ed) Handbook on atherosclerosis. Elsevier, Amsterdam
2. Adams CWM, Poston RN (1986) Advances in the pathology of atherosclerosis. In: Fidge NH, Nestel PJ (eds) Proceedings of the VIIth international symposium on atherosclerosis. Exc Med, Amsterdam, pp 525-529
3. Abdulla YH, Adams CWM, Morgan RS (1967) The reaction of connective tissues to implantation of purified sterol, sterol esters, phosphoglycerides, glycerides and free fatty acids. J Pathol Bacteriol 94: 63-71
4. Adams CWM, Bayliss OB, Turner DR (1975) Phagocytes, lipid-removal and regression of atheroma. J Pathol 116: 225-238
5. Adams CWM, Bayliss OB, Morgan RS (1977) Permeability in atherosclerosis: fluorescence test in green light with trypan blue. Atherosclerosis 27: 353-359
6. Aschoff L (1924) Lectures on pathology. Hoeber, New York, pp 131-153
7. Baranowski A, Adams CWM, High OB, Bowyer DB (1982) Connective tissue responses to oxysterols. Atherosclerosis 41: 255-266
8. Campbell GR, Campbell JHC, Burnstock G (1981) Differentiation and phenotypic modulation of arterial smooth muscle cells. In: Schwartz CJ, Werthessen NT (eds) Structure and function of the circulation, vol 3. Plenum, New York, pp 357-399
9. Caplan BA, Schwartz CJ (1973) Increased endothelial turnover in areas of in vivo Evans' blue dye uptake in the pig aorta. Atherosclerosis 17: 401-417
10. Caro CG (1973) Transport of materials between blood and wall in arteries. In: Porter R, Knight J (eds) Atherogenesis: initiating factors. CIBA Found Symp 12: 127-164
11. Constantinides P (1966) Plaque fissures in human coronary thrombosis. Atherosclerosis 6: 1-17
12. Duguid JB (1926) Atheroma of the aorta. J Pathol Bacteriol 29: 371-387
13. Duguid JB (1952) The arterial lining. Lancet II: 207-208
14. Falk E (1985) Unstable angina with fatal outcome: dynamic coronary thrombosis leading to infarction and/or sudden death. Circulation 71: 699-708
15. Friedman M, Byers SO (1962) Excess lipid leakage: a property of very young vascular endothelium. Br J Exp Pathol 43: 363-372
16. Friedman MH, Deters OJ, Bargeron CB, Hutchins GM, Mark FF (1986) Shear-dependant thickening of the human arterial intima. Atherosclerosis 60: 161-171

17. Geiringer E (1951) Intimal vascularisation and atherosclerosis. J Pathol Bacteriol 63: 201-211
18. Hajjar DP, Fabricant CG, Minick CR, Fabricant J (1986) Virus-induced atherosclerosis. Herpes-virus infection alters cholesterol metabolism. Am J Pathol 122: 62-70
19. Hauss WH, Junge-Hulsing G, Hollander HJ (1962) Changes in metabolism of connective tissue associated with ageing and arterio-atherosclerosis. J Atherosclerosis 2: 50-61
20. High OB, Adams CWM (1980) The role of macrophages and giant cells in advanced human atherosclerosis. Atherosclerosis 36: 441-447
21. Keohane S, Poston RN, Adams CWM (1987) Coronary artery dilatation in atherosclerosis (to be published)
22. Leary T (1941) The genesis of atherosclerosis. Arch Pathol 32: 507-555
23. Legrand YJ, Fauver F, Arbeille B, Leger D, Mouhli H, Gutman N, Muh JP (1986) Activation of platelets by microfibrils and collagen. Lab Invest 54: 566-573
24. Lendrum AC (1963) The hypertensive diabetic kidney as a model for so-called collagen diseases. Can Med Assoc J 88: 442-552
25. Mitchell JRA, Adams JH (1977) Aortic size and aortic calcification. Atherosclerosis 37: 437-446
26. Mitchinson MJ, Hothersall DC, Brooks PN, De Burbure CY (1985) The distribution of ceroid in human atherosclerosis. J Pathol 145: 177-183
27. Osborn GR (1963) The incubation period of coronary thrombosis. Butterworths, London
28. Poole JCF, Florey HW (1958) Changes in the endothelium of the aorta and the behaviour of macrophages in experimental atheroma of rabbits. J Pathol Bacteriol 75: 245-251
29. Poston RN, Davies DF (1974) Immunity and inflammation in the pathogenesis of atherosclerosis - a review. Atherosclerosis 19: 353-367
30. Roberts WC, Levy RI, Fredrickson DS (1970) Hyperlipoproteinemia: a review of the five types with first reports of necropsy findings in type 3. Arch Pathol 90: 46-56
31. Robertson AL, Khairallah PA (1973) Arterial endothelial permeability and vascular disease. Exp Mol Pathol 18: 241-249
32. Rose G, Prineas RJ, Mitchell JRA (1967) Myocardial infarction and the intrinsic calibre of coronary arteries. Br Heart J 29: 248-256
33. Ross R, Lebanoff SJ (1971) The smooth muscle I. In vivo synthesis of connective tissue proteins. J Cell Biol 50: 159-167
34. Ross R, Vogel A (1978) The platelet derived growth factor. Cell 14: 203-210
35. Ross R (1986) The pathogenesis of atherosclerosis - an update. N Engl J Med 314: 488-500
36. Rus HG, Niculescu F, Constantinescu E, Cristea A, Vlaicu R (1986) Immuno-electron microscopic localization of the terminal C5b-9 complement complex in human atherosclerotic fibrous plaque. Atherosclerosis 61: 35-42
37. Virchow R von (1856) Gesammelte Abhandlungen zur wissenschaftlichen Medizin. Muller, Berlin
38. Wilson J, Adams CWM, Brander WL (1978) The antiocclusive effect of coronary dilatation with age. Atherosclerosis 29: 503-507
39. Wright HP, Evans M, Green R (1975) Aortic endothelial mitosis and Evans blue dye uptake in cholesterol fed rabbits. Atherosclerosis 21: 105-113
40. Zimmerman M, McGeachie J (1986) Quantitation of the relationship between aortic endothelial intercellular cleft morphology and permeability to albumin. Atherosclerosis 61: 35-42

Non-Arterial Deposition of Lipids and Lipoproteins: Significance in Relation to Atherogenesis

K. W. Walton

Introduction

Professor F. Gotthard Schettler has had a longstanding interest in seeking better means of identifying those at risk of atherosclerosis and thereby instituting effective preventative or prophylactic measures. For example, 32 years ago he published a paper entitled *"Ist der sogenannte Greisenbogen der Hornhaut ein Hinweis auf Atherosklerose?"* [1]. He has also had an enduring interest in the mechanisms of atherogenesis.

For these reasons, it seemed that an appropriate contribution to a *Festschrift* to mark his 70th birthday might be a review of work done, since his early paper, on non-arterial lesions associated with atherosclerosis (not only the corneal arcus but also lesions at other sites) which might have significance in relation to mechanisms involved in atherogenesis.

Atherosclerosis has been defined by a Study Group of the World Health Organisation (WHO) [2] as: "a variable combination of changes of the intima of arteries (as distinct from arterioles) consisting of the focal accumulation of lipids, complex carbohydrates, blood and blood products, fibrous tissue and calcium deposits, and associated with medial changes".

However, it is now well-recognised that severe atherosclerotic arterial disease can be accompanied by a variety of non-arterial lesions with similar pathological features, and in particular, a "focal accumulation of lipid, complex carbohydrates" etc., like that seen in arteries. For example, in addition to the corneal arcus, concomitant localised lesions of an essentially similar kind can occur in: skin and tendons (xanthomata); heart valves; and arterial bypass grafts derived from autogenous veins or even from synthetic (plastic) materials.

Extra-Arterial Lesions Accompanying Atherosclerosis

Corneal Arcus in Man

The occurrence of a corneal arcus has been held to reflect broadly the incidence of atherosclerosis, while both arcus formation and atherosclerosis are related to plasma low-density lipoprotein (LDL) levels. This is seen in older age-groups of many populations. For example, the incidence of arcus senilis and of atherosclerosis both increase with age [3, 4], in parallel with increase of LDL levels [5, 6]. But these associations can even be seen at younger ages. For instance, children with

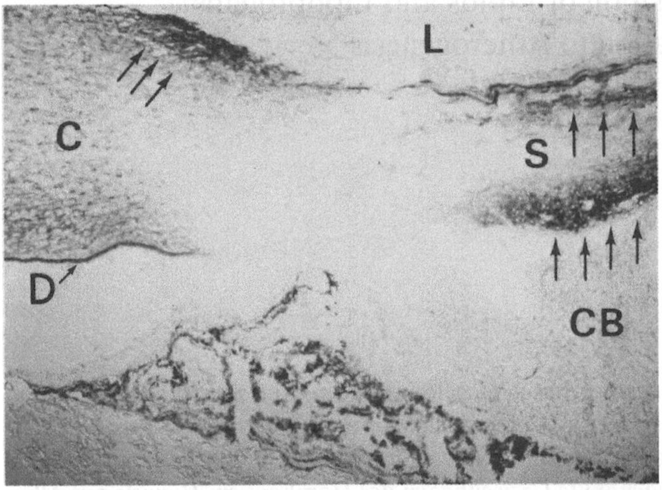

Fig. 1. Frozen section from anterior segment of human eye with severe corneal arcus. Note heavy lipid deposition (red in original, *black areas marked by small arrows* in picture) involving sclera *(S)*, overlying ciliary body *(CB)* and throughout full thickness of cornea *(C)* but especially marked at the margin of the limbus *(L)* and in Descemet's membrane *(D)*. Haematoxylin, oil red O and light green (ORO/LG) × 50

familial hyperlipidaemias with early and gross elevation of LDL, may show an arcus juvenilis in association with precocious atherosclerotic cardiovascular disease [7].

A personal study [8] of these associations was conducted in two parts. In one part, 104 (63 M, 41 F) consecutive cases of sudden death (age range 20–93 years), referred for coroner's autopsies, were examined for the presence/absence of a corneal arcus and its severity was noted, but the eyes were not examined histologically. In these subjects, the extent and severity of atherosclerosis in the aorta, coronary, cerebral, renal and femoral arteries was graded as proposed by the WHO Study Group [2].

In this series, no arcus was seen in anyone below 45, although some young males showed early atherosclerosis in the aorta, coronary or other arteries. In males aged 45–55, and in females a decade older, an early arcus was apparent. At older ages in both sexes, the severity of the arcus advanced and a broad association with the advance of atherosclerosis in general was noted. But no correlation was found between arcus formation and the presence or severity of atherosclerosis in any *one* arterial territory.

This part of the study thus confirmed Schettler's earlier conclusion [1], and later ones of others [3–6, 9–11], that the arcus is of limited value for the assessment (say) of risk of developing coronary heart disease.

In the second part of this study [8], the eyes were examined histologically and immuno-histologically in 16 subjects (11 M, 5 F; age range 45–92 years) presenting at routine necropsy with an arcus; and from 4 subjects (3 M, 1 F; age range 21–44) with no visible corneal change.

In eyes showing corneal arcus formation of varying severity, it was found that in early lesions, lipid deposition was confined to the cornea and sclera, but later, lipid

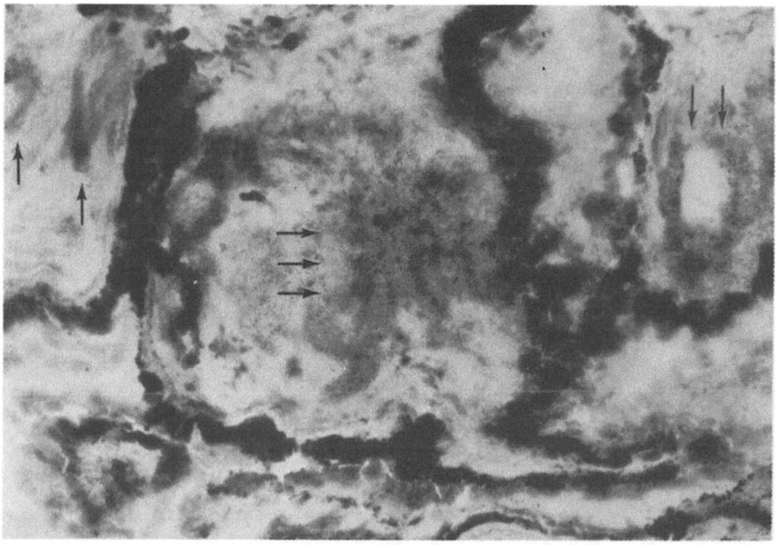

Fig. 2. Frozen section of eye, from same case as in Fig. 1, at higher magnification, to show portion of ciliary body and ciliary processes with pigmented epithelial cells bordering ciliary processes and extracellular lipid as droplets in core of ciliary processes (red in original, *grey* in picture and *indicated by arrows*) (ORO/LG) ×500

was also seen in the ciliary body, ciliary processes (see Figs. 1 and 2) and in the iris. At all these sites the lipid was almost entirely extracellular and apparently bound to collagen or deposited in the ground substance, while fat-filled cells were scanty or absent.

Immuno-histology showed a diffuse distribution (presumptively in the interstitial fluid of the ground substance) of albumin and immunoglobulin G (relatively small molecular weight plasma proteins) in the cornea, ciliary body and iris in all the cases. In the absence of arcus formation, no larger molecular weight plasma proteins were detected at these sites.

On the other hand, in older subjects with an arcus, fibrinogen-related antigen (FRA), immunoglobulin M and apolipoprotein B (apo B) antigen were seen in these positions, the apo B being closely related to the sites where lipid was present (see Figs. 2, 3, 7 and Fig. 13 of [8] for colour illustrations of this). This identity of distribution of lipid and apo B, indicating the presence of intact plasma apo B-containing lipoproteins (LpB) in the tissue, was supported by the similarity of the lipid composition of a cornea affected by arcus formation to that of plasma LDL (see Table 1). The entry of LpB and other macromolecular plasma proteins into the tissue bounding the anterior chamber of the eye suggested that arcus formation (like atherosclerosis) is influenced by alteration of vascular permeability as well as by hyperlipidaemia.

This proposition was examined further in an animal model.

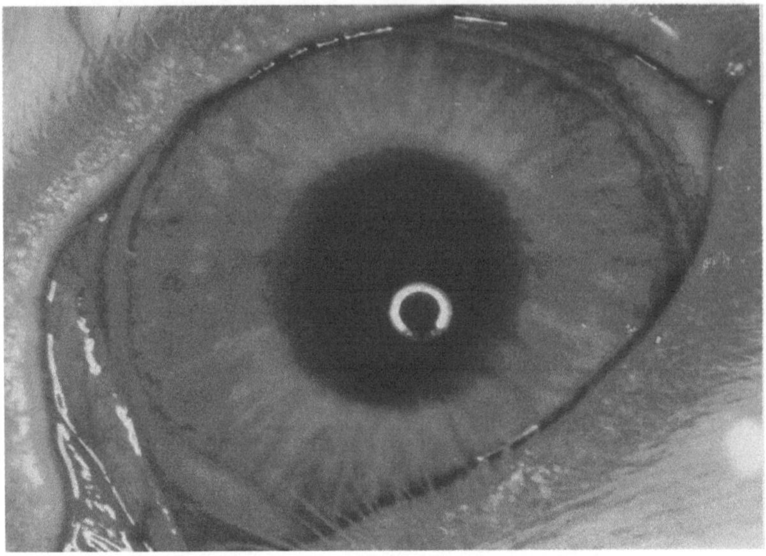

Fig. 3. Naked eye appearance of eye of albino rabbit maintained on cholesterol diet for 20 weeks, showing lipid deposits in iris as whitish streaks radiating from pupil

Table 1. Lipids in cornea affected by arcus, as compared with plasma LDL[a] (lipid composition as weight per cent of dry tissue)

	Cornea (%)	LDL (%)
Sterol esters	57	50
Triglycerides	2	8
Free sterol	13	13
Unestified fatty acid	>1	1
Phospholipids	28	28

[a] Data kindly supplied by Dr. C. M. van Gent, Gaubius Institute, Leyden, Netherlands, and republished with permission.
Note: corneal total lipid: 1.71 mg in 31.50 mg dry tissue.

Corneal Arcus in the Lipid-Fed Rabbit

When hyperlipidaemia is induced in rabbits by lipid feeding, lipid deposition in the eye, as in man, accompanies the development of lipid-filled arterial lesions. In a companion study [12] to the one referred to above, the eyes of 30 rabbits maintained on lipid-supplemented diets for varying periods were examined histologically and immuno-histologically. The eyes of an additional eight animals lipid-fed for limited periods and then returned to a normal diet, were also similarly examined.

In rabbits, because of anatomical differences in the vascular supply to the iris (the

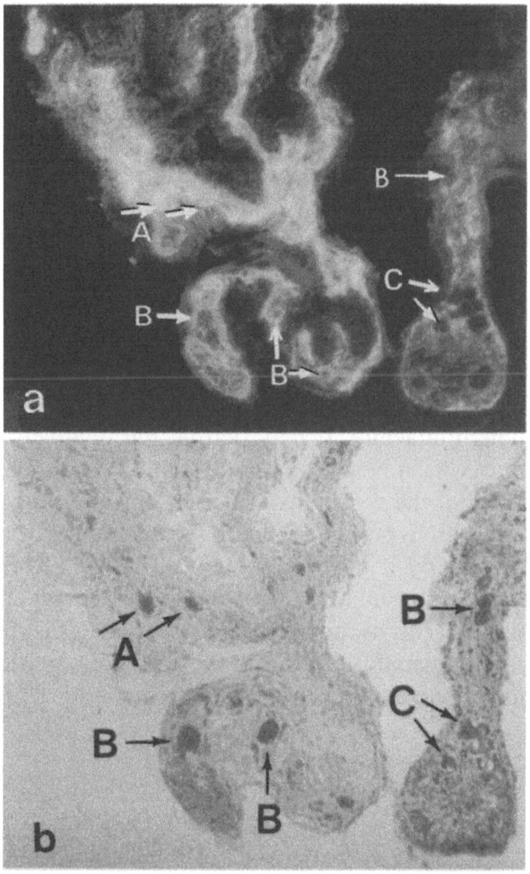

Fig. 4 a, b. Consecutive frozen sections of eye from rabbit on lipid-supplemented diet for 14 weeks, to show portions of two ciliary processes. ***a*** Section treated with fluorescein-labelled anti-rabbit LDL (anti-apo B). Note extensive distribution of specific fluorescence (*white* in picture, bright green in original). ***b*** Corresponding field from section stained with ORO/LG. Note distribution of extracellular lipid (*grey* in picture, red in original) corresponding to fluorescence in ***a***. But note that fat-filled cells at *A* give bright fluorescence; those at *B* give weaker fluorescence; and those at *C* fail to fluoresce, suggesting different stages of catabolism of apo B of LpB taken up by cells. ×75

presence of large numbers of highly vascular ciliary processes extending from the ciliary body to the pupillary margin of the iris) lipid deposition in the iris appears earlier and is more conspicuous than corneal involvement. This is particularly easily seen in albino animals in whom the iris is unpigmented (see Fig. 3).

Immuno-histology showed that, as in man, the lipid was initially in the form of LpB (see Fig. 13 of [12]). But in the rabbit there appeared to be a more exuberant cellular response to the deposited lipoprotein, with the formation of numerous fat-filled cells. These showed variable reactivity with labelled anti-LpB (see Fig. 4) probably representing various stages of intracellular degradation of apo B (the immuno-reactive site). The extent and severity of the eye lesions correlated with the intensity of hyperlipidaemia but was only broadly related to the severity of arterial lesions in the same animals. Some evidence of regression of the eye changes was observed in animals removed from lipid-supplemented diets.

Significance of Altered Vascular Permeability in Eye Lesions. As in man, the importance of vascular dilatation and hyperaemia (factors altering vascular permeability) in localising lipid deposition has previously been shown in the lipid-fed rabbit model. For example, it has been observed [13] that unilateral exposure of one eye to intense light; implants into one anterior chamber; and other procedures causing hyperaemia of one eye, produced more intense lipid deposition in the treated than in the contralateral control eye in these experimental animals.

It seems possible that variability in vascular permeability, from similar causes, may explain known anomalies in the incidence of the arcus in man. For instance, a high prevalence of arcus formation has been noted in Negro populations in Africa [15–17] and in the USA [18] without accompanying evidence of arterial disease or hyperlipidaemia. It may be that the relatively high prevalence of low-grade conjunctivitis in Negro populations and exposure to intense sunlight (producing hyperaemia of the conjunctival vessels and those of the superficial limbal plexus) might outweigh hyperlipidaemia in producing the arcus in these populations.

Similarly, it has been shown [14] in the lipid-fed rabbit that abrasion of the cornea centrally, (i. e. at a normally avascular site not affected by lipid deposition) results in local vascularisation and the accumulation of lipid. The parallelism was pointed out between this effect and the lipid keratopathy following corneal trauma or keratitis in humans.

Xanthomata

Cutaneous xanthomata occur in man in association with both primary and secondary hyperlipidaemias and are characteristically distributed in skin at sites of pressure or minor trauma (elbows, knees, buttocks); and in skin liable to creasing or folding (palmar creases, eyelids). Xanthomata also occur in tendons subjected to friction near joints (finger tendons) or to weight stress (Achilles tendon). If treatment is effective in reducing hyperlipidaemia, xanthomata decrease in size with loss of their lipid.

Lesions similar to human xanthomata occur spontaneously in lipid-fed rabbits, but appear on the feet and have also been observed by some authors [19, 20] to occur in the skin over the nape of the neck. It was suggested by Anitschkow [21, 22], who first observed xanthomata in lipid-fed animals, that their localisation might be due to altered vascular permeability.

In personal experiments [23, 24] it was observed that while xanthomata occurred spontaneously on the feet of cholesterol-fed rabbits maintained in cages with a wire-mesh floor, nodules in this position were absent or less conspicuous in animals on the same diet but kept in cages with a solid floor well-padded with straw. As for nodules elsewhere, it was noted that firm lumps (later shown to be xanthomata) developed in the nuchal skin of a cholesterol-fed rabbit precisely where it was customarily grasped as the animal was lifted out of its cage by the scruff of the neck. But if this method of handling animals was avoided, no nodules developed at this site. These observations suggested that trauma to the feet or to the nuchal skin, respectively, in these animals was a localising factor - possibly by causing the release of compounds altering vascular permeability locally and allowing the escape of lipoprotein-rich plasma into the tissues. They also suggested a means to put this hypothesis to the test.

The theory was supported when it was then shown that: similar xanthoma-like nodules (see Figs. 13-19 of [23]) could be induced at elective sites in the skin of cholesterol-fed rabbits by the repeated intracutaneous injection of histamine or bradykinin; that isologous radioactively labelled rabbit LDL localised selectively in these areas, which also showed increased vascular permeability as shown by Evan's blue localisation; and that rabbit LDL could be identified immuno-histologically in the same areas, at first extracellularly in the dermis, and later within fat-filled cells (Fig. 5) which finally formed xanthoma-like clusters. Identical injections of histamine or bradykinin in animals on normal diets failed to produce comparable skin lesions.

Early induced lesions in moderately hyperlipidaemic animals regressed when histamine injections were stopped. But induced lesions in animals with gross hyperlipidaemia, and spontaneous lesions near inflammatory foci or at pressure sites (e.g. foot pads) persisted and became indurated. The degree of fibrosis within the nodule, as well as continuity of altered permeability and hyperlipidaemia, influenced the degree of resolution which occurred. In man, similarly, a sustained fall in plasma lipids leads to reduction in size and loss of lipid from xanthomata, but fibrous scars persist at the sites of long-standing lesions.

These results led to the conclusion that skin xanthomata are granulomas of a specialised kind which develop in hyperlipoproteinaemic rabbits (and, by analogy, in man) because of the leakage of lipoprotein-rich plasma into the dermal connective tissues at sites of increased vascular permeability, with binding of the lipoprotein to tissue components and later uptake by tissue histiocytes and macrophages.

With regard to human tendons, it has recently been found (Walton, unpublished) that the lipid deposits commonly found in the Achilles tendon (Fig. 6 a) of even normolipidaemic subjects over the age of 65, and tendon xanthomata in younger hyperlipidaemic subjects, can be shown to consist of extracellular collagen-bound LpB (Fig. 6 b) and that nearby small arterioles contain similar deposits in their walls. These findings suggest that a similar mechanism to that outlined above for the skin lesions applies also to tendon xanthoma formation.

Lipid Deposits in Heart Valves

Surveys on lipid accumulation in heart valves [25, 26] have shown that: (a) no lipid accumulates in tricuspid or pulmonary valves, regardless of age; (b) little or no lipid is seen in the mitral and aortic valves before the age of 20 but the incidence of lipid deposits in these valves then increases rapidly and is almost invariable after the age of 55, in both sexes; (c) the extent of mitral and aortic valve involvement roughly parallels the extent of involvement of the aorta by raised atherosclerotic lesions, and is increased by hypertension.

Examination of the process by histology and immuno-histology [27] shows it to

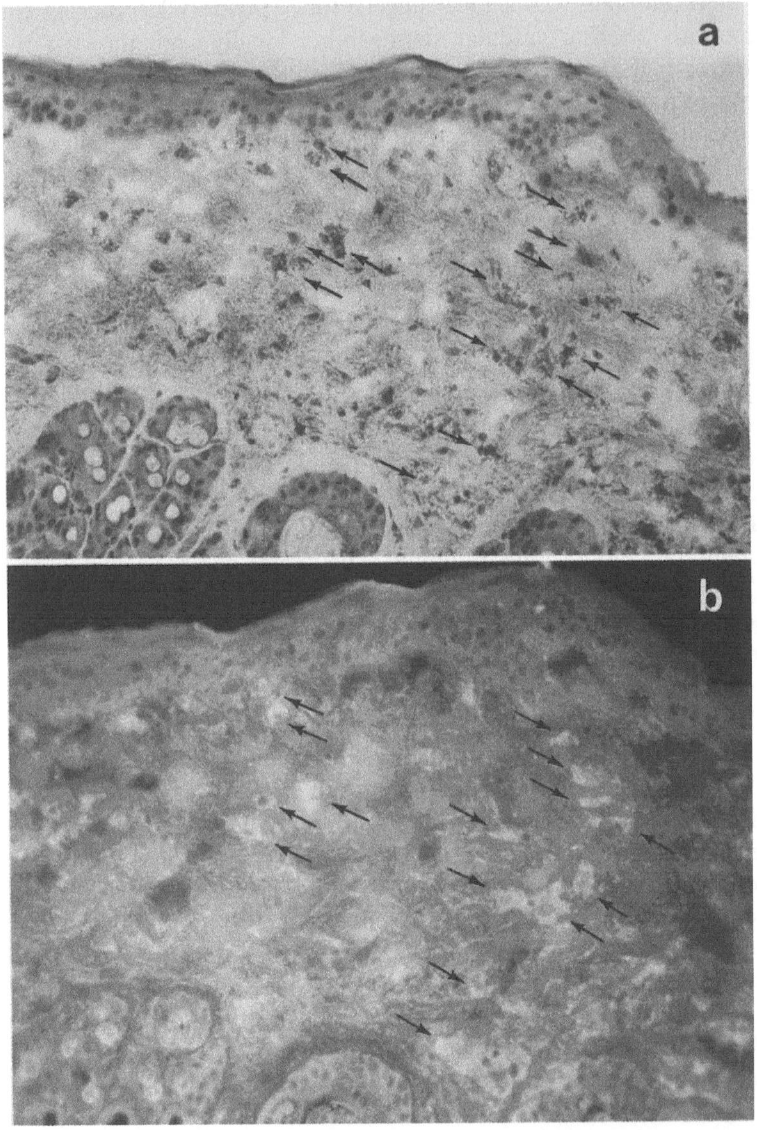

Fig. 5 a, b. Consecutive frozen sections of intracutaneous injection site in skin of cholesterol-fed rabbit after 10 days of daily 10 μg histamine injections. ***a*** Section stained with ORO/LG to show diffuse distribution of collagen-bound lipid droplets in dermis (*grey* in picture, red in original) and lipid-filled cells (*black* in picture and *indicated by arrows,* deep red in original). ***b*** Corresponding field from section treated with fluorescein-labelled anti-rabbit LDL (anti-apo B). Note diffuse specific fluorescence in dermis (*grey* in picture, dull green in original and contrasting with blue autofluorescence of epidermis and skin adnexae) and bright specific intracellular fluorescence (*white* in picture, intense green in original) corresponding with distribution of fat-filled cells in ***a***. ×420

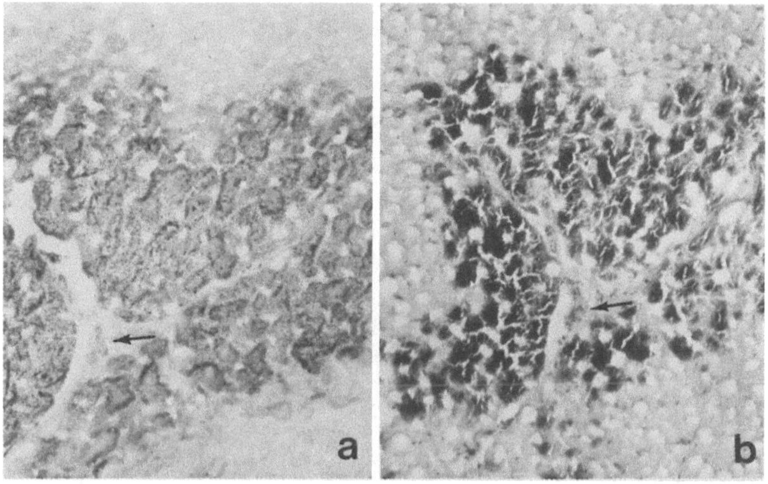

Fig. 6 a, b. Corresponding fields from transverse section through Achilles tendon of normolipidaemic male, aged 72. ***a*** Section stained with ORO/LG to show lipid (*grey* in picture, red in original) bound to collagen arranged in bundles around Y-shaped septum contained small arteriole *(arrow)*. ***b*** Section treated with horseradish peroxidase-labelled anti-apo B to show close correspondence of distribution of reaction product (*black* in picture, brown in original), indicating presence of apo B, with that of lipid as seen in ***a***. × 190

resemble atherosclerosis in other parts of the vascular tree, not only in being in direct continuity with atherosclerosis of the aorta, and in morphology and time-relations of development, but also in that LpB can again be shown to be the principal vehicle for lipid transport into the lamina propria of the valves. Moreover, in affected valves, lipid (LpB) is seen to be distributed, extending from surfaces directly opposed to the pressure resulting from valve closure into the valve substance (see Figs. 2-6 of [27]). This suggests that plasma is actually forced into the valves, where its LpB and FRA become entrained, emphasising the importance of 'ultra-filtration' pressure in determining the sites of accumulation of LpB in atherosclerotic lesions.

Lipid Deposits in Vascular Grafts

Patients with peripheral arterial disease severe enough to warrant vascular bypass surgery are susceptible to atherosclerosis in general, as shown by a high mortality from coronary or cerebral artery disease in the same individuals. There has, nevertheless, been some controversy as to whether 'true' atherosclerosis (which occasions the original necessity for grafting) can recur in the grafts [28, 29].

In recent personal studies conducted with surgical colleagues [30, 31], the changes in 29 vein grafts which had been in position for between 2 days and over 12 years; and those in 39 synthetic grafts (32 Dacron and 7 Teflon) varying in duration between 2 months and 18 years, from patients of this kind were examined histologically and immuno-histologically.

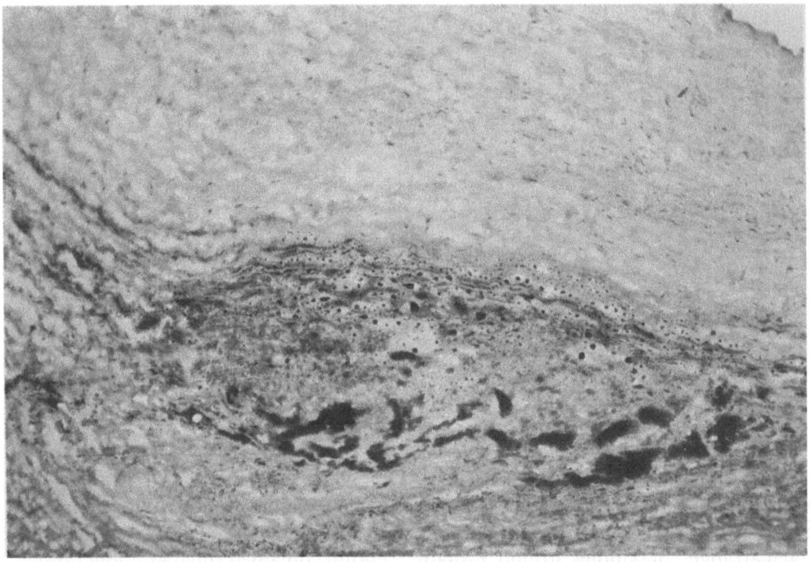

Fig. 7. Frozen section of autogenous vein graft, stained with ORO/LG, to show lipid bound to collagen in depth of thickened graft on either side of 'atheroma-like' lesion containing lipid as droplets, as large lipid aggregates and in fat-filled cells. Lumen of graft in *upper right hand corner.* × 190

It was concluded that, in both vein and plastic grafts, the lesions which developed, after 2 or more years, were indistinguishable from 'genuine' atherosclerosis. This was because, once again, lipid/LpB and FRA were present in distributions closely resembling those seen in arteries and the grafts developed complications (such as thrombosis, calcification and aneurysmal dilatations) similar to those in atherosclerotic vessels. Not surprisingly, the most advanced lesions and the most severe complications were seen in patients with the most adverse 'risk' factors (diabetes, hypertension, hyperlipidaemia, etc.).

In vein grafts, which rapidly developed a diffuse and uniform thickening ('arterialisation') due to marked intimal proliferation, the atherosclerosis-like changes occurred in this newly-formed connective tissue (Fig. 7). But these grafts frequently showed additional irregularly distributed thickening due to the deposition of mural thrombus and its organisation and fibrosis. These areas also often contained lipid which was similarly identified as LpB. At the fibrotic stage, platelet antigens were no longer detectable in these areas, suggesting that the lipid originated from insuded LpB rather than from platelets, as postulated by some proponents [32, 33] of the thrombogenic theory of atherosclerosis.

Similarly, the initial porosity of plastic prostheses was shown to alter because they are rapidly permeated by thrombus which becomes progressively organised and converted, first to loose connective tissue and then to dense collagen, providing a conduit partially permeable by plasma. Immuno-histology showed the involvement of fibrinogen, fibrin, platelets and plasminogen in the early stages and also the permeability to plasma proteins of the established conduit. Once more lipid, identifiable as LpB, was detected in organised thrombi (Fig. 8) in these plastic grafts but again in the absence, at this stage, of detectable platelet antigens.

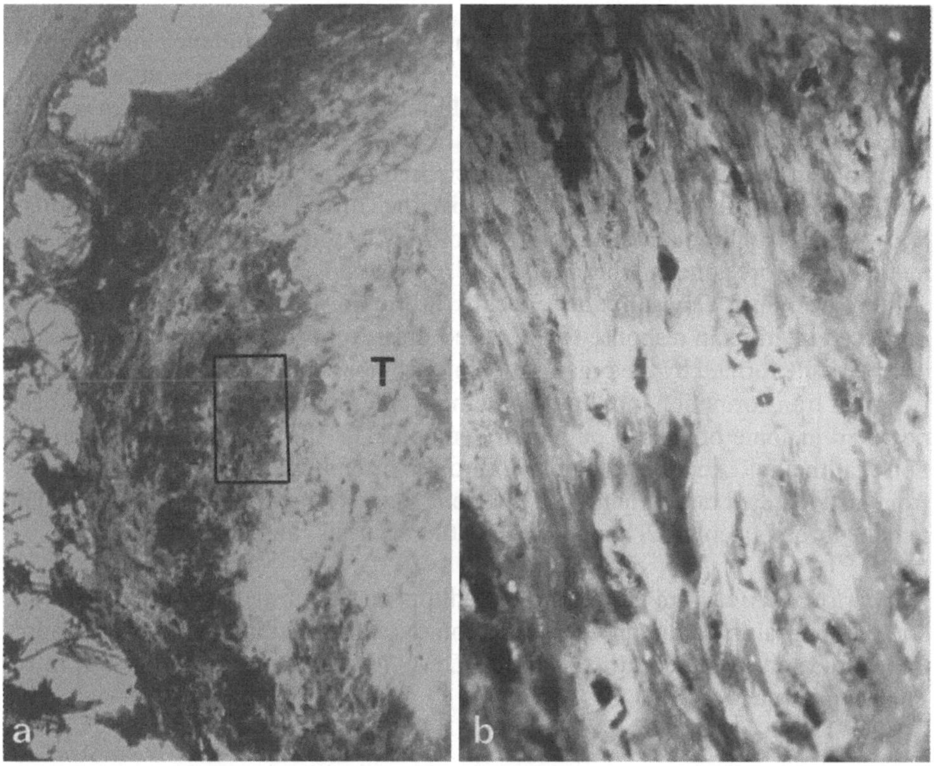

Fig. 8. ***a*** Frozen section of old thrombosed Dacron graft (duration 9 years) showing low-power view of extensive lipid infiltration (*black* in picture, red in original) of the fibrous tissue permeating the graft (many of the plastic fibres of which have fallen out of the section during processing) and of portions of the adherent and partially occluding thrombus *(T)*. Note the area enclosed by a *rectangle*. ***b*** Higher power view of corresponding frozen section of graft shown in ***a***, treated with anti-apo B. Note specific fluorescence (*white* in pucture, green in original) in area corresponding with lipid-infiltrated area outlined by rectangle in ***a***. ***a*** × 60; ***b*** × 375

A study of the development of the atherosclerosis-like changes in vein and plastic grafts indicated that the lesions in both arise initially as extracellular deposits of LpB and FRA in areas of the mesenchymal proliferation which characterises (in vein grafts) the response to altered (arterial) blood pressure, or (in both vein and plastic grafts) the end-product of the organisation of thrombi. It is possible that LpB and FRA are entrained in this tissue by interaction with proteoglycans or other components known to be abundant in newly forming connective tissues.

Discussion

From this review of atherosclerosis-associated non-arterial lesions, it is submitted that the (by now) 'classical' definition of atherosclerosis previously quoted is too restrictive in that the basic pathological process, which we call atherosclerosis when if affects arteries, is *not* confined to the intima of arteries but also occurs in other connective tissues in proximity with the circulation and permeated by a plasma insudate.

It is also suggested that the identity of the constituents of, and the close morphological similarity between, non-arterial and 'true' arterial lesions suggests a common mechanism of formation for both kinds of lesions which has significance in relation to mechanisms of atherogenesis. This is because acceptance that an insudative mechanism operates, not only in the specialised connective tissues of the arterial wall, but also in the tissues of the eye (to give the corneal arcus) and in skin or tendons (to give xanthoma), allows analysis of how certain 'risk factors' operate and mutually reinforce one another *at the level of the arterial wall* [34].

Moreover, lipid deposition also occurs: in the newly formed connective tissue produced in grafts in response to the raised pressure within them; and in the connective tissue formed by the organisation of thrombi in both vein and plastic grafts. A similar transformation into lipid-containing atherosclerosis-like lesions has been observed in some organised pulmonary emboli [35]. The unequivocal demonstration that the lipid, in some organising thrombi or emboli at all these sites, derives from insuded LpB rather than from platelets, suggests that the lipid/insudative [36] and the thrombogenic [32] hypotheses of atherogenesis can be reconciled.

Acknowledgements. I am grateful to the editors and publishers of Atherosclerosis, and the Journal of Pathology for permission to reproduce illustrations which originally appeared in these journals, and to Dr. C. M. van Gent for permission to republish his data (Table 1).

References

1. Schettler FG (1954) Ist der sogenannte Greisenbogen der Hornhaut ein Hinweis auf Atherosklerose? Dtsch Med Wochenschr 79: 915
2. World Health Organization (1958) Classification of atherosclerotic lesions. WHO Tech Rep Ser 143
3. Rodstein M, Zeman FD (1963) Arcus senilis and arteriosclerosis in the aged. Am J Med Sci 245: 70
4. McAndrew GM, Ogston D (1965) Arcus senilis in middle-aged men. Br Med J 1: 425
5. Shanoff HM, Little JA (1964) Studies of male survivors of myocardial infarction due to "essential" atherosclerosis. III. Corneal arcus: Incidence and relation to serum lipids and lipoproteins. Can Med Assoc J 91: 835
6. Rifkind BM (1965) The incidence of arcus senilis in ischaemic heart disease: its relation to serum lipid levels. Lancet 1: 312
7. Khachadurian AK (1964) The inheritance of essential familial hypercholesterolaemia. Am J Med 37: 402
8. Walton KW (1973) Studies on the pathogenesis of corneal arcus formation. I. The human corneal arcus and its relation to atherosclerosis as studied by immunofluorescence. J Pathol 111: 263
9. Beaumont JL, Anguera RG, Lenegre T (1960) La signification clinique du gerontoxon (arcus corneae). Bull Soc Med Hop, Paris 76: 637
10. Pomerantz HZ (1962) The relationship between coronary heart disease and certain physical characteristics. Can Med Assoc J 86: 57
11. Hickey N, Maurer B, Mulcahy R (1970) Arcus senilis: its relation to certain attributes and risk factors in patients with coronary heart disease. Br Heart J 32: 449
12. Walton KW, Dunkerley DJ (1974) Studies on the pathogenesis of corneal arcus formation.

II. Immunofluorescent studies on lipid deposition in the eye of the lipid-fed rabbit. J Pathol 114: 217
13. Friedman M, Byers SO (1959) Some local factors affecting iridic lipid infiltration in hypercholesteremic rabbits. Am J Physiol 187: 842
14. Cogan DG, Kuwabara T (1959) Ocular changes in experimental hypercholesteremia. Arch Ophthalmol 61: 219
15. Davidson JC, Kolbe R (1965) Arcus senilis and ischaemic heart disease. Lancet 1: 707
16. Bersohn I, Politzer WM, Blumsohn D (1969) Arcus senilis corneae - its relationship to serum lipids in the South African Bantu. S Afr Med J 43: 1025
17. Cook GC, Kanyerezi BR (1970) Corneal arcus in the Ugandan African. Amer Heart J 79: 718
18. Macaraeg PVJ, Lasagna L, Snyder B (1968) Arcus not so senilis. Ann Intern Med 68: 345
19. Parker F, Odland GF (1968) Experimental xanthoma. Am J Path 53: 537
20. Parker F, Peterson N, Odland GF (1966) A comparison of cholesterol ester fatty acid patterns in the blood and in evolving xanthoma and atheroma during cholesterol-feeding of rabbits. J Invest Dermatol 47: 253
21. Anitschkow N (1913) Über die Veränderungen der Kaninchenaorta bei experimenteller Cholesterinsteatose. Beitr Path Anat 56: 379
22. Anitschkow N, In: Cowdry EV (ed) (1933) Arteriosclerosis. Macmillan, New York, pp 271-322
23. Walton KW (1973) The role of altered vascular permeability in the induction of experimental xanthomata. Nutr Metab 15: 59
24. Walton KW, Thomas C, Dunkerley DJ (1973) The pathogenesis of xanthomata. J Pathol 109: 271
25. McManus JFA, Lupton CH (1963) Lipid deposits in the aortic cusp of the mitral valve. Their relationship to atheroma and atherogenesis. Arch Pathol 75: 674
26. Sell S, Scully RE (1965) Aging changes in the aortic and mitral valves. Histologic and histochemical studies, with observations on the pathogenesis of calcific aortic stenosis and calcification of the mitral annulus. Amer J Pathol 46: 345
27. Walton KW, Williamson N, Johnson AG (1970) The pathogenesis of atherosclerosis of the mitral and aortic valves. J Pathol 101: 205
28. Editorial (1972) Atheroma in venous bypass grafts. Lancet 1: 241
29. Fievez M (1972) Vein grafting for atheroma in the lower limb. Lancet 1: 594
30. Walton KW, Slaney G, Ashton F (1985) Atherosclerosis in vascular grafts for peripheral vascular disease. Part 1. Autogenous vein grafts. Atherosclerosis 54: 49
31. Walton KW, Slaney G, Ashton F (1986) Atherosclerosis in vascular grafts for peripheral vascular disease. Part 2. Synthetic arterial prostheses. Atherosclerosis 61: 155
32. Duguid JB (1960) The thrombogenic hypothesis and its implications. Postgrad Med J 36: 226
33. Chandler AB, Hand RA (1961) Phagocytosed platelets - a source of lipids in human thrombi and atheroclerotic plaques. Science 134: 946
34. Walton KW (1975) Pathogenic mechanisms in atherosclerosis. Am J Cardiol 35: 542
35. Sevitt S, Walton KW (1986) Atherosclerotic lesions from the reduction of pulmonary emboli. Atherosclerosis 59: 193
36. Virchow R von (1862) Gesammelte Abhandlungen zur Wissenschaftlichen Medizin. Hirsch, Berlin

On the Role of Lipoprotein Antibody Immune Complexes in Atherogenesis

A. N. Klimov

Introduction

One of the relatively new trends in the investigation of causes and conditions of atherosclerosis development is the study of the role of immunological factors in the formation of atherosclerotic lesions of the arteries.

Somewhat earlier we formulated the autoimmune theory of the pathogenesis of atherosclerosis [6, 7, 12]. According to this theory the following chain of events underlies the development of this disease: (a) the formation of autoantibodies to apolipoprotein B-(apo B) containing lipoproteins (LP) due to one cause or another; (b) the formation of a circulating LP antibody immune complex in the blood; (c) an increase of vascular permeability as a result of general manifestations of the immunocomplex disease or as a result of local injury of the arterial wall due to fixation of LP antibody immune complex and, in consequence, a sharp influx both of the complex itself and of free apo B-containing LP into the intima of arteries; (d) uncontrolled uptake by arterial wall macrophagal cells of LP antibody immune complex and the transformation of these cells into foam cells; (e) the development of a local atherosclerotic lesion, destruction of cells and fibers, the disintegration products of which find their way into regional lymph nodes along the lymph efflux; (f) the formation of antibodies to these vascular antigens, their fixation upon the changed vascular structures (formation of the autoimmune complex in situ), a new local impairment of the arterial wall and further progression of the atherosclerotic process.

The theory put forward attributes the key role in the development of atherosclerosis to the LP antibody immune complexes; the formation of such complexes leads to an initiation and/or aggravation of the atherosclerotic process. In other words, atherosclerosis is regarded as a disease of immune complexes. In this review we shall confine ourselves to the discussion of only those aspects of this theory which concern LP antibody immune complexes.

The Production of Autoantibodies to LP and the Formation of LP Antibody Immune Complexes

Autoantibodies to LP were detected for the first time in myeloma patients, and it was presumed that it was the formation of autoimmune complexes with LP as an antigen that brought about the development of xanthomas and atherosclerotic plaques in such patients [1, 13, 14]. Somewhat later such immune complexes or free antibodies to LP were detected in adult persons without any signs of ischemic heart disease (IHD) and in IHD patients [8, 10, 17]. They were also found in animals with experimental hyperlipidemia [5, 10, 11]. The antigens in such complexes were apo B-containing LP [very low- (VLDL) or low-density lipoproteins (LDL)]; the antibodies in the majority of cases belonged to the IgG class (with the exception of myeloma patients in whom IgA and IgM were also detected). It is significant that LP-IgG immune complexes were not detected in 10–15-year-old children. In healthy subjects of 16–30 years of age immune complexes were detected in 50%, and after the age of 30 in approximately 60% of cases; in IHD patients, regardless of age, immune complexes were detected in over 70% of cases. However, in contrast to the myeloma patients, in healthy adults or in patients with IHD, immune LP-IgG complexes circulate in the blood at significantly lower concentrations.

For a long time it was considered that the LP-IgG immune complex in the blood existed in excess antigen, taking into consideration the rather high concentration of apo B-containing LP in the plasma. However, the data of Szondy et al. [17], who detected a sufficiently high frequency of free antibodies to LP in IHD patients together with LP antibody immune complexes attest to the fact that the complexes mentioned may circulate in the blood in antibody excess, at least in some patients. In this case evidently, the antigen may be only a certain subfraction of apo B-containing LP, carrying a definite antigenic determinant which is absent in other LP of this class.

The causes leading to the formation of autoantibodies to LP are not known. There are a number of hypotheses regarding the pathogenesis of autoimmune disease which may be divided into two groups. The first group of hypotheses presumes that the cause of development of autoimmunity is due to a high molecular compound acquiring autoantigenic properties because of its particular modification. In this respect, LP is quite a "suitable" compound, since it is difficult to name other high molecular compounds circulating in the blood which are subjected to such significant changes depending on the external and internal environmental conditions. Variations in the composition, conformation of protein components, the possibility that complexes are formed with other compounds (haptenes, inherent and alien antigens), partial degradation in the blood and tissues under the action of proteolitic enzymes, lipid peroxidation, and other modifications taking place normally and pathologically are practically without limit for LP and any one of them may lead to the appearance of autoantigenic properties in LP. The possibility of producing, in principle, autoantibodies to modified LP was shown in experiments in which specific antibodies to methylated, ethylated, acetylated, carbamylated [16], or glycosylated [2] LDL appeared after immunization of animals with the modified homologous LDL mentioned above. Of particular interest is the possibility of obtaining an immune response to glycosylated LDL, since such LP are detected in the blood of patients with diabetes [15]. The possibility of antibody production to alien antigens that have found their way into the organism cannot be excluded; these antibodies may cross-react with LP.

The other group of hypotheses describing the pathogenesis of autoimmune diseases places function impairment of the immunocompetent system at the basis of these diseases, i. e., loss of tolerance to some unchanged proteins. It is quite possible that the development of autoimmune reaction to LP may also be accomplished in such a way, regardless of whether loss of tolerance to LP takes place according to the mechanisms described by the hypothesis of forbidden clones, by the hypothesis of T-suppressor insufficiency, or by the hypothesis of normal self-discernment impairment. Moreover, in cases of myeloma, antilipoprotein antibodies appear due to some pathology of the immunocompetent system. In this respect the data on T-suppressor activity decrease in patients with IHD when autosensitization to LP is detected [8] also deserves attention.

Fixation of LP Antibody Immune Complex in the Vascular Wall and Its Injuring Action

Deposition of LP antibody immune complex in the arterial wall was first demonstrated with the help of immunomorphological methods. According to analysis of parallel sections it was found that apo B-containing LP, IgG, and C_3 fraction of complement are deposited in one and the same place of aortic intima of rabbits with experimental atherosclerosis [18], and also the intima of human coronary arteries [7]. This is regarded as proof that all these components, partially or completely, enter the arterial wall as parts of one complex. It is important to note that the detection of autoimmune LP-IgG complex in rabbit aorta coincided with the disappearance of such a complex from the circulation, and also with a decrease of complement concentration and apo B-containing LP in the blood.

We also managed to isolate LP antibody immune complex from the tissue fluid of an affected human aorta [10]. This complex was situated in the aorta wall, both in a water-soluble form and in a fixed state. It should be noted that the complex isolated from the aorta possessed a somewhat greater hydrated density in comparison with the plasma immune complex, that, evidently, is connected with the metabolic changes of this complex in the vessel wall.

In order to elucidate whether LP antibody immune complex produces an injuring effect upon the endothelial lining, experiments were carried out in which we studied the influence of VLDL-IgG complex upon the penetration of ^{125}I-LDL into the rabbit carotid artery during perfusion in situ. In these experiments VLDL-IgG complex in antigen excess was added to citrated autologous blood with which perfusion was performed. It was established that after only 45 min of perfusion with blood that contained VLDL-IgG complex there is severe damage of the endothelial cells and a sharp increase of influx into the intima of ^{125}I-LDL, which was added to the perfusate during the last 15 min of perfusion, in comparison with the carotid artery perfused with blood not containing the immune complex [7].

Thus the available data attest to the fact that LP antibody autoimmune complex is deposited in the arterial wall and may produce an injuring effect upon the endothelial lining.

Uptake of LP Antibody Immune Complex by Macrophagal Cells and Their Transformation into Foam Cells

It is well-known that the physiological function of immune complex formation is to eliminate the antigen from the blood and other media as soon as possible. The elimination of immune complexes is performed by the reticuloendothelial system, an integral part of which is the macrophage. Hence, one may presume that LP antibody complex will not be an exception either, and that the production of antibodies to LP must lead to an accelerated elimination of the latter from the circulation. Such a presumption was expressed for the first time by Noseda et al. [14] who detected the LP antibody immune complex in the blood of a patient with myeloma and pronounced hypolipidemia. Hypolipidemia in this patient was regarded by the authors as a result of fast elimination from the blood of LP of the immune complex. Subsequently, Ho et al. [4] showed that in patients with myeloma and hyperlipidemia, in whom antibodies to LP had been detected, the rate of cholesterol elimination from the circulation and its excretion from the organism, as well as the rate of cholesterol synthesis, were significantly increased. The authors presumed that LP cholesterol of immune complexes, unlike cholesterol of free LP, is not able to inhibit cholesterol synthesis in tissues, and that leads to the development of hypercholesterolemia (autoimmune hyperlipidemia). Groszek et al. [3] also detected an increased elimination of chylomicrons and VLDL from the circulation during normal activity of lipoprotein lipase and decreased activity of hepatic lipase in a patient with benign gamma-globulinopathy and xanthomatosis. The patient had an immune complex containing LP rich in triglycerides as an antigen. The rates of cholesterol synthesis and catabolism, and lipid concentration in the blood plasma in this patient were normal.

It was established in our experiments that LP-IgG immune complexes (human VLDL or LDL plus rabbit antibodies to apo B of man) intravenously administered to healthy rabbits disappeared from the circulation significantly faster than free LP; an increase in antibody content in the immune complex brought about an acceleration of its elimination from the circulation [9]. That is, direct data was obtained that LP as an integral part of the immune complex is eliminated from the circulation significantly faster than free LP.

When studying the uptake of LP antibody complex by human lung fibroblasts and mouse peritoneal macrophages in vitro it turned out that such a complex was taken up less actively by fibroblasts, and considerably more actively by macrophages than free LP. Macrophages took up a complex prepared in antibody excess particularly actively [8, 9]. These data permit the conclusion that it is mainly cells of the macrophagal type that are responsible for quick elimination of LP-IgG complex from the circulation. The data that following administration of such a complex to rabbits, the relative uptake of LP by the spleen was greater than after administration of LP not bound with antibodies also attest to a pre-eminent uptake of LP antibody complex by cells of the reticuloendothelial system. Other studies showed that an accelerated elimination of LP antibody complex from the circulation is carried out by macrophages, chiefly with the help of receptors to the Fc fragments of antibodies, though nonspecific endocytosis (endocytic uptake without participation of B, E receptors) also plays a certain role in the uptake of the immune complex mentioned [9].

Thus, the available data convincingly attest to the fact that LP antibody complexes forming in the organism are very quickly eliminated from the circulation. At the same time, as mentioned above, such complexes are detected in the majority of patients with IHD and also in rabbits with experimental hypercholesterolemia though in relatively low concentrations. Possible explanations of such an inconsistency may be: (a) a decelerated elimination of immune complexes from the circulation due to a functional insufficiency of the monocyte-macrophage system (e.g., due to its saturation with lipids); (b) composition peculiarities of the immune complexes which impede their uptake by cells of the reticuloendothelial system; (c) a continuous formation of such immune complexes at a rate which is not less than that of their elimination from the circulation.

In our experiments it was demonstrated that in rabbits with experimental hypercholesterolemia and LP antibody complexes or free antibodies to LP in the blood, the intravenously administered LDL-IgG complex was eliminated from the circulation significantly faster than free LDL, as was the case in healthy rabbits. The blood monocytes of rabbits with experimental hypercholesterolemia also retained the ability for active uptake of immune complexes: during incubation in vitro the monocytes took up LP of immune complexes on average 28% more actively than free LP. Thus, the reticuloendothelial system of rabbits with hypercholesterolemia and LP antibody complexes or free antibody to LP in the blood retained the ability to actively take up immune complexes. Therefore, the presence of immune complexes in the blood cannot be explained by the fact that the reticuloendothelial system in these animals is not able to eliminate immune complex in general or by the fact that this ability is weakened.

Of the two remaining possible explanations of the presence of autoimmune complexes in the blood, we believe the assumption that immune complexes are constantly formed in the organism at a sufficiently high rate to be the most probable. The data on the presence of high concentrations of LP antibody immune complexes in the blood of patients with gamma-globulinopathy accompanied by acceleration of cholesterol [4], chylomicron, and VLDL [3] catabolism due to the fast elimination of such complexes by the reticuloendothelial system attest in favour of this presumption.

After the data on an active uptake of LP antibody complexes by macrophages were obtained, there arose the question: can an uptake of such complexes by macrophages lead to an accumulation of cholesteryl ester in the cells and transformation of the latter into foam cells? It is known that the appearance of foam cells in the intima of arteries is a characteristic morphological sign of a developing atherosclerotic process.

The experiments carried out in our laboratory showed that a 72-h incubation of mouse peritoneal macrophages with the LDL-IgG complex actually led to a transformation of macrophages into foam cells with an accumulation of a large number of lipid vacuoles, residual bodies, and cholesterol crystals in their cytoplasma. Macrophage incubation with free LDL did not lead to a formation of foam cells. The cholesteryl ester content in the macrophages incubated with the immune complex was approximately 60 times higher than that in cells incubated with free LDL or with lipoprotein-free serum, and reached a level typical for foam cells (60.8 μg cholesteryl ester/mg cell protein). The concentration of unesterified cholesterol in these cells increased to a considerably lesser degree [9].

Conclusion

Thus, the data obtained attest to the fact that the formation of LP antibody immune complex may lead to fast elimination of such a complex from the circulation due to its active uptake by cells of the reticuloendothelial system, in particular by macrophages. Excessive uptake of such immune complexes by macrophages of the arterial wall may lead to transformation of the latter into foam cells, which play an important role in the formation of atherosclerotic lesions of the arteries.

We consider the formation of LP antibody immune complexes to be a peculiar case of modified LP with an increased affinity for the cells of the reticuloendothelial system. At the same time the formation of these complexes may also be regarded as an additional way of elimination of „alien" LP from the blood:

Apo B-containing LP ⟶ Uptake by mesenchymal cells through B, E receptors
↓
Modified apo B-containing LP ⟶ Formation of LP antibody immune complexes
↓
Uptake by macrophages of arterial wall ⟵ (Formation of LP antibody immune complexes)
↓
Formation of foam cells
⋮
↓
Atherosclerosis development

This scheme illustrates the participation of modified apo B-containing LP in atherogenesis.

When evaluating the role of immune complexes in atherogenesis, one should bear in mind the fact that immune complexes of any nature, even those which contain non-LP antigen, may produce an injuring effect upon the endothelium of vessels. However, immune complexes, including LP as antigen, play a specific role in this process due to the atherogenicity of the antigen. Besides, it is probable that the production of anti-LP antibodies may lead to a disturbance of lipid metabolism and to development of "autoimmune hyperlipidemia" [1] of an atherogenic character. However, this presumption requires further study.

References

1. Beaumont JL (1970) Autoimmune hyperlipidemia. An atherogenic metabolic disease of immune origin. Rev Eur Etud Clin Biol 15: 1037-1041
2. Curtiss LK, Witztum JL (1983) A novel method for generating region-specific monoclonal antibodies to modified proteins. Application to the identification of human glycosylated low density lipoproteins. J Clin Invest 72: 1427-1438
3. Groszek E, Abrams JJ, Grundy SM (1981) Normolipidemic planar xanthomatosis associated with benign monoclonal gammapathy. Metabolism 30: 927-935
4. Ho KJ, De Wolf VG, Siler W, Lewis LA (1976) Cholesterol dynamics in autoimmune hyperlipidemia. J Lab Clin Med 88: 769-779

5. Ioffe VI, Zubzhitsky Yu N, Nagornev VA, Klimov AN (1973) Immunological characteristics of experimental atherosclerosis. Bull Exp Biol Med 75, no 6: 72-76 (in Russian)
6. Klimov AN (1974) Immunobiochemical mechanisms of atherosclerosis development. Proc Acad Med Sci USSR 2: 29-36 (in Russian)
7. Klimov AN (1985) Autoimmune theory of pathogenesis of atherosclerosis. Proc 16th FEBS congress, Part A, VNU Science, pp 233-249
8. Klimov AN (ed) (1986) Immunoreactivity and atherosclerosis. Meditzina, Leningrad (in Russian)
9. Klimov AN, Denisenko AD, Popov AV et al. (1985) Lipoprotein-antibody immune complexes. Their catabolism and role in foam cells formation. Atherosclerosis 58: 1-15
10. Klimov AN, Denisenko AD, Zubzhitsky Yu N, Gerchikova EA (1978) Detection of autoimmune complex lipoprotein-antibody in human blood plasma and aorta wall. Proc Med Chem 24: 539-543 (in Russian)
11. Klimov AN, Petrova-Maslakova LG, Nagornev VA, Magracheva EYa (1975) Isolation and identification of autoimmune lipoprotein-antibody complex from blood serum of rabbit with experimental atherosclerosis. Proc Med Chem 21: 526-531 (in Russian)
12. Klimov AN, Zubzhitsky Yu N, Nagornev VA (1979) Immunochemical aspects of atherosclerosis. Atheroscler Rev 4: 119-156
13. Lewis LA, Page IH (1965) An unusual serum lipoprotein-globulin complex in a patient with hyperlipemia. Am J Med 38: 286-297
14. Noseda G, Riesen W, Schlumpf E, Morell A (1972) Hypo-β-lipoproteinemia associated with auto-antibodies against β-lipoproteins. Eur J Clin Invest 2: 342-347
15. Schleicher T, Deufel T, Wieland OH (1981) Nonenzymatic glycosylation of human serum lipoproteins. Elevated E-lysine glycosylated low density lipoprotein in diabetic patient. FEBS Lett 129: 1-4
16. Steinbrecher UP, Fisher M, Witztum JL, Curtiss LK (1984) Immunogenicity of homologous low density lipoprotein after methylation, ethylation, acetylation, or carbamylation: generation of antibody specific for derivatized lysine. J Lipid Res 25: 1109-1116
17. Szondy E, Horvath M, Mezey Z et al. (1983) Free and complexed anti-lipoprotein antibodies in vascular diseases. Atherosclerosis 49: 69-77
18. Zubzhitsky Yu N, Nagornev VA, Petrova-Maslakova LG (1974) Immunological and immunomorphological study of experimental atherosclerosis in rabbits. Proc Acad Med Sci USSR 2: 57-60 (in Russian)

Role of Different Agents Affecting Endothelial Cells in the Process of Atherosclerosis – In Vitro Examinations

H. Jellinek, E. Csonka, A. Somogyi, and E. Takács

The history of atherosclerosis research now stretches over more than a century. The advent of new techniques always opened new fields of research. Therefore current atherosclerosis research makes use not only of the new morphological facilities offered by the various electron microscopic techniques but also of the refined and sophisticated methods of biochemistry, genetics, cytology, cell biology, molecular biology, etc. This broader approach to the problem appears to have enlarged considerably the scope of atherosclerosis research which is no longer merely the study of a specific condition but rather that of the general biology and pathology of the arterial system at various hierarchical levels, from molecules to the vessels of various calibers and structures.

One of the specialized fields of research concentrates on the endothelial cells forming the internal layer of the arteries irrespective of their size and caliber. These cells are a particular type of the cells of epithelial origin. Among various special features, it has the unique capability of involvement in the transport of objects from the size of a small molecule (or ion) up to that of a whole cell (e.g., macrophage). It has also been discovered that endothelial cells are *actively* involved in all these transport processes in contrast to the classical concept of their being merely passive barriers between the circulating blood and the organism.

This unique function of the endothelial cells explains why the study of the permeability of their cytoplasmic membrane has become an exciting field of research. In our Institute, in vivo vessel permeability studies have been carried out since 1961 [19]. The in vivo examination of this problem involves very considerable technical difficulties, therefore we started to make use of the tissue culture method.

Our colleagues in the tissue culture laboratory of our Institute were the first to report (in 1973) on the successful cultivation and maintainance of pure lines of endothelial cells (from the minipig) in vitro [4–6]. This result was also presented at the Heidelberg Symposium in 1973 by Björkerud. The basic principles of the procedure were later successfully adapted to aortas of human embryos, calves, and rats. A further important step was the cultivation of endothelium on collagen membranes, making preparation procedures for electron microscopy more convenient [8]. A recent achievement is a method for preparing endothelial cell cultures from small, vulnerable aortas [29].

With this technique we have been able to study directly the effect of certain risk factors on the endothelial cell. Since these cells are known to interact with an extremely broad spectrum of materials, structures, and even cells, it seems that the number of factors presenting potential hazards to endothelium might be very considerable.

The present paper is a report on our studies on in vitro cultured endothelial cells of different origin.

Interaction of Smooth Muscle and Endothelial Cells

Exponentially growing and stationary endothelial cells have been known to stimulate and to inhibit the proliferation of smooth muscle cells, respectively. Little information is, however, available on the effect of smooth muscle cells on the endothelial cells. For this purpose a cocultivation procedure has been developed in our laboratory which allows us to grow the two spatially separated cells in the same medium [12, 13]. We have examined the proliferation-stimulating effect of smooth muscle cells on the endothelial cells and vice versa in intra- and interspecific combinations, using bovine, pig, or rat aortic cell cultures. The effect was registered as the incorporation of labeled thymidine detected by liquid scintillation counting. The results are summarized in Fig. 1.

The smooth muscle cells usually had an inhibitory effect on the proliferation of endothelial cells except for the pig smooth muscle cells which had a stimulatory effect in both inter-, and intraspecies combinations. Schumacher et al. [28] isolated a substance from smooth muscle cells which had an inhibitory effect on the endothelial cells. The inhibitory effect of smooth muscle cells in our experiments may be explained on the same basis. Smooth muscle cells of the pig were found, however, to stimulate the growth of endothelial cells from the same as well as from the other species. In this case we may suppose the existence of a nonspecific stimulant.

On the other hand the endothelial cells stimulated smooth muscle cell proliferation in a species-specific way. In an interspecies combination, either inhibition or no effect was observed. Both data in the literature and the present results suggest that the equilibrium-regulating interactions of stimulatory and inhibitory substances produced by one and the same cells may be of considerable biological importance

The effect of smooth muscle cells on endothelial cell proliferation

smooth muscle \ ENDOTHELIAL CELL	BOVINE	RAT	PIG
bovine	⬇	⬇	⬇
rat	⬇	O	⬇
pig	⬆	⬆	⬆

The effect of endothelial cells on smooth muscle cell proliferation

endothelial \ SMOOTH MUSCLE	BOVINE	RAT	PIG
bovine	⬆	O	⬇
rat	⬇	⬆	⬇
pig	⬇	O	⬆

⬆ stimulation ⬇ inhibition O no effect

Fig. 1. Interaction between endothelial and smooth muscle cells. The effect of proliferation activity of different cell types in cocultivation with other cell types as measured by ^{3}H-thymidine incorporation

and they may play an important role in the regulation of neovascularization or in the re-endothelization of denuded intimal areas.

Viruses as Risk Factors

Cells coating the interior of the vessels are exposed not only to the normal components of the blood but also to anything (ions, molecules, particles, etc.) that may be present in the circulation under pathological conditions. Many viruses are known to produce one or repeated periods of viremia. Some of them have also been supposed as playing a role in the pathogenesis of atherosclerosis, by altering the fine structure of the cell membrane and hence the cell membrane permeability [16, 24]. Fabricant et al. succeeded in producing severe atherosclerosis in chickens by a strain (MDV) of herpes virus [14]. The same virus was also found to affect the normal metabolism of the medial smooth muscle cells [15]. In biopsy samples obtained from the aorta in association with surgical operations on atherosclerotic patients the presence of herpes virus virions in the endothelium as well as in the smooth muscle cells was frequently demonstrable [18]. Several viruses were successfully grown in cultured endothelial cells [17].

It is known that some enveloped nononcogenic viruses modify the cytoplasmic membrane of the cell so as to develop a lectin-binding capability similar to that of malignantly transformed cells [25]. Using this phenomenon as an indicator, it was demonstrated that cultured cells of vessel wall origin (endothelium, smooth muscle, adventitial fibroblasts) developed lectin binding as early as 6 h after the infection with the virus. Smooth muscle cells and fibroblasts reacted only after 24 and 72 h, respectively [7]. The same phenomenon may also appear in vivo under appropriate conditions. Some other enveloped viruses may also be tested further for their possibly similar effect on cells of vascular origin. Our observations may contribute to the better understanding of the capillary lesions in virus-induced eruptions and some accidental, local permeability changes in the vessels of patients with unidentified infections caused by enveloped viruses.

Morphological examination of the endothelial or smooth muscle cells infected by measles failed to reveal any conspicuous cytopathogenic effect, inspite of the measurable replication of the virus. In some cases, however, - especially in smooth muscle cell cultures - some syncytium formation was observed, probably due to the replication of the virus (Fig. 2 a). In infected endothelial cells we could demonstrate the presence of lysosomes containing viral nucleocapsids (Fig. 2 b).

The decisive evidence for virus replication in cells of the vessel wall was obtained by titrating the supernatant of the cultures 8 days after infection. As shown in Table 1 replication of virus was demonstrable as an increase of the virus titre.

The vaccinal strain Leningrad-16 (Batch No. 021-1969) of the measles virus used as inoculum was maintained and titrated in a transformed line of pig aortic smooth muscle cell culture highly sensitive to the virus [10]. Titration of the virus replicated in the different vessel wall cells and in the human embryonic skin fibroblasts was also performed in the transformed cell line. Good replication of the virus was observed in smooth muscle cells of rat, pig, and calf origin, while endothelial cells of similar origin appeared to support virus replication only to a lower degree (Table 1).

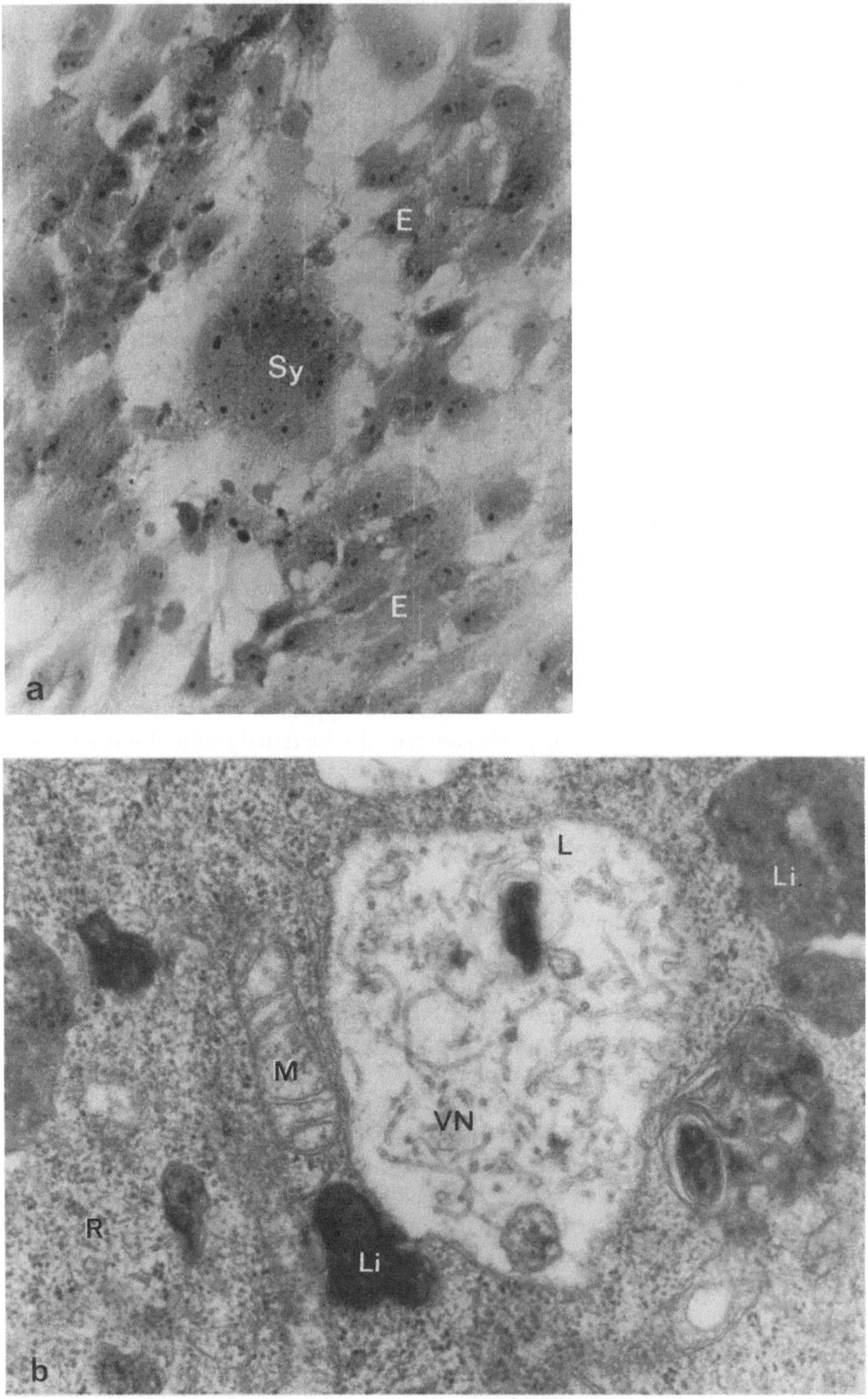
E
Sy
E
a
L
Li
M
VN
R
Li
b

Table 1. The mean virus yield in the standard human embryonic skin fibroblast cell microplate cultures (controls) was taken to be 100%. The mean yields obtained under identical conditions in all other cell types tested were compared to the controls

Tissue culture	Virus yield (%)
Human embryonic skin fibroblast	100
Bovine aortic endothelial culture	56
Bovine aortic smooth muscle culture	100
Pig aortic endothelial culture	67
Pig aortic smooth muscle culture	100
Rat aortic endothelial culture	78
Rat aortic smooth muscle culture	100

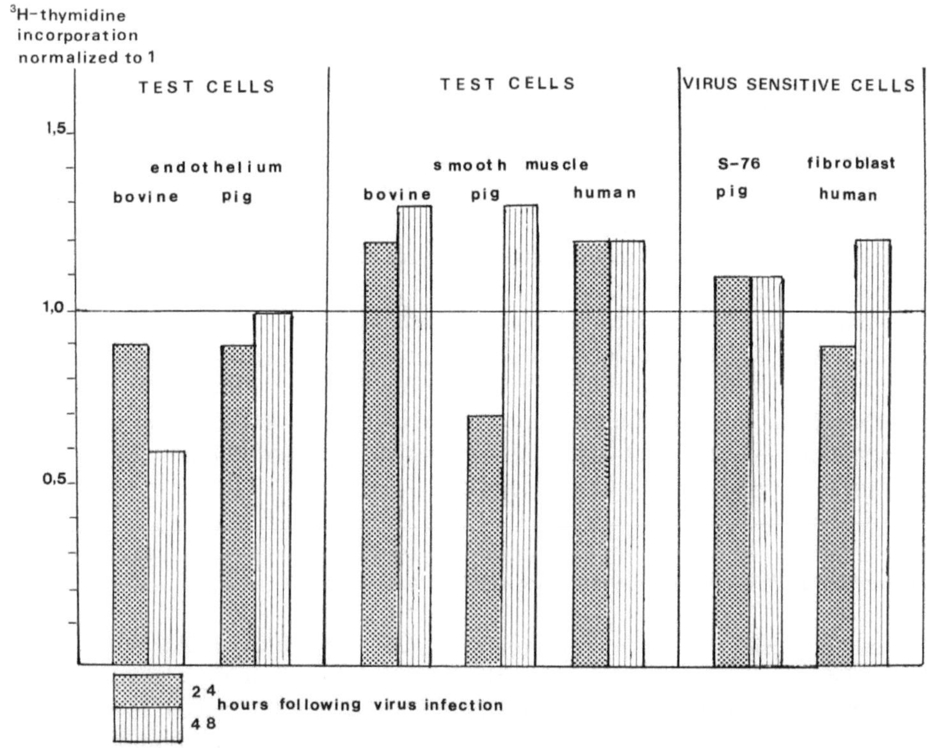

Fig. 3. Effect of measles virus on the proliferation of different aortic endothelial and smooth muscle cells 24 and 48 h after infection

◁ ***Fig. 2 a, b.*** Bovine aortic endothelial cell infected with measles virus. ***a*** Syncytium formation caused by the virus. *E*, endothelial cells; *Sy*, syncytium. Azan stain, ×480. ***b*** Measles virus nucleocapsid in the lysosome of a virus infected cell. *L*, lysosome; *VN*, viral nucleocapsid; *M*, mitochondrium; *R*, ribosome; *Li*, lipid droplet. ×30000

The effect of the early phases of measles virus replication was examined on the proliferation of endothelial and smooth muscle cells of different species (Fig. 3).

As shown by ^{3}H-thymidine incorporation, virus replication inhibited the proliferation of the endothelial cells of all species tested, while it uniformly stimulated the replication of the smooth muscle cells relative to the control.

The present studies, as well as the data available in the literature, show that viruses may replicate in different cells cultured from the vessel wall. This suggests that viruses may affect the structure, integrity, functions, and/or permeability of the vascular cell membrane, thus representing a direct or indirect risk factor to the vessel as a structure. The possibility of herpes-induced smooth muscle cell proliferation in the vessel wall is also mentioned by Fabricant [15] and by Benditt [3]. Our results represent additional evidence for the potential role of viruses as risk factors in atherosclerosis.

Effect of Lipofundin on Cells of the Vessel Wall

Lipofundin-S 20% (Braun, Melsungen) is a soybean oil preparation containing lipoprotein particles stabilized to the average size of the chylomicron granules. Using this preparation as a tracer we have studied the changes in the permeability of cells of vascular origin [20–22]. In vivo experiments in rats have shown Lipofundin to induce proliferation of the medial smooth muscle cells [23]. To examine the possible mechanism of this effect cultured vascular cells were also treated with Lipofundin.

Two hours after Lipofundin addition the cells were shown to engulf Lipofundin droplets. After 72 h the droplets were already present in the lysosomes (Fig. 4a, b).

The proliferation-stimulating effect of Lipofundin was studied by ^{3}H-thymidine incorporation. Only the results of some preliminary studies are available but these suggest unequivocally that Lipofundin stimulates the proliferation of both the endothelial and the smooth muscle cells.

Interaction of Protein Macromolecules with Endothelial Cells

Endothelial cells produce a plasminogen activator which could result in an increased plasmin level in circulating blood [2, 9]. There are many plasma constituents which may interfere with plasmin binding to endothelial cells. It is well-documented that thrombin binds tightly to endothelial cells, and antithrombin III may influence this interaction [1]. Therefore we examined the relative binding nature of these components. Interaction of human plasmin and human alfa-thrombin with cultured minipig aortic endothelial cells was studied using ^{125}I-labeled enzyme. Our results show that plasmin binds tightly to endothelial cells with a K_d value of approximately 10^{-9} *M* and there is no uptake of plasmin by cells. The thrombin

Fig. 4 a, b. Lipofundin-treated bovine aortic endothelial cells. ***a*** The cells had engulfed the Lipofundin droplets 2 h after treatment. *LF*, Lipofundin droplets; *N*, nucleus; *n*, nucleolus; *J*, junction. × 10000. ***b*** The Lipofundin droplets are present in the lysosomes 72 h after treatment. *L*, lysosome; *LF*, Lipofundin; *MF*, microfilaments; *WP*, Weibel-Palade body. × 30000 ▷

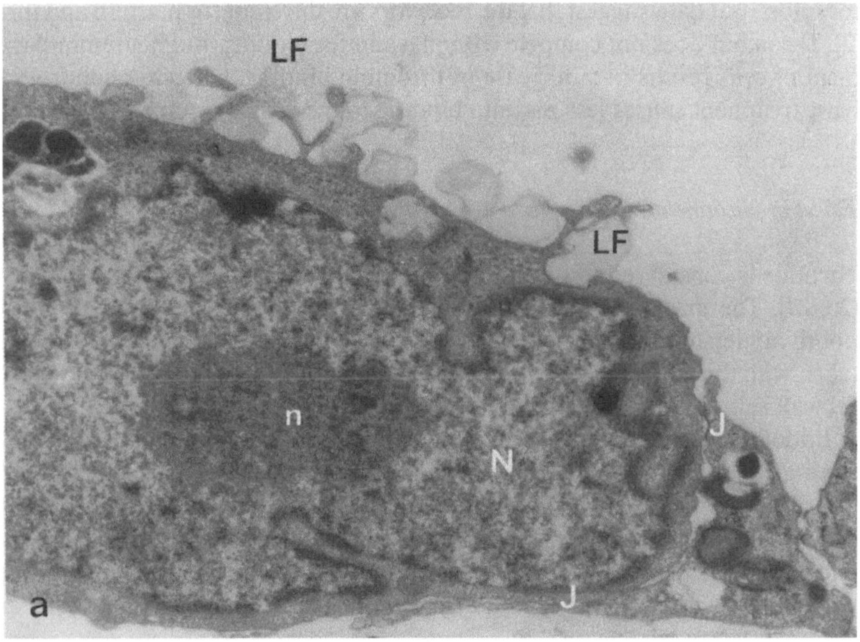
LF
LF
n
N
J
J
a

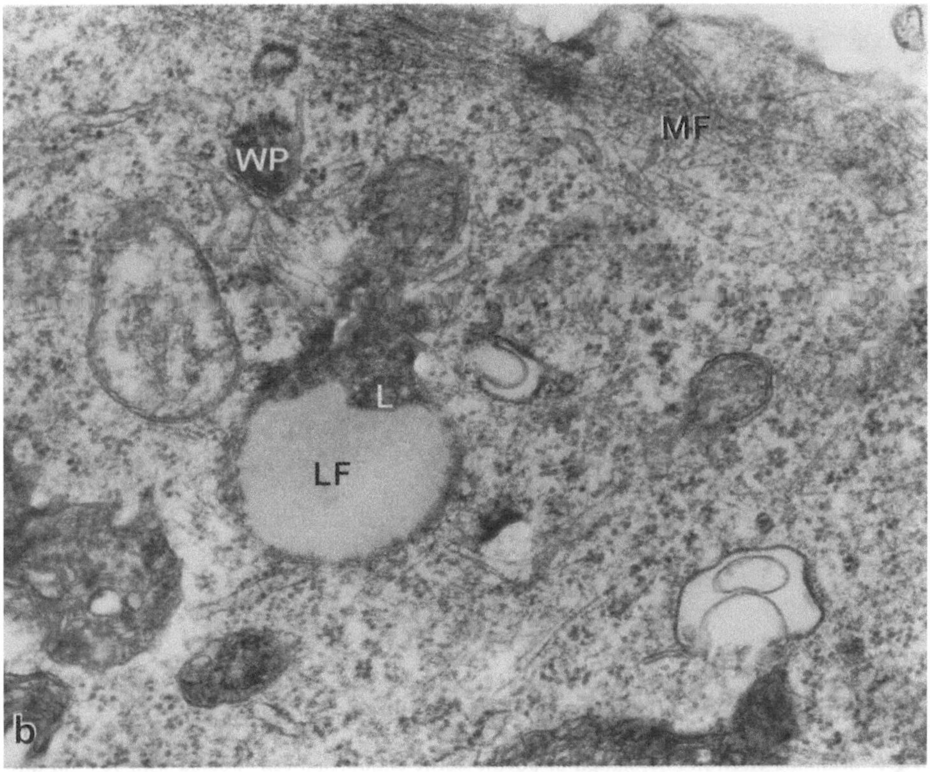
MF
WP
L
LF
b

binding was characterized by a K_d value of 3×10^{-8} *M*. In terms of endothelial cell receptors, our data suggest that the receptors are different for plasmin and thrombin [2]. Thrombin does not compete with plasmin for binding and neuraminidase treatment of cells results in a decrease of thrombin binding, whereas chondroitin ABC lyase treatment causes less plasmin binding to the cells.

Effect of Nicotine on Cells of the Vessel Wall

Nicotine is considered to be an important risk factor in all cardiovascular changes [26, 27]. The mechanism of action of this 162,23 daltons, highly toxic alcaloid is poorly understood in the pathogenesis of atherosclerosis. Our studies were undertaken with the aim of seeing if there was a specific effect of this alcaloid on the vessel wall cells in addition to its high toxicity.

Endothelial, smooth muscle, and adventitial fibroblast cells cultured from vessels were treated with different final concentrations (from 10^{-4} *M* to 10^{-9} *M*) of nicotine. The effect of the alcaloid on the cytoskeletal system was examined as an indicator of the protein synthesizing and polimerizing activity of the cell. The cytoskeleton was visualized in a polimerization microscope and quantitative estimations were done by means of an Opton cytophotometer. An increase of the total amount

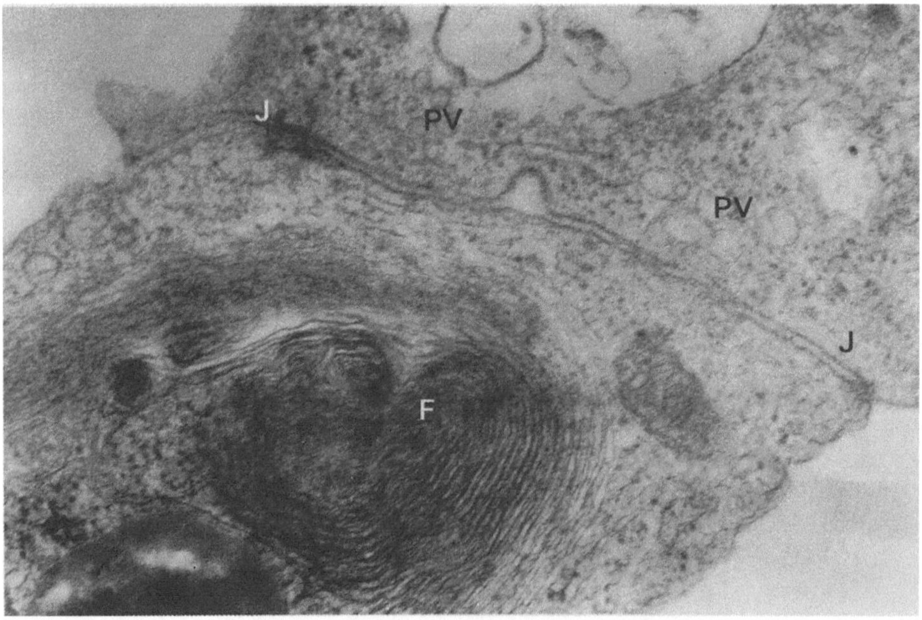

Fig. 5. Bovine aortic endothelial cells treated with 10^{-4} *M* final concentration of nicotine. *PV*, pynocytotic vesicle; *J*, junction; *F*, fingerprint-like body. × 30000

Fig. 6. Scanning electron micrograph of bovine aortic endothelial cells treated with 10^{-4} *M* final ▷ concentration nicotine. *Above:* Control cells. *Below:* Toxic effect of nicotine. × 3000

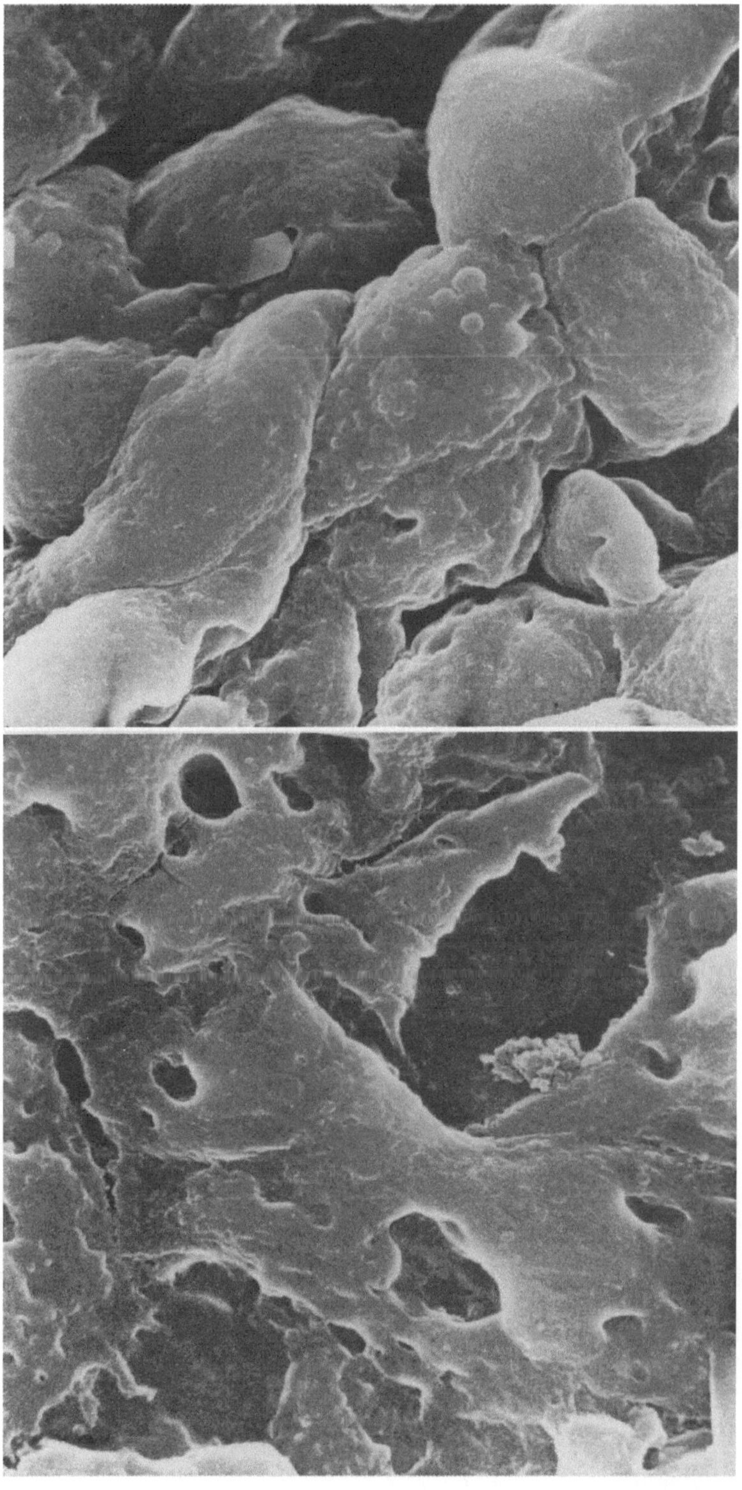

of cytoskeleton was observed in the smooth muscle and endothelial cells in parallel to the increase of the amount of nicotine present. No such effect was seen in the fibroblasts [11].

The effect of nicotine treatment was also evaluated by measuring the incorporation of ^{3}H-thymidine by the cells. In the concentration range 10^{-6} M-10^{-7} M, nicotine stimulated the incorporation in all, and particularly in the smooth muscle, cells. When the nicotine concentration was increased further the incorporation decreased, probably due to the toxic effect of the drug.

Morphological examinations of the cells by transmission and scanning electron microscopy revealed a cytotoxic effect of nicotine only at a final concentration of 10^{-4} M (Figs. 5 and 6).

In contrast to the toxic effect, the cytoskeleton synthesis and proliferation-stimulating effects may be considered as specific ones since the latter were induced by very low concentrations (10^{-6} M-10^{-7} M) of nicotine. This appears to be of some importance in human pathology since the final concentration of nicotine in the blood of heavy smokers is usually about 10^{-6} M. Thus apparently both the smooth muscle proliferation-stimulating and the toxic effects of nicotine may contribute to the early severe atherosclerotic lesions and to the progress of other vascular lesions in heavy smokers.

References

1. Bauer PI, Machovich R, Arányi P, Büki KG, Csonka E, Horváth I (1983) Mechanism of thrombin binding to endothelial cells. Blood 61: 368-372
2. Bauer PI, Machovich R, Büki KG, Csonka E, Koch AS, Horváth I (1984) Interaction of plasmin with endothelial cells. Biochem J 218: 119-124
3. Benditt EP, Barett T, McDougall JK (1983) Viruses in the etiology of atherosclerosis. Proc Natl Acad Sci USA 80: 6386-6389
4. Csonka E, Kádár A, Kerényi T, Jellinek H (1973) Morphology of cultured endothelial and smooth muscle cells of different origin. Acta Morphol 14: 18
5. Csonka E, Kerényi T, Koch AS, Jellinek H (1975) In vitro cultivation and identification of aortic endothelium from miniature pig. Arterail Wall 3: 31-37
6. Csonka E (1977) Techniques for culturing arterial endothelial cells. In: Manning GW, Haust MD (eds) In: Atherosclerosis. Plenum, New York, pp 719-723
7. Csonka E, Koch AS, Nemes L (1979) Measles virus induced lectin binding in cultured, aortic cells. Arterial Wall 5: 3-6 1979
8. Csonka E, Szemenyei K, Miskulin M, Robert AM (1980) Morphological examination of aortic endothelial and smooth muscle cells grown in vitro on collagen membranes. Artery 8: 253-258
9. Csonka E, Bauer PI (1982) Effect of plasmin on aortic endothelial cells. Acta Biochim Biophys Acad Sci Hung 17: 70 (abstract)
10. Csonka E, Koch AS, Kádár A, Óváry I (1984) Examination of a spontaneously transformed aortic smooth muscle cell line. I. Morphological examinations. Acta Morphol Hung Acad Sci 32: 195-205
11. Csonka E, Somogyi A, Augustin J, Haberbosch W, Schettler G, Jellinek H (1985) The effect of nicotine on cultured cells of vascular origin. Virchows Arch (Pathol Anatol) 407: 441-447
12. Csonka E, Jellinek H (1986) Aortic endothelial and smooth muscle cell interaction in culture. Acta Morphol Hung Acad Sci (to be published)
13. Csonka E, Koch AS, Bauer PI, Büki KG (1986) Interspecific interaction of aortic endothelial and smooth muscle cells. Acta Morphol Hung Acad Sci (to be published)
14. Fabricant CG, Fabricant J, Litrenta MM, Minick CR (1978) Virus induced atherosclerosis. J Exp Med 148: 335-340

15. Fabricant CG, Hajjar DP, Minick CR, Fabricant J (1981) Herpes virus infection enhances cholesterol and cholesteryl ester accumulation in cultured arterial smooth muscle cells. Am J Pathol 105: 176-184
16. Foster KA, Gill K, Micklem KJ, Pasternak CA (1980) Survey of virally mediated premeability changes. Biochem J 190: 639-646
17. Friedman HM, Macarak EJ, MacGregor RR, Wolfe J, Kefalides NA (1981) Virus infection of endothelial cells. J Infect Dis 143: 266-272
18. Györkey F, Melnick JL, Guinn GA, Györkey P, DeBakey ME (1984) Herpes viridae in the endothelial and smooth muscle cells of the proximal aorta in atherosclerotic patients. Exp Mol Pathol 40: 328-336
19. Jellinek H, Nagy Z, Hüttner I, Bálint A, Kóczé A, Kerényi T (1969) Investigations of the permeability changes of the vascular wall in experimental malignant hypertension by means of colloidal iron preparation. Br J Exp Pathol 50: 13
20. Jellinek H (1977) The use of twin tracer technique for the study of the movement of exogenous particles through the hypoxic arterial wall and their uptake by adventitial lymphatics. Folia Angiol 25: 156
21. Jellinek H (1977) Evidence of the specificity of the colloidal iron tracer technique and demonstration of partial injury of the aortic wall by twin tracer technique. Folia Angiol 25: 261
22. Jellinek H (1977) Twin tracer technique to follow up the increases permeability. Prog Biochem Pharmacol 13: 111
23. Jellinek H, Hársing J, Füzesi Sz (1982) A new model for arteriosclerosis. An electron microscopic study of the lesions induced by i. v. administered fat. Atherosclerosis 43: 7-18
24. Pasternak CA, Micklem KJ (1981) Virally induced alterations in cellular permeability: a basis of cellular and physiological damage? Biosci Rep 1: 431-448
25. Poste G, Reeve P, Alexander DJ, Terry G (1972) Studies on the cytpathogenicity of Newcastle Disease virus: effect of lectins on virus infected cells. J Gen Virol 17: 81-89
26. Schettler G (1983) The major problem in man. In: Schettler FG, Gotto AM, Middelhoff G, Habenicht AJR, Jurutka KR (eds) Proceedings of VIth international symposium on atherosclerosis. Springer, Berlin Heidelberg New York, pp 3-11
27. Schievelbein H, Heinemann G (1983) Nicotine and atherosclerosis. In: Schettler FG, Gotto AM, Middelhoff G, Habenicht AJR, Jurutka KR (eds) Proceedings of VIth international symposium on atherosclerosis. Springer, Berlin Heidelberg New York, pp 899-902
28. Schumacher BL, Grant D, Eisenstein R (1985) Smooth muscle cells produce an inhibitor of endothelial cell growth. Arteriosclerosis 5: 110-115
29. Thiery J, Csonka E (1984) New method for culturing endothelial cells from small vessels. In: Röhlich P, Bácsy E (eds) Tissue Culture and Res Akadémiai Kiadó, pp 491-496

On the Delayed Experimental Pathologic Involvement of Cerebral Arteries in Hypercholesterolemic Monkeys, Rabbits and Spontaneously Hypertensive Rats

G. Weber, L. Resi, and P. Tanganelli

Delayed development of atherosclerotic lesions of cerebral arteries compared to other arterial areas has been observed in man at autopsy [13, 15, 18] as well as in animal models: rhesus and cynomolgus monkeys [24]; New Zealand rabbits fed an atherogenic diet [9, 23], even if subjected to aortic coarctation [25]; and spontaneously hypertensive rats (SHR) fed a rat atherogenic diet [26].

As in man, the development of atherosclerotic lesions at the cerebral level in animal models is delayed but not completely inhibited: in basilar arteries in rabbits, lesions have been described 1 year after the beginning of an atherogenic diet [28]; the progression of the lesions was much slower than in other arterial areas (e.g., carotid or renal arteries); in monkeys on an atherogenic diet the appearance of experimental atherosclerotic lesions in cerebral arteries developed early if Goldblatt-type hypertension was provoked [8, 17].

In cynomolgus and rhesus monkeys fed an atherogenic diet for 8-12 months, the carotid arteries were extensively affected by intimal lesions which were filled with foam cells [24]. However, a scanning electron microscopic (SEM) examination revealed no lesions in the basilar, vertebral, and middle cerebral arteries of the same atherosclerotic monkeys. During a transmission electron microscopic (TEM) examination, these intracranial arteries showed no, or only minimal, circumscribed (spot) lesions, without foam cells, in the presence of some extracellular lipid and basilar membrane fragments in the edematous subendothelial space. Necrobiosis of endothelial cells was sometimes noted. The few smooth muscle cells which are physiologically present in the subendothelial space of the cerebral arteries of primates [1, 2, 22] frequently appeared in these lesion areas surrounded by a nest of basement membrane beads but they did not contain lipid droplets.

In New Zealand rabbits fed an atherogenic diet [23], aortic and carotid lesions were already present when the cerebral arteries were not at all involved at light microscopic or TEM examination.

In New Zealand rabbits subjected to aortic coarctation and submitted to a hypercholesterolemic diet for a 4-month period [25] our preliminary observations at the aortic and carotid levels were similar to those described by Pick and Hollander in monkeys [8, 17]: while the aortic intimal lesions appeared already severe at gross examination and were histologically atheromatous, the carotid lesions showed only a few lipid droplets in the smooth muscle cells, disseminated in a subendothelial "edematous" space; the cerebral arteries did not show any intimal lesions. Kurozumi et al. [10] found no foam cell lesions in the intima of cerebral arteries at some distance from branching sites, but insudation of plasma and foam cells in intimal cushions at branching sites. We did not make the latter observation in our study.

In spontaneously hypertensive rats (SHR) subjected to a short-term atherogenic (cholesterol-sodium cholate) diet [26] there were no gross atherosclerotic lesions. At histological level, both in aortic and carotid arteries, the lesions appeared similar to the ones described by Still and O'Neal [20]. The cerebral arteries, however, had no lesions in the wall. The endothelial cells in these arteries appeared well distended over the elastic membrane, the superficial portion of which had a "moth-eaten" appearance as previously described by Staubesand and Seydewitz [19]. The cytoplasm of the endothelial cells contained many dense, osmiophilic bodies.

Even the observations conducted at the intimal level on aortic, carotid, and cerebral arteries of growing SHR before and after the onset of hypertension (4-6 weeks and 8-12 weeks of age, respectively) revealed no lesions of cerebral arteries in any of the examined age-groups [27]. No lesions were observed in aortas of SHR aged 4 and 6 weeks; in rats aged 8 weeks disseminated lesions were evident in the intima: the subendothelial space was expanded due to a characteristic edematous substance whose appearance seemed to correspond to the one described by Limas et al. [12]. The endothelial layer appeared almost continuous, even though in some places it was much thinner and attenuated; some monocytic cells could be seen adhering to the endothelial cells. In carotid arteries similar lesions were already visible at 6 weeks and they reached a more severe degree at 12 weeks. Some of the endothelial cells appeared affected by regressive necrobiotic lesions. At cerebral arteries level, we noted only a few areas in which adherence of monocytes was noticeable in one of the rats of the 12-week group.

It appears clear from all the data quoted that development of experimental pathologic lesions of intracranial cerebral arteries is delayed in comparison to the aortic and carotid ones. In the search for an explanation, we have posed the question as to whether some endothelial cell surface characteristics could help to explain the delayed intimal involvement of a part of the lesions, supposing that the cerebral endothelium has different morphologic and permeability properties from noncerebral endothelium (cf. [16]).

A great variability in the endothelial glycocalyx reactivity has already been noted: not only (as described by Gerrity et al. [3]) in the "blue" and "white" areas of the aorta of minipigs and in different regions of the aorta of pigeons [11], but also in rabbits in which almost completely positive aortic intimal areas have been recorded alongside almost completely negative areas [6]. We have repeatedly observed a great variability in findings by making use of the Bernhard and Avrameas concanavalin A (*Canavalia ensiformis* agglutinin - Con A) reaction (Fig. 1).

Enzymic removal of sialic acid from the surface of arterial endothelium resulted in increased adhesion of circulating platelets [7] and of leukocytes [4].

Moreover Görög and Born [5] have described a greatly accelerated movement of low-density lipoprotein (LDL) from circulating blood into the arterial wall after removal of neuraminidase sialic acid from the endothelial glycocalyx of rabbit carotid arteries. As sialic acid depletion also means that there is a changed electric charge, we wonder whether alteration of the surface charge, besides increasing cerebrovascular permeability [15], could also help to explain, for instance, the lack of macrophage adhesion and hence the lack of foam cells in the intimal "insudative"-type lesions observed in intracranial cerebral arteries of hypercholesterolemic monkeys.

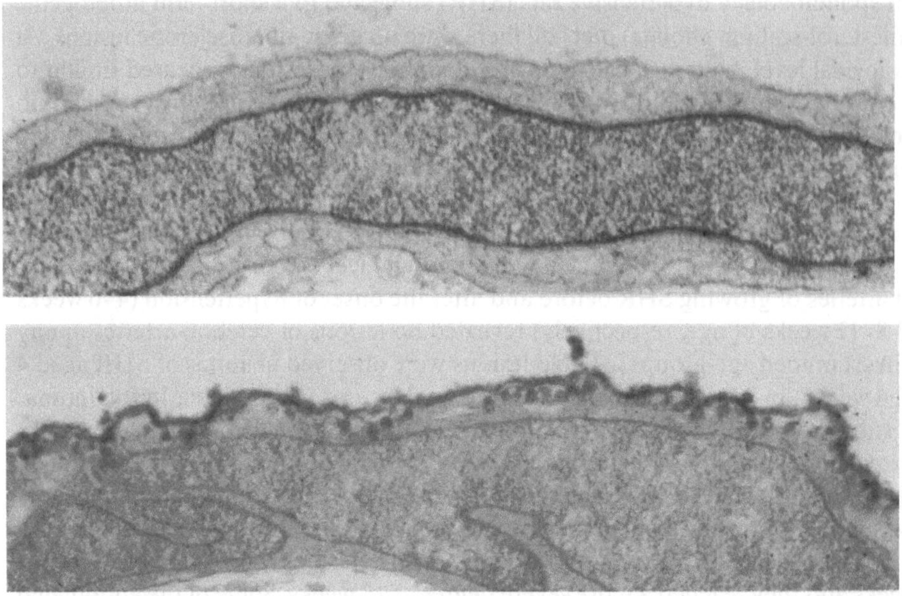

Fig. 1. Rabbit aorta on a normocholesterolemic diet. The luminal endothelial surface shows, in the same ultrathin section, different reactivities using the Bernhard and Avrameas Con A method. (T EM × 24000, × 17500)

So as not to limit the range of our observations to the results of the Con A reaction (according to the Bernhard and Avrameas method), we are now making use of various biotinylated lectins in order to try to localize different saccharide residues on the endothelial cell luminal plasma membrane of arterial vessels. Aortic, carotid, basilar, and middle cerebral artery samples of rabbits (normocholesterolemic or after a 2-4-month hypercholesterolemic diet), according to the biotin-avidin affinity methods used by Nag [16], were submitted to: Con A, wheat germ agglutinin (WGA), soybean agglutinin (SBA), and peanut agglutinin (PNA). After these reactions alpha-D-mannosyl, sialic acid, alpha-*N*-acetylgalactosaminyl, and beta-D-galactosyl residues were stained. Sialic acid invariably occured in a terminal position, while galactose was most frequently found either in a subterminal or terminal position; mannose, on the other hand, generally occupied a more proximal place in the "score" of branching polysaccharides [21]. After the Con A reaction only those residues were stained which had the appropriate configuration of substitution (mannosyl and glucosyl residues in the alpha-D-pyranose configuration). Before SBA, PNA, and WGA staining, some artery samples were also submitted to neuraminidase pretreatment for removal of sialic acid residues.

From our preliminary data, which still need further investigation before they are complete, it appears that mannosyl residues, being sialic acid, are less well-represented at the arterial endothelial surface also in rabbits on a hypercholesterolemic diet. Regional differences are now less relevant than previously observed with the Con A reaction according to Bernhard and Avrameas. It must be noted that an obvious lack of reactivity is evident in the intracranial arteries in some surface areas, chiefly in rabbits on a 4-month hypercholesterolemic diet. Sialic acid residues are

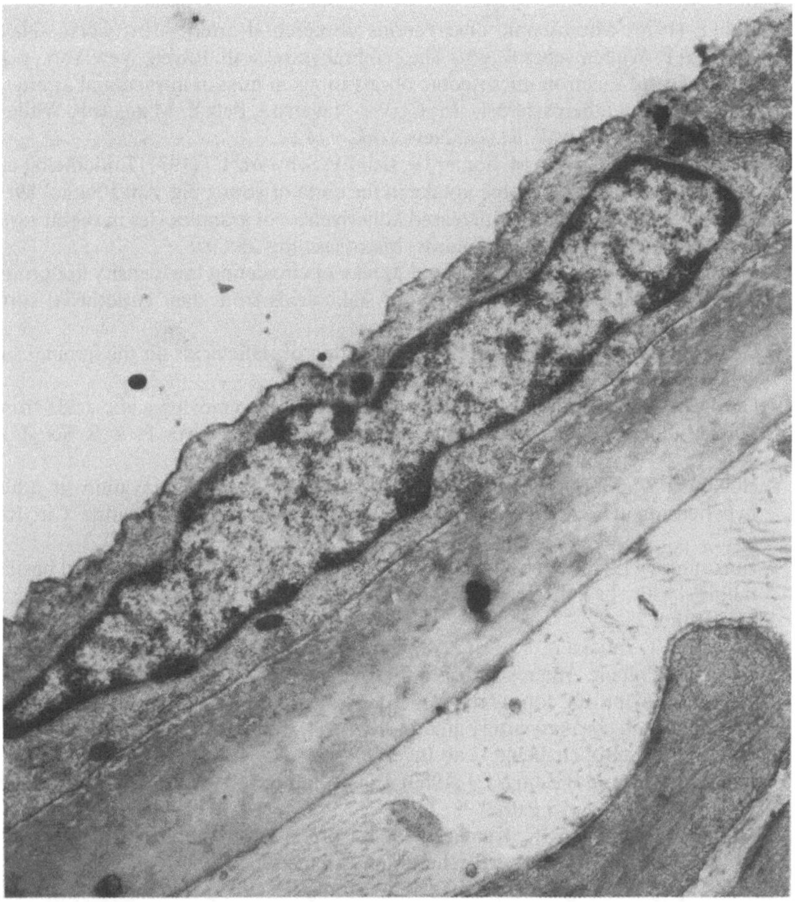

Fig. 2. Rabbit on a 2-month hypercholesterolemic diet. No lesion is detectable at basilar artery level. The PNA reaction of the luminal endothelial surface does not appear very pronounced nor uniform, clearly showing discontinuities. (T EM × 15000)

greatly decreased after neuraminidase. Disseminated areas are characterized by a lack of WGA reactivity and are increased in rabbits on a 2-month hypercholesterolemic diet. As for the galactosyl residues, their reactivity is much lower at every arterial level examined. The weak PNA reactivity of the intracranial endothelial cells appears higher than in the carotid and aortic ones (Fig. 2).

We are currently investigating the densitometric measurements of these different lectin reactivities (work still in progress), but even with this reservation it does not seem after all possible, even after having made use of biotinylated lectins in rabbits, to give too much relevance to the glycocalyx reactivity to help explain the delayed atherosclerotic involvement of the cerebral arteries. At any rate, it seems that the state (and thickness) of the glycocalyx or other specific cell surface characteristics (e.g., arrangements of microvilli) or different cell shapes or dimensions still need to be investigated further in order to understand their role in the delayed atherosclerotic involvement of the cerebral in hypercholesterolemia and/or hypertension.

References

1. Dahl E (1976) Microscopic observations on cerebral arteries. In: Cervos-Navarro J, Betz E, Matakas F, Wüllenweber R (eds) The cerebral vessel wall. Raven, New York, p 15
2. Dahl E (1976) Electron microscopic observations in human intracranial arteries: changes seen with aging and atherosclerosis. In: Cervos-Navarro J, Betz E, Matakas F, Wüllenweber R (eds) The cerebral vessel wall. Raven, New York, p 61
3. Gerrity RG, Richardson M, Somer JB, Bell FP, Schwartz CJ (1977) Endothelial cell morphology in areas of in vivo Evans blue uptake in the aorta of young pig. Am J Pathol 89: 313
4. Görög P, Born GVR (1982) Increased adhesiveness of granulocytes in rabbit earchamber blood vessels perfused with neuraminidase. Microvasc Res 23: 380
5. Görög P, Born GVR (1982) Increased uptake of circulating low-density lipoproteins and fibrinogen by arterial walls after removal of sialic acids from their endothelial surface. Br J Exp Pathol 63: 447
6. Görög P, Born GVR (1983) Uneven distribution of sialic acids on the luminal surface of aortic endothelium. Br J Exp Pathol 64: 418
7. Görög P, Schraufstatter I, Born GVR (1982) Effect of removing sialic acids from endothelium on the adherence of circulating platelets in arteries in vivo. Proc R Soc Lond [Biol] 214: 471
8. Hollander W, Madoff I, Paddock J, Kirkpatrick B (1976) Aggravation of atherosclerosis by hypertension in a subhuman primate model with coarctation of the aorta. Circ Res [Suppl 2] 38: 63
9. Kurozumi T (1975) Electron microscopy on permeability of the aorta and basilar artery of the rabbit - with special reference to the changes of permeability by hypercholesterolemia. Exp Mol Pathol 23: 1
10. Kurozumi T, Tanaka K, Yae Y (1978) Hypertension-induced cerebral atherosclerosis in the cholesterol-fed rabbit. Atherosclerosis 30: 137
11. Lewis JC, Taylor RG, Jones ND, St Clair RW, Cornhill JF (1982) Endothelial surface characteristics in pigeon coronary artery atherosclerosis. I. Cellular alterations during the initial stages of dietary cholesterol challenge. Lab Invest 46: 123
12. Limas C, Westrum B, Limas CJ (1980) The evolution of vascular changes in the spontaneously hypertensive rat. Am J Pathol 98: 357
13. Mathur KS, Kashyap SK, Kumar V (1963) Correlation of the extent and severity of atherosclerosis in the coronary and cerebral arteries. Circulation 27: 929
14. McGarry P, Solberg LA, Guzman MA, Strong JP (1985) Cerebral atherosclerosis in New Orleans: comparisons of lesions by age, sex, and race. Lab Invest 52: 533
15. Nag S (1984) Cerebral endothelial surface charge in hypertension. Acta Neuropathol (Berl) 63: 276
16. Nag S (1985) Ultrastructural localization of monosaccharide residues on cerebral endothelium. Lab Invest 52: 553
17. Pick R, Johanson PJ, Glick G (1974) Deleterious effects of hypertension on the development of aortic and coronary atherosclerosis in stumptail macaques *(Macaca speciosa)* on an atherogenic diet. Circ Res 35: 472
18. Solberg LA, McGarry PA, Moosy J, Strong JP, Tejada C, Löken AC (1968) Severity of atherosclerosis in cerebral arteries, coronary arteries, and aortas. Ann NY Acad Sci 149: 956
19. Staubesand J, Seydewitz V (1981) Über eine Besonderheit der Membrana elastica interna kleiner Gehirnarterien. Therapiewoche 31: 4528
20. Still WJS, O'Neal RM (1962) Electron microscopy study of experimental atherosclerosis in the rat. Am J Pathol 40: 21
21. Stoddart RW, Collins RD, Jacobson W (1980) Lectin staining of carbohydrates of haemic cells: the cells of normal blood and bone marrow and of myeloid leukaemias. J Pathol 131: 321
22. Suzuki M (1974) Atherosclerotic lesions of the cerebral arteries in young persons. In: Schettler G, Weizel W (eds) Atherosclerosis III. Springer, Berlin Heidelberg New York, p 492
23. Weber G, Cesari S, Fabbrini P, Petrelli L, Resi L, Tanganelli P (1983) On delayed cerebral atherosclerosis. Ultrastructural and ultrahistochemical observations in the cholesterol-fed rabbits. G Arterioscler [Suppl] 1: 47
24. Weber G, Fabbrini P, Resi L, Sforza V, Tanganelli P, Vesselinovitch D, Wissler RW (1983) An

ultrastructural comparison of diet-induced atherosclerosis of arteries supplying the central nervous system in cynomolgus and rhesus monkeys. Appl Pathol 1: 121

25. Weber G, Mattei FM, Fabbrini P, Resi L, Cesari S, Petrelli L, Tanganelli P (1984) Osservazioni preliminari, a livello ultrastrutturale, sulla reattività delle arterie cerebrali di coniglio New Zealand a stimoli aterogeni combinati (dieta ipercolesterolica e ipertensione). Boll Soc Ital Biol Sper 60: 553
26. Weber G, Alessandrini C, Centi L, Gerli R, Novelli MT, Petrelli L, Resi L, Salvi M, Tanganelli P (1986) On delayed development of intimal lesions in cerebral arteries of spontaneously hypertensive rats (SHR) subjected to a short-term atherogenic diet (a TEM study). Appl Pathol, (in press)
27. Weber G, Alessandrini C, Centi L, Gerli R, Novelli MT, Petrelli L, Resi L, Salvi M, Tanganelli P (1986) Delayed intimal lesions development in cerebral arteries versus aorta and carotid of spontaneously hypertensive rats (SHR). Exp Mol Pathol 44: 340
28. Wilson RB, Miller RA, Middleton CC, Kinden D (1982) Atherosclerosis in rabbits fed a low cholesterol diet for five years. Arterioclerosis 2: 228

Enzyme-Acylalcohol-Alcohol Interactions in the Arterial Wall

J. Patelski, T. Szwajca, and K. Świdzińska

Introduction

Complex enzyme-acylalcohol-alcohol systems and interactions are involved in the metabolism and accumulation of lipids in the arterial wall. They result in, and from, linked sequences of reversible transacylations depending on physiochemical conditions in this and other tissue compartments.

The results previously obtained for human and experimental atherosclerosis and for the in vitro multi-reactant systems [3, 4, 7, 8] were considered in connection with the acylenzyme mechanism [2] of both decomposition and synthesis of acylalcohols. However, no experimental evidence was produced for the acylenzyme formation.

The present paper is concerned with the enzyme-acylalcohol relationships and formation of the acylenzyme complex in the arterial wall.

Material and Methods

Lipolytic enzyme activities and lipid composition were determined in human arteriosclerotic femoral and iliac arteries. Correlations for the enzyme specific activities (milliunits per 1 mg protein) and metabolic activities (specific activity per tissue metabolite concentration) and for the activity ratios were calculated [3].

In vitro formation of the acylenzyme complex was investigated as follows. Acetone-butanol powders from pig thoracic aortas and aqueous extracts from the powders [7] were used.

For separation of proteins by thin-layer chromatography (TLC), silica gel 60 F_{254} plastic sheets, 20×20 cm (Merck, FRG) were used. They were impregnated (2×20 cm) with the aqueous extract, dried in a cold air stream and immersed in 99% ethanol-water mixture, 99:5 vol., respectively. Resolution followed at approximately 20 °C for 5 h. Subsequently the sheets were dried and cut into strips of equal width (3 cm). Protein fractions were visualised using the Ninhydrin-cadmium reagent. Corresponding areas of uncoloured strips were rinsed out into test tubes and protein was eluted with the phosphate buffer (Na_2HPO_4, NaH_2PO_4) at pH 7.00 and ionic strength $\mu = 0.146$ mol/litre, i.e. equal to that of isotonic solution of sodium chloride (3×1 ml). Other strips with the separated proteins and the eluted fractions were used for enzyme examinations. Protein was determined by means of the microbiuret method according to Itzhaki and Gill [1].

To test the formation of the acylenzyme complexes, the individual strips with separated proteins were sprayed with different substrate solutions (palmitic, stearic, oleic and linoleic acid, oleylcholesterol, diacylglycerophosphocholine and triacylglycerol - Sigma, USA - 2.5×10^{-4} mol/litre in the phosphate buffer). Subsequently the Ninhydrin reaction was used to prove the reactive and non-reactive fractions.

In order to watch the energetic changes in time or conformational activity of the isolated enzyme, the technique of recording dynamic absorbancy of the enzyme and acylenzyme (oleylenzyme) complex was worked out as reported earlier [9] and was used as follows. The enzyme and enzyme-substrate solutions (1:1 vol.) in quartz cuvettes (1 cm) were placed in an electric rotor (~33 rpm) adapted for irradiating consecutive samples, in order to stop the protein changes at different time. The samples were exposed to UV light (Hanau mercury lamp with S-500 burner, 238-579 nm wavelength, $I_0 = 6.65 \times 10^{14}$ quanta/cm$^2 \cdot$s) at 0.076 s intervals (1.824 s per rotation/24 samples). Subsequently, absorbancy was measured in a VSU 2-P spectrophotometer (Zeiss, Jena) at 222 nm.

The absorbancy *(A)* values have been ploted against time *(t)*, $A = f(t)$ demonstrating the enzyme energy levels in the form of periodically variable functions. These are expressed by the equations $y = b \sin (\pi/a)x$ and $y = |b \sin (\pi/a)x|$ for the enzyme and oleylenzyme, respectively, where y is absorbancy, x is time, b is the function amplitude and $2a$ is the function period. Formation of the acylenzyme results in a reduced sinusoidal maximum and a different course of the function.

Results and Discussion

Relationship Between the Lipolytic Enzyme Activities and Lipid Composition of the Arterial Wall

Correlations for enzyme-specific and metabolic activities and for the activity ratios are shown in Fig. 1. Positive interactions within two groups of results with either glycerol ester hydrolase (GEH, EC 3.1.1.3) and acyl-CoA:cholesterol acyltransferase (ACAT, EC 2.3.1.26) [2, 5] or phosphatide acylhydrolase (PAH, EC 3.1.1.4) and cholesterol ester hydrolase (CEH, EC 3.1.1.13) activities in the numerator (3, 4, 7, 8) and negative interactions between the groups may be distinguished.

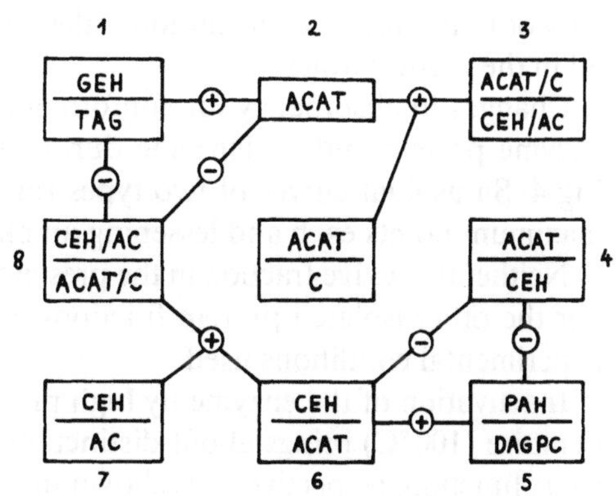

Fig. 1. Interactions of enzyme-specific and metabolic activities and their ratios. ⊕ ⊖, correlations ($r > 0.7$, $P \leq 0.05$). For details and abbreviations, see text

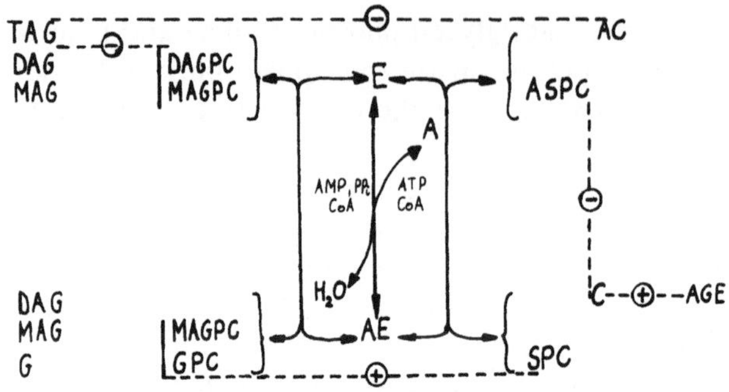

Fig. 2. Enzyme-acylalcohol-alcohol system and interactions in the arterial wall. *A*, acid (acyl); *E*, enzyme; *G*, glycerol; *GPC*, glycerophosphocholine; *SPC*, sphingophosphocholine. For other abbreviations, see text. ⊕ ⊖, correlations ($r > 0.7$, $P \leq 0.05$)

Higher synthesis and accumulation than decomposition of acylcholesterols (ACs) and diacylglycerophosphocholine (DAGPC) at enhanced decomposition of triacylglycerols (TAGs), and vice versa, is in agreement with data obtained in experimental animals [5, 6].

Interactions of the acylalcohols and alcohols expressed in terms of the acylenzyme-mediated transacylations of substrate products are shown in Fig. 2. Different solubility and reactivity of acylalcohols and alcohols involved in the arterial transacylations at the same reacting groups [3] and approximate activity ranges of the enzyme(s) present may be expected to affect accumulation and transportation of the compounds. In this regard, the compounds of mixed function such as monoacylglycerophosphocholine (MAGPC), monoacylglycerol (MAG) and diacylglycerol (DAG), acting as both fatty acyl donors and acceptors [4, 7, 8], may be of major importance.

Formation of the Acylenzyme Complex

Five protein fractions were separated from the aqueous extracts from acetone-butanol powders of pig aorta (Fig. 3). Fraction No. 2 was found to form acylenzyme complexes in the presence of both free and esterified fatty acids, as indicated by the negative Ninhydrin reaction (Fig. 3). The reactive fraction represents approximately 20% of total protein concentration, the latter amounting to approximately 2.2 mg/ml in the crude extract.

Changes in absorbancy (or conformation) of both the isolated fraction No. 2 or enzyme protein and acylenzyme during a given period of time, are presented in Fig. 4. Sinusoidal curves of two types for periodically variable functions with two maximum points each and lessening amplitudes can be seen.

Neither the active fraction in the presence of the corresponding alcohol solutions, nor the other isolated protein fractions and albumin revealed such activity in the experimental conditions used.

Inactivation of the enzyme by high proton concentration (pH 4.5) and high temperature (100 °C) brings about distinct changes and perturbations in the course of sinus function, respectively, as shown in Figs. 5 and 6.

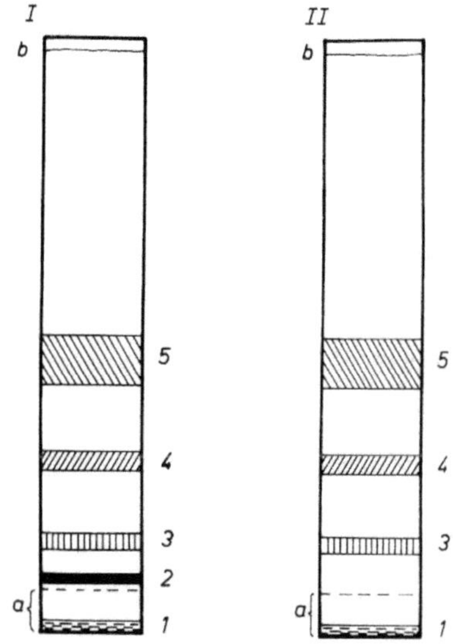

Fig. 3. Proteins extracted with water from acetone-butanol powders of pig aortas and separated by TLC: before *(I)* and after *(II)* the treatment with substrate. *1-5*, protein fractions; *a*, area impregnated by the aqueous extract; *b*, front of the solvent

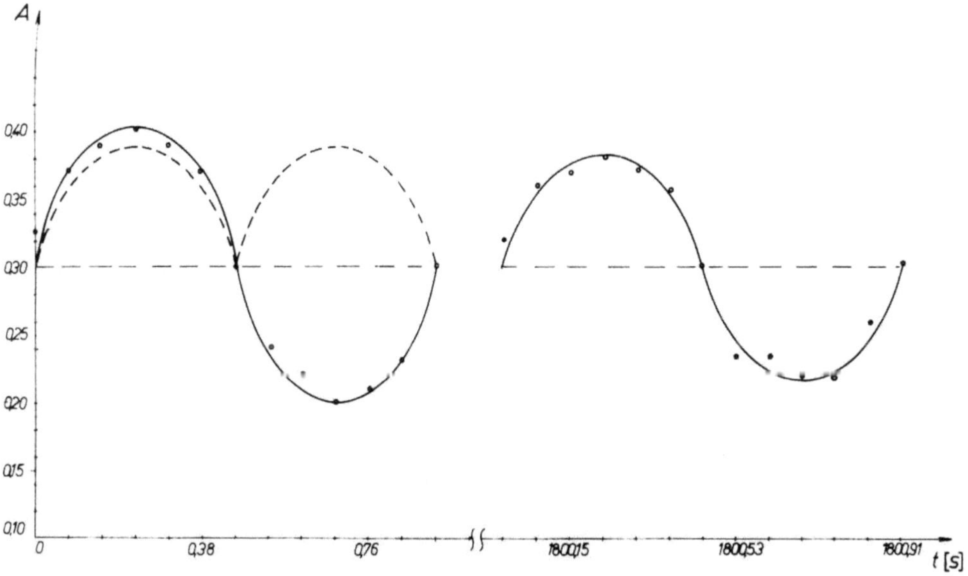

Fig. 4. The changes in absorbancy of the enzyme protein during a given period of time. Protein concentration: 2.4×10^{-5} g/ml, phosphate buffer $\mu = 0.1465$ mol/litre, pH 7.00, $\lambda = 222$ nm. ——, without substrate; -----, with substrate

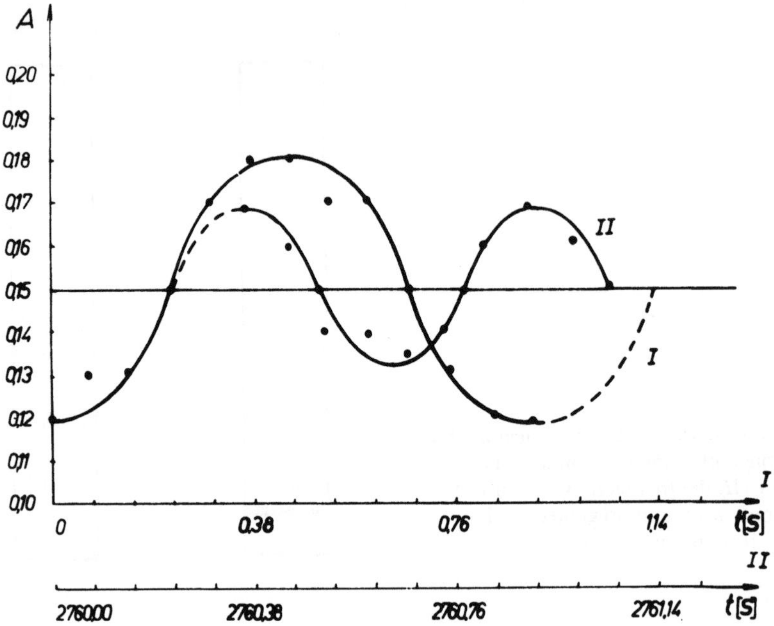

Fig. 5. The effect of reduced pH on the dependence of absorbancy of the enzyme during a given period of time. Protein: 2.5×10^{-4} g/ml, phosphate buffer $\mu = 0.1465$ mol/litre; *I*, pH 7.00; *II*, pH 4.5, changed to 7.00

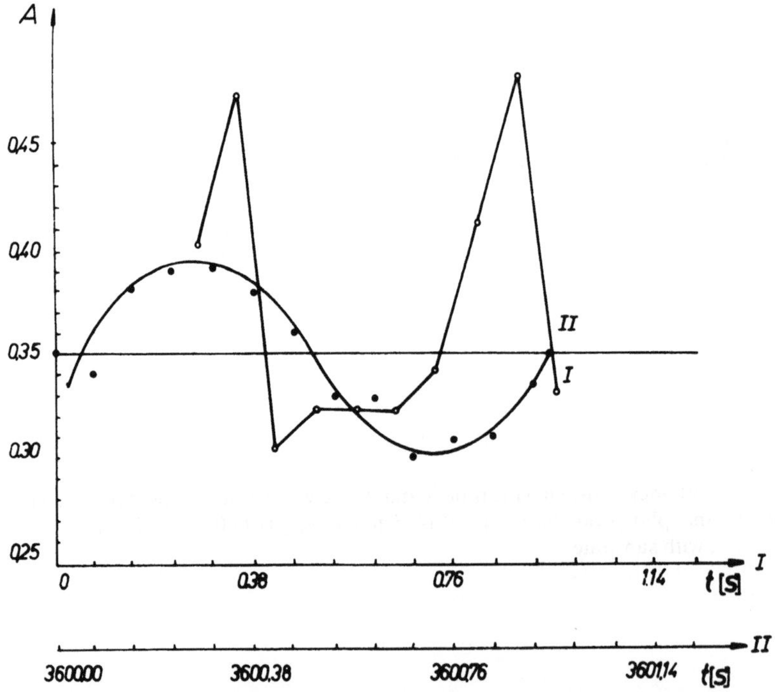

Fig. 6. The effect of temperature on the dependence of absorbancy of the enzyme during a given period of time. Protein: 0.8×10^{-5} g/ml, phosphate buffer $\mu = 0.1465$ mol/litre, pH 7.00; *I*, 20 °C; *II*, after inactivation at 100 °C

The results indicate formation of the acylenzyme complex and support the common mechanism of enzyme-catalysed hydrolysis and transacylations of lipids in the arterial wall.

In the isolated enzyme, energy must have been absorbed from the input ultraviolet wave to fix the conformational changes. The curves obtained for the enzyme and acylenzyme show the conformational activity according to sinus functions with the two extreme points for maximum reactivity in two elementary processes within the period of 0.912 s.

The very fast step in enzyme action is important for the linked transacylation sequences and interactions in the enzyme-acylalcohol-alcohol systems. A better understanding of the mechanism of lipid metabolism and accumulation will depend upon the measurement of the rates of the elementary processes in a physiological environment and under the influence of different agents.

Acknowledgement. This work was supported by grant W. 10.8.4.13.04 from the Ministry of Health and Social Welfare in Poland.

References

1. Itzhaki F, Gill DM (1964) A micro-biuret method for estimating protein. Anal Biochem 9: 401
2. Kraut J (1977) Serine proteases: structure and mechanism of catalysis. Annu Rev Biochem 46: 331
3. Patelski J (1980) Enzyme systems of the arterial wall: relationship between enzyme activities and lipid composition. Artery 8: 368
4. Patelski J, Pioruńska-Stolzmann M (1985) Effects of substrate fatty acids on products of lecithin hydrolysis and acyl-CoA-independent transacylation with cholesterol by aortic enzyme preparations. Enzyme 34: 217
5. Patelski J, Bowyer DE, Howard AN, Gresham GA (1968) Changes in phospholipase A, lipase and cholesterol esterase activity in aorta in experimental atherosclerosis in the rabbit and rat. J Atheroscler Res 8: 221
6. Patelski J, Bowyer DE, Howard AN, Jennings IW, Thorne CJR, Gresham GA (1970) Modification of enzyme activities in experimental atherosclerosis in the rabbit. Atherosclerosis 12: 41
7. Patelski J, Pioruńska-Stolzmann M (1979) Cholesterol ester: lysolecithin transacylation in the aorta. Enzyme 24: 342
8. Patelski J, Pioruńska A, Pioruńska-Stolzmann M (1986) Oleylglycerol hydrolysis and acyl-CoA-independent transacylation with cholesterol by enzyme preparations from pig aorta. Enzyme 35: 13
9. Szwajca T, Świdzińska K, Patelski J (1984) New approach to the properties of enzyme protein and its reaction with fatty acid as a substrate in the arterial wall (in Polish). In: XVI congress of the Polish Physiological Society, Katowice, 1984, abstract p 347

The Effect of Balloon De-Endothelialization on Arterial Enzymes and Metabolic Intermediates in Rabbits

T. Zemplenyi, D. W. Crawford, D. F. Tidwell, and M. A. Cole

Experimental, pathologic, and clinical evidence indicates that endothelial injury or loss of endothelium may produce thickening of the arterial tunica intima, and thus facilitate the deposition of lipoproteins and the development of atherosclerotic lesions. The underlying mechanism for intimal thickening appears to be exposure of medial smooth muscle cells (SMC) to mitogens such as growth factors derived from platelets, monocytes, and perhaps even the endothelium itself [1], which induce proliferation of SMC and their migration into the intima. Exposure to low-density lipoproteins or to hypoxic conditions also seems to induce SMC proliferation [2, 3]. The nutrition and oxygenation of comparatively thin arteries, such as aortas of small animals or even peripheral arteries of larger mammals, depends primarily on diffusion from the arterial lumen and the oxygen supply may become impaired by intimal thickening. The aim of the present investigation has been to find out whether in such arteries intimal thickening produced by balloon catheter de-endothelialization would result in metabolic changes believed to favor atherogenesis.

Materials and Methods

A total of 16 white New Zealand male rabbits weighing 3000–3300 g prior to successful de-endothelialization (see below) were used. Male rabbits of the same age served as controls. The endothelium was removed from the abdominal aortas and both ilio-femoral arteries of the experimental rabbits using an appropriately preformed 3 French Fogerty balloon catheter (American Edwards Model 12-080-3F). The catheter was inserted into the right carotid artery of anesthesized animals and pushed downwards into the aorta. The balloon was inflated to a pressure of 30–40 mm Hg and pulled twice through the abdominal aorta and once through the ilio-femoral arteries under X-ray control.

Enzyme and metabolic intermediate measurements in the aorta were done after 11 weeks in nine rabbits and after 19 weeks in six rabbits. (One animal died 14 weeks following de-endothelialization and was not used for the study.) Prior to killing the animals the right femoral artery was exposed surgically under light oxygen-nitrous-oxyde-methoxyflurane mixture anesthesia in order to measure oxygen tension profiles across the artery [4]. This measurement lasted an average 4–5 min. Afterwards the anesthesia was made more complete, the abdominal cavity was opened and the abdominal aorta quickly separated from the surrounding tissue while the animal was usually still alive. The abdominal aorta was then quickly removed, opened, cleaned of blood and adventitial tissue (except for a small portion used for histology) and cut longitudinally into two parallel segments. One was immediately freeze-clamped using a clamp precooled in liquid nitrogen, and further processed for metabolic intermediate measurements (see below). The procedure - from removing the aorta until freezing - lasted, on average, 3 min. The other segment of the aorta was chopped into small pieces, and, using a Polytron homogenizer with a PT-10 generator, an approximately 4% homogenate (w/v) in ice-cold saline was prepared. It was extracted by rotation for 10 min at 4 °C and centrifuged at 5000 *g* for 10 min. The pellet was re-extracted overnight, centrifuged in an identical way and the supernatant fractions from both extractions were combined. Enzyme activities and metabolic intermediates were determined in aliquots from each aorta separately, as described before [5, 6].

Results

As shown in Table 1, in the abdominal aortas the activity of lactate dehydrogenase (LDH), lipoamide dehydrogenase, and the lysosomal β-glucuronidase was significantly increased 11 weeks following de-endothelialization. The number of samples in which activity measurements for *N*-acetyl-β-glucosaminidase (NAGA), the other lysosomal hydrolase, were available was only half of those for β-glucuronidase (five samples); this limited number may be the reason that for NAGA only a trend toward increased activity could be detected. The same may also be true for the lack of significant difference in isocitrate dehydrogenase (ICDH) activity, in spite of a trend toward higher activity (117.9 versus 57.2) in the de-endothelialized aortas. No significant differences in the aortic level of lactate, pyruvate or glucose were detected in the experiments of 11 week duration.

Table 1. Abdominal aorta enzyme activities in experimental (E) and control (C) rabbits 11 weeks following de-endothelialization

Enzyme	Group	*n*	Activity/100 µg DNA (mean ± SEM)	Significance *P*
Lactate dehydrogenase	C	5	578 ± 104	< .05
	E	5	1209 ± 226	
Malate dehydrogenase	C	9	2399 ± 429	NS
	E	8	2494 ± 414	
Isocitrate dehydrogenase	C	4	57.2 ± 15.4	NS
	E	5	117.9 ± 16.8	
Lipoamide dehydrogenase	C	7	82.9 ± 13.7	< .05
	E	8	164.0 ± 27.9	
β-Glucuronidase ($\times 10^3$)	C	10	829.4 ± 138.0	< .001
	E	9	2544.0 ± 306.0	
N-Acetyl-β-glucosaminidase (NAGA) ($\times 10^3$)	C	5	2324.0 ± 341.0	NS
	E	5	4101.0 ± 964.0	

NS, not significant.

Table 2. Abdominal aorta enzyme activities in experimental (E) and control (C) rabbits 19 weeks following de-endothelialization

Enzyme	Group	*n*	Activity/100 μg DNA (mean ± SEM)	Significance *P*
Lactate dehydrogenase	C	4	352 ± 124	NS
	E	6	454 ± 116	
Malate dehydrogenase	C	5	1004 ± 269	NS
	E	6	1285 ± 240	
Lipoamide dehydrogenase	C	9	68.27 ± 5.34	< .05
	E	5	96.00 ± 14.15	
β-Glucuronidase ($\times 10^3$)	C	5	1411 ± 383	< .05
	E	6	3191 ± 585	
N-Acetyl-β-glucosaminidase ($\times 10^3$)	C	5	2028 ± 423	NS
	E	6	3507 ± 654	

NS, not significant.

Table 2 shows that similarly to the experiments of shorter duration, the activity of lipoamide dehydrogenase and β-glucuronidase was significantly increased in the abdominal aortas 19 weeks following de-endothelialization although the number of aortas available at the end of the 19-week period was only limited. The activity of LDH and NAGA also revealed a similar trend toward increase compared to control aortas. The activity of malate dehydrogenase (MDH), when expressed on the fat-free dry-weight basis (not shown in the Table) revealed a significant ($P < 0.005$) decrease compared with control animals. This is of some interest because the level of lactate was significantly elevated in the abdominal aortas 19 weeks after de-endothelialization, calculated on the aortic DNA content basis (261.4 ± 94.0 versus 118.2 ± 33.0 nmol/100 μg DNA).

Discussion

For reasons outlined in the introduction one could expect that intimal thickening would result in local hypoxia of the arterial wall. Indeed, in human aortas with advancing age and associated progressive diffuse intimal thickening the activity of LDH, as demonstrated both histochemically and biochemically [7, 8] increases in the mid-zone aortic layers, and this increase is mainly attributable to the enhanced activity of the anaerobic (electrophoretically slow moving) forms of LDH isoenzymes [9]. Previous work also indicated that a common denominator of various types of vascular injury has been a decline in tricarboxylic acid cycle (TCA) enzymes and an increased activity of lysosomal hydrolases [8]. A similar pattern emerged from studies in which atherosclerosis-susceptible and atherosclerosis-resistant human or animal arteries or arterial segments were compared. Such a pattern was considered an indirect evidence of the important role of vascular injury and vascular hypoxia in atherogenesis [8, 9].

In view of the above background information the present study produced several rather unexpected results. The findings of the first experimental series indicate that in contrast to the senescent human aorta with its chronically and progressively thickened tunica intima, the thickening of the abdominal aorta produced acutely in rabbits by de-endothelialization leads not only to an initial elevation of the activity of LDH and lysosomal hydrolases but also enhances the activity of lipoamide dehydrogenase and most likely also of many other enzymes involved in arterial metabolism. One can hypothesize that this type of injury, namely "denudation" of the endothelial lining, exposes the SMC to the immediate action of growth factors mentioned in the introduction. The resulting cell proliferation together with the associated vigorous metabolic activity becomes expressed in the rise of activity of enzymes involved in anabolic and catabolic reactions.

The results obtained in the second experimental series - although with a limited number of animals - indicate that with time and slowing of cell proliferation the difference in enzyme activities between experimental and control aortas becomes less marked except for the lysosomal β-glucuronidase and probably other lysosomal hydrolases as well. Re-endothelialization of the tunica intima may be another essential contributing factor in this regard [10]. Unfortunately, the activities of the rate-limiting glycolytic enzymes such as pyruvate kinase and phosphofructokinase were extremely low and impossible to evaluate: however, the elevated aortic level of lactate in the experiment of longer duration (second experimental series) may be an indicator of impaired tissue oxygenation in the aortas with intimal thickening.

As stated before, all in all, the changes produced by de-endothelialization of the abdominal aortas resulted in much less pronounced metabolic changes than expected. One possible explanation comes from our results in the de-endothelialized ilio-femoral arteries with oxygen tension profiles measured across the arterial wall using the microelectrode technique mentioned in Methods (results to be published separately). For the interpretation of the present data it appears enlightening that it was detected that the negative effect of intimal thickening on tissue oxygenation has been counteracted by an adaptive proliferation of adventitial and medial nutrient channels - vasa vasorum - within the arterial wall. In good agreement, the oxygen tension profiles revealed augmentation of oxygen delivery to the adventitia and outer layers of the media of the arterial wall.

Finally, it has to be mentioned that in a subsequent experimental series (to be published in detail) in which animals with de-endothelialized aortas were on a cholesterol regimen for 6 weeks, the activity of LDH and pyruvate kinase increased significantly, the activity of TCA enzymes declined significantly and the activity of lysosomal hydrolases became increased by 250%.

Summary

The abdominal aortas of nine rabbits were studied for 11 weeks, and of six rabbits for 19 weeks following balloon catheter-induced de-endothelialization. The activity of the enzymes investigated (LDH, lipoamide dehydrogenase, ICDH, β-glucuronidase, NAGA) exhibited either a significant increase or at least a clear tendency toward increase as compared with control aortas. The activity of malate dehydrogenase revealed a decreased activity, and the aortic level of lactate was increased but only in the experimental series of longer (19 weeks) duration.

The enhanced activity of the enzymes 11 weeks following de-endothelialization possibly mirrors vigorous metabolic activity associated with proliferation of smooth muscle cells exposed to platelet-derived and other growth factors.

Experimental intimal thickening of shorter duration does not seem to lead to arterial wall hypoxia. Related experiments indicate that tissue oxygenation in such arteries is preserved by a protective proliferation of vasa vasorum.

Acknowledgement. Supported by Grant-in-Aid 643 from AHA-GLAA.

References

1. Ross R, Raines E, Bowen-Pope D (1982) Growth factors from platelets, monocytes and endothelium: their role in cell proliferation. Ann NY Acad Sci 397: 18-24
2. Fisher-Dzoga K, Vesselinovitch D, Wissler RW (1974) The effect of estrogen on the rabbit aortic medial tissue culture cells. Am J Pathol 74: 52A
3. Paule WJ, Zemplenyi T, Rounds DC, Blankenhorn DH (1976) Light and electron microscopic characteristics of arterial smooth muscle cell cultures subjected to hypoxia or carbon monoxide. Atherosclerosis 25: 111-123
4. Crawford DW, Back LH, Cole MA (1980) In vivo oxygen transport in the normal rabbit femoral arterial wall. J Clin Invest 65: 1498-1508
5. Zemplenyi T (1977) Metabolic intermediates, enzymes and lysosomal activity in aortas of spontaneously hypertensive rats. Atherosclerosis 28: 233-246
6. Zemplenyi T, Fronek K (1981) Chemical sympathectomy by 6-hydroxydopamine and arterial enzymes and lactate in the rabbit. Exp Mol Pathol 34: 123-130
7. Adams CWM (1967) Vascular histochemistry. Lloyd-Luke, London
8. Zemplenyi T (1968) Enzyme biochemistry of the arterial wall as related to atherosclerosis. Lloyd-Luke, London
9. Zemplenyi T (1975) Vascular metabolism, vascular enzymes and the effect of drugs. In: Kritchevsky D (ed) Pharmacology of hypolipidemic agents. Springer, Berlin Heidelberg New York pp 291-348 (Handbook of experimental pharmacology, vol 41)
10. Falcone DJ, Hajjar DP, Minick CR (1984) Lipoprotein and albumin accumulation in reendothelialized and deendothelialized aorta. Am J Pathol 114: 112-120

Epidemiology, Risk Factors

Coronary Heart Disease Epidemiology - Perspectives

F. H. Epstein

Epidemiology is, according to one of its definitions, the basic science of preventive medicine. Coronary heart disease epidemiology has made spectacular strides during the past 30 years and has provided the groundwork for the prevention of this disease in the community and in individuals, primarily in terms of the risk factor concept. In fact, the term "risk factor" which has become a household word, originated in the course of epidemiological studies into the precursors of coronary heart disease. Now, in the mid-1980s, it is time to take stock as we are at the crossroads with regard to two major questions: (a) to what extent is current knowledge sufficient for the prevention of premature coronary heart disease; (b) what further research is needed to improve the predictive power of risk factos? The second question relates both to refining prediction in terms of known or suspected risk factors and to the discovery of new risk factors. To the extent that risk factors are causally related to the disease, answers to the second question will not only improve the ability to characterise high-risk groups but will also contribute to knowledge concerning the etiology of coronary heart disease and atherosclerosis. Thus, it will improve both predictive and preventive power.

Fundamental to these discussions are the concepts "population strategy" and "high-risk strategy". It is assumed that the two strategies are not alternatives but are complementary. It is also assumed that current knowledge about the major risk factors, i.e. serum lipids, blood pressure and smoking, is sufficient to make a major impact on preventing premature disease at the community level, i.e. in terms of the population strategy. The need is to act on these risk factors, as recommended by many agencies as well as individual experts around the world, amongst whom Gotthard Schettler stands courageously and forcefully in the front line. In terms of the high-risk strategy, individual predictive power leaves a good deal to be desired, remarkable though it is in comparison with the predictability of other chronic diseases. In this essay, a good deal of attention will be given to this matter.

Anyone attempting to look into the future will be aware of the hazards involved and his own limitations of vision. Nevertheless, the aim will be to present more than a purely personal view. Perspectives are necessarily based on the past and present. It would be difficult, in an essay such as this, to provide an adequate bibliography of the history of coronary heart disease epidemiology upon which the thoughts to be presented are based. The assumption is made, therefore, that the broad areas covered have become common knowledge amongst atherosclerosis research workers. If correct, this in itself would be an indication of the degree to which epidemiology has assumed an established position in this field of investigation.

Geographical Pathology

Geographical Pathology was the title of a textbook, published by Hirsch of Berlin in the year 1860. The Council for International Organizations of Medical Sciences (CIOMS) defined the term as "comparative studies between different ethnic, national and social groups". One of the cornerstones of current knowledge is the recognition that coronary heart disease shows great international differences in frequency. These are probably due in large part to differences in nutrition, reflected in serum cholesterol levels when countries with high industrial development are compared with largely agrarian parts of the world. Industrialised Japan is an exception but it still has a low fat consumption. The Seven Country Study, initiated by Keys, is the single, most convincing example of this statement. On the other hand, there are differences between industrial countries which are, at best, only partially explained by differences in nutrition, serum lipids, smoking habits and blood pressure. The same applies to differences within the same country. A further and most important example is differences between social classes within the same country, risk being usually lowest in the highest classes, likewise explained only in part by differences in the major risk factors. Quite probably the lower coronary heart disease risk in women is due not only to biological reasons. Searching for the causes of these differences is certainly a research priority and will no doubt lead to the discovery of new risk factors or confirmation of merely suspected influences. Similarly, the differences between countries in secular trends require explanation and will lead to new insights which are sought in the MONICA project of the World Health Organisation and the ARIC project in the United States. These gaps in knowledge in no way undermine existing knowledge concerning the major risk factors but bridging them will complement it.

Old and New Risk Factors

The causal relationship between coronary heart disease and the three major risk factors (serum lipids as influenced by nutrition, blood pressure and smoking) is firmly established and it will be taken for granted. On the other hand, there is a need to improve the predictive power in terms of serum lipid fractions. A beginning was made with the discovery, or rather re-discovery, of high-density lipoprotein (HDL) but it is still not clear whether HDL plays an active role in anti-atherogenesis or merely mirrors a more fundamental mechanism. The HDL subfractions, the apolipoproteins, the intermediate-density lipoproteins, isoforms of apolipoproteins and other expressions of genetic polymorphisms, the very low-density lipoproteins all require investigation from the point of view of their predictive value, singly and in combination. It is known that receptors can be influenced by nutritional habits but the phenomenon must be quantified and the interpersonal variability in response determined. Why do some people have stronger connective tissue reaction to intracellular lipid infiltration than others? Exactly how do hypertension and smoking damage arteries and the myocardium? Answers to all of these questions would be important to epidemiologists, provided that tests could be developed which are sufficiently simple and accurate to be used under field conditions and provided that those shown to be at increased risk can be protected by preventive measures. For these and other reasons, epidemiologists must work together with scientists in other research fields.

More should be known about metabolic balance. Predisposition to coronary disease seems to be associated with a low energy intake, contrary to expectation. It also plays a role as to where in the body fat accumulates. Physical activity protects but what is the mechanism? Nothing ranks second to the need for a much better definition and measurement of the factors concerning haemostasis-thrombosis and the degree to which they can be influenced by living habits such as eating and smoking. If it were known why diabetics are at greater risk, important new insights into the fundamental processes of atherogenesis and myocardial effects could be gained. There can be little doubt that individual susceptibility to the disease is partially determined by a number of hormones but corresponding studies are difficult and have been neglected. Last but not least, there is more and more evidence that constellations of psychosocial influences are independent risk factors for coronary heart disease but the responsible mechanism must be discovered in order to make optimal use of the preventive potential inherent in this knowledge.

From the point of view of the high-risk strategy of prevention, there is a paramount need for a major effort to disentangle genetic from environmental factors in the genesis of coronary heart disease. The question is of limited importance for prevention at the community level - the population strategy - because environmental rather than genetic factors are overwhelmingly responsible for regional and, probably, social variations in disease frequency, even though genetic factors may play a more general role in variations of lipid and blood pressure levels between populations and in disease susceptibility or resistance, as possibly in Japan. Recent studies have shown that certain genetic polymorphisms, sometimes located on chromosome 11, are more common in patients with coronary disease than in controls. Isoforms of apolipoprotein E have been associated with serum lipid concentrations. The independent predictive power of these genetic variations remains to be established. Up to now, these studies of genetic markers have been related mostly to those connected with serum lipids but it is likely that there are genetic factors affecting atherogenesis which are unrelated to serum lipids. Furthermore, genetic factors involved in the regulation of blood pressure must not be forgotten. Apart from the advances in molecular genetics, there are the results of family studies which indicate that familial aggregations of coronary heart disease are mediated only in part by the familial resemblance in the major risk factors. There is obviously a need for close collaboration between epidemiologists, population geneticists and molecular geneticists to make the most of these exciting new developments. It is conceivable that the major risk factors exert maximal influence only in persons with specific genetic predispositions. If this were true, the specificity and sensitivity of prediction would be much enhanced.

The overall problem of improving predictive power of tests can be generalised (Table 1). At present, the multiple logistic function, incorporating the risk factors serum cholesterol, blood pressure and smoking, can concentrate half of the new events of coronary heart disease (50 out of a 100) among the 200 men in the top quintile of the risk function, giving a predictive power of 25% (50 events out of 200). The addition of a hitherto unknown risk factor X would not enhance prediction

Table 1. Predictive power of tests for coronary heart disease (CHD) in middle-aged men, CHD incidence 10% in 10 years

	MLF	MLF+ Risk factor X	Optimal test
All men	1000	1000	1000
Men with CHD	100	100	100
All men with positive test	200	360	100
Men with CHD and positive test	50	75	90
Predictive power of positive test (%)	25	21	90
Sensitivity (%)	50	75	90
Specificity (%)	83	68	99

MLF, multiple logistic function; risk factor X, independent of MLF and singly of equal predictive power.

because both the numerator and the denominator have been increased (75/360 = 21%) [1]. Though the sensitivity of the test has been improved by "capturing" 75 of the 100 new events in a positive test, specificity has been decreased. An "ideal" test might have a predictive power of 90%, with equally high or higher sensitivity and specificity. Such a situation was called utopian almost 20 years ago [2]. Today, a predictive power of 50% has possibly come within our reach if new risk factors can be found which are more closely related to the mechanisms of the disease than those presently available. This would put additional wind into the sails of the high-risk strategy. It would also reduce the present dilemma of preventive treatment which lies in having to treat prophylactically a considerable number of high-risk individuals who will not benefit from the treatment, i. e. who would not develop premature clinical disease even without preventive therapy. However, contrary to the view of some workers, there would still be a primary need for the population strategy at the community level.

Lastly, under this heading, the question arises as to what types of new studies are required to provide answers to these problems. The retrospective case-control studies and prevalence studies in the community still have their place. However, in order to obtain reliable estimates of predictive power, the long and hard method of prospective studies is indispensable. In the design of new studies, the inclusion of families will permit optimal use of genetic markers. A powerful study design lies in the use of cases and controls who are representative of the community, rather than the time-honoured selection of hospitalised patients or so-called volunteers. The bias inherent in such study subjects often makes the interpretation of data difficult, if not impossible.

Old and New Disease End Points

Improving predictive power for coronary heart disease, as just discussed, is all very well and good but what is coronary heart disease in this context? Before leaving the subject of risk factors, it should be remembered that the various clinical manifestations of the disease (history of myocardial infarction, angina pectoris, latent ECG changes) are powerful risk factors in themselves. For better prediction, priority must be given to the development of relatively simple non-invasive or harmless invasive tests of myocardial function or latent myocardial damage not adequately expressed by ECG changes. It is likely that many of those persons who escape premature clinical disease in the face of elevated "major" risk factors do so because they have little myocardial dysfunction or damage. It would clearly be of much practical importance to identify such people and determine their absolute disease risk. Furthermore, there are still gaps in our knowledge concerning the epidemiology of angina pectoris, as opposed to myocardial infarction with survival. There is a great need to discover the reason why women are relatively protected against coronary disease, which requires, among other things, better measures of the extent of coronary atherosclerosis, myocardial damage and myocardial function in women as compared to men. Finally, there is the greatest urgency to study the end point of sudden death. There are still no predictive tests specifically for sudden death and it almost seems a matter of chance whether the victim of a heart attack dies suddenly or survives. Perhaps some hope lies in predictive tests incorporating measures of thrombogenesis but, more likely, factors relating to the state of the heart itself carry more promise.

Intervention Studies

During the past 15 years intervention studies have been in the forefront of epidemiological research. What is their future? If the emphasis is on primary prevention through changes in life styles, future studies should probably be community based, along the lines of the projects in North Karelia, Finland, those in the United States (Stanford, Minnesota, Rhode Island) and also the recent *"Deutsche Herz-Kreislauf-Präventionsstudie"* in the Federal Republic of Germany. Populations employed in industry and by Government also fall into this category. It is questionable whether large, randomised intervention studies in high-risk groups, like the MRFIT Study, useful though they are, should be done again because they are limited by the ability to motivate participants effectively and by the loss of statistical power on account of concomitant changes in the reference groups. However, if it is a question of testing the preventive potential of pharmaceutical agents, the need for randomised trials is inescapable. In the future there will be increasing use of intervention studies in which the end point for evaluation will not be clinical events like myocardial infarction but methods for measuring the regression (or lack of progression) of atherosclerotic lesions. This applies to both pharmacological or life style interventions and their combinations. Such studies provide objective evidence of effectiveness and are more economical in numbers. On the other hand, their results cannot be directly extrapolated to the general population without collateral data from other types of studies.

Health and Behaviour

The prerequisite for the preservation of health is a constructive attitude towards health on the level of the individual, the family and the community. Research into the determinants of healthy behaviour is a priority for preventive medicine in general and preventive cardiology in particular. Given proper knowledge and a positive attitude, what is needed to turn these into action towards healthier living habits? Apart from the strictly behavioural aspects of the problem and the matter of motivation, it is not adequately known how much change in behaviour is needed to cause changes in risk factors which will result in measurable reductions of disease risk. It is the hope that relatively little behaviour change leads to relatively large changes in risk but it is not certain whether more drastic alterations in life style may be needed. The reasons for faulty behaviour affecting health are only partially known and little attention has been given to the possibility that effective health messages may not be the same for people from different social classes.

Primary and Secondary Prevention

For primary prevention, the fundamental need is for action on the basis of existing knowledge, notwithstanding the requirements of further research into more powerful prediction and improved health behaviour, as previously discussed. There is a need for model programmes with built-in research components, as well as action on the national level. For secondary prevention, the situation is less clear-cut. The possibilitites of pharmaceutical intervention are by no means exhausted. There is the question as to what extent risk factors towards a first infarct are also risk factors for a recurrence. It is likely that there are risk factors which are largely specific for reinfarction, in addition to those related to the progression of atherosclerosis. In this connection, it should be kept in mind that primary and secondary prevention are a continuum as far as prevention of atherosclerosis, as opposed to its myocardial consequences, is concerned. Last but not least, there remains a good deal to be learned about the optimal methods for rehabilitation.

Strategies of Prevention

Prevention is ultimately concerned with individual people. However, it has already been stated that the high-risk strategy misses a large proportion of people who will develop clinical disease because the predictive power towards this end is going to be insufficient, even with the improvements to be expected from future research. Therefore, a combination of the high-risk with the population strategy is needed to make a major dent in the epidemic proportions of the disease in most industrialised countries. This is, in fact, the recommendation of the World Health Organisation [3], apart from the advice issued by a number of other responsible bodies and individual experts. The population strategy is aimed at everybody, including people of all ages. The most important target for the population strategy is young people because the ultimate aim is not the present generation but a new generation with a healthier way of life and, consequently, a lower prevalence of risk factors.

Concluding Remarks

Perspectives for future epidemiological research into the prevention of premature coronary heart disease have been outlined. To achieve these ends, epidemiology must lean heavily on progress in other fields of atherosclerosis research and clinical cardiology. In this short essay, it would have been impossible to provide a bibliography of the relevant research pertaining to these areas, recognising that the future must take account of current knowledge. A comprehensive review of this essential background is provided in a recent book [4] which also contains an extensive chapter on the epidemiology and prevention of the disease caused by atherosclerosis and its complications [5].

In closing, the outlook is not only on the prevention of coronary heart disease but on the preservation of health more generally. There is increasing evidence to suggest that the measures which protect against premature coronary heart disease will also help to preserve health on a much broader front through the prevention of other, major chronic diseases [5]. There is good reason to think that these preventive measures not only prolong life but, at least equally importantly, will reduce the amount of invalidism which is often associated with advancing age.

References

1. Epstein FH (1979) Predicting, explaining and preventing coronary heart disease. Mod Concepts Cardiovasc Dis 48: 7-12
2. Epstein FH (1967) Predicting coronary heart disease. JAMA 201: 795-800
3. Prevention of coronary heart disease (1982) Report of a WHO expert committee. Technical report series 678. World Health Organization, Geneva
4. Olsson AG (ed) (1986) Atherosclerosis - the biology and clinical science. Churchill Livingston, Edinburgh (to be published)
5. Epstein FH, Hanefeld M (eds) (1986) Epidemiology and prevention. In: Olsson AG (ed) Atherosclerosis - the biology and clinical science. Churchill Livingston, Edinburgh (to be published)

Obesity and Cardiovascular Disease

P. Björntorp

Introduction

The problem of obesity and cardiovascular disease has had an interesting development through extreme opinions prevailing during different periods. First, it seemed clear that obesity was associated with increased mortality, mainly explainable by increased cardiovascular disease. This opinion was based mainly on material from insurance statistics [1], and it is obvious that criticism can be directed from a scientific standpoint against the lack of random recruitment of subjects to such populations. Insurance holders choose to be insured and are therefore a preselected group with unknown specific characteristics.

After this initial phase came modern prospective studies, based on truly nonselected populations, recruited at random from the population and studied over a number of years. The criticism of the previous work now seemed to be not only justified, but also correct, as no increased risk of cardiovascular disease and premature mortality was observed for obesity (for review see [2]). It was even suggested that moderate obesity might be a sign of good health, because the curve describing the relationship between body mass index (BMI), a measurement of general obesity, and mortality was U- or J-shaped. This meant that not only the fattest but also the leanest subjects were at a high risk of premature mortality.

This situation was difficult to understand because obesity, when examined, was regularly followed by a number of established factors increasing the risk cardiovascular disease such as hypertension, hyperlipidemia, diabetes mellitus, and hyperinsulinemia. Although it should be clear that the risk-factor discussion only implies statistical associations, there is a lot of information available linking these risk factors causally to cardiovascular disease.

Another phase in the development of knowledge in this area occurred when information became available indicating that an association between obesity and cardiovascular disease could be found, if large enough populations were examined for long enough periods of time. For example, in the large Framingham study, 20 years or more were required before the association became clear [3]. This kind of observation suggests that an association between obesity and cardiovascular disease, if present, cannot be very strong.

At this point it should be made clear that the term cardiovascular disease has not always been well defined. There are several observations in the literature suggesting that obese subjects, perhaps mostly severely obese subjects, suffer an increased risk of sudden death [2]. Excluding massive pulmonary embolism, there is reason to suspect that the remaining cardiac deaths might, to a large extent, be due to fatal arrythmias, which might have background causes other than ischemic heart disease. Thus, there might well be at least two causes of cardiac mortality in obesity with completely different background. The following discussion will focus only on cardiovascular disease, defined as ischemic heart disease, with its probable background of coronary atherosclerosis.

A number of factors increasing the risk of cardiovascular disease are thus regularly present in obese subjects, but it still seemed that long periods of time were required before these risk factors could "precipitate" cardiovascular disease. In nonobese populations these risk factors are known from numerous studies to be associated with cardiovascular disease after a much shorter time.

At this point a number of possible explanations come to mind. Obesity might only be an indicator of parallel phenomena causing cardiovascular disease, or it might protect against the risk factors mentioned. Smoking, one of the strongest risk factors, is less prevalent among obese subjects. The increased risk might only be found in a subgroup of the obese population.

Obesity, Smoking, and Cardiovascular Disease

The U- or J-shaped BMI-mortality curves discussed above suggested that the relationship between body weight and mortality was not the same throughout the whole population, a subgroup of lean subjects actually being at high risk. Closer analyses showed that these lean subjects were smokers, who are known to be lean and to have a high mortality from a number of diseases [3]. Furthermore, in a large sample covering a majority of the Norwegian population [4], detailed analysis of the relationship of BMI to individual diseases were possible. There appear to be typical low-BMI and high-BMI diseases. The former include various pulmonary diseases, often known to be smoking associated, such as pulmonary carcinoma and emphysema, and chronic bronchitis, as well as insulin-dependent diabetes mellitus. Obesity-related diseases include cardiovascular disease, stroke, non-insulin-dependent diabetes mellitus, and a number of carcinomas such as of the colon and of the female genitalia. Analysing the relationship of BMI to cardiovascular disease only shows that the curve describing this relationship is more rectilinear, parts of the increased total mortality in the lean population having disappeared. The remaining increased risk here might be due to lean smokers who have died of cardiovascular disease. Interpretation of these findings thus suggests that there might be two populations of subjects with cardiovascular disease, one consisting of lean smokers, and the other consisting of other subjects where obesity related factors play an important role. This then suggests that cardiovascular disease may be independent of obesity in a subgroup (smokers), while in the remaining population obesity might be important.

Obesity Subdivisions

Transectional Studies. There are observations suggesting that the increased risk of cardiovascular disease in obese subjects is found only in a subgroup of the obese population. In this regard it is useful to return to transectional studies of the prevalence of factors increasing the risk of cardiovascular disease in different subgroups of the obese population. Almost 40 years ago Vague [5] described a subdivision of human obesity according to the distribution of surplus adipose tissue. He started out from the normal, physiological distribution of adipose tissue in both sexes, where women have a characteristic distribution of adipose tissue in the gluteal-femoral regions, which men usually do not have. Obese women usually have an exaggeration of this physiological distribution, with accumulation of excess adipose tissue in the gluteal-femoral regions, while obese men accumulate excess fat in their main depots, which are localized in the upper part of the body. These patterns are not, however, exclusive to the respective sexes. Occasionally men with gluteal-femoral obesity are seen, these mostly being severely obese, and it is not infrequent to find women with fairly pronounced upper-body obesity. However, Vague [5] labelled these obesities android and gynoid respectively, indicating that they were typically but not exclusively found in men and women respectively.

Further extensive work demonstrated that a number of factors increasing the risk of cardiovascular disease were associated with android rather than gynoid obesity. These included hypertension, hyperlipidemia, and diabetes mellitus, and Vague actually observed a greater prevalence of atherosclerotic disease among android-obese subjects. More recent work has fully confirmed Vague's pioneering work [6, 7], and in addition has focused attention on the abdominal adipose tissue regions as the adipose tissues most closely associated statistically with the risk factors. Furthermore, sex by itself and degree of overweight have been excluded in the analysis.

The closest associations have been found with simple measurements of waist circumference, analysed in relation to hip circumference (W:H ratio) to control for frame size of different individuals. This simple measurement is actually more effective at determining the increased risk associated with abdominal obesity than more complicated measurements such as skin folds, or other regional thickness measurements, as well as fat-cell size or number determinations. However, recent studies indicate that intraabdominal fat mass, measured with computerized tomography might be the measurement most closely related to the risk factors associated with obesity [8].

Longitudinal Studies. Knowing this strong association of factors increasing the risk of cardiovascular disease with the W:H ratio in transectional studies, it was logical to perform an analysis of this ratio as a prospective indicator of the risk of cardiovascular disease. The results of such studies show that the W:H ratio is indeed a good indicator of risk of cardiovascular disease, as well as of stroke, diabetes mellitus, and premature mortality among men, and for the same diseases (diabetes not analysed) in women [9-11]. The measurement of abdominal obesity was the only obesity quantitation which was a significant indicator of risk among the men, and the strongest of various obesity measurements in the women. Similar studies, with essentially the same results, have also been published recently [12].

Thus, these recent studies demonstrate that only one type of obesity is associated with cardiovascular disease, namely android obesity, the type which from numerous previous studies is known to be associated with factors increasing the risk of cardiovascular disease. This fact may make it possible to explain the statistical findings described above that show that obesity only appears as a factor increasing the risk of cardiovascular disease after a long period of observation. The association is present only in a subpopulation, and the effect becomes "diluted" in the total obese population.

Mechanisms

A natural question is of course how android obesity is causally associated with morbidity and mortality. It should first be mentioned that the distribution of adipose tissue is not the only android characteristic of this group. Muscle mass, morphology and function [13], as well as various endocrine features [14], also show android characteristics. Different possibilities exist to explain the morbidity caused by android obesity. One of these is the characteristics of adipose tissue itself. It turns out that abdominal adipose tissue is highly lipolytic, producing excess circulating free fatty acids (FFA) upon stimulation [15]. Interestingly, the most sensitive adipose tissue regions in this regard seem to be the omental and mesenteric regions, drained by the portal circulation (Rebuffé-Scrive, personal communication, 1986). Excess circulating FFA might have a number of unwanted effects, both in the portal and the general circulation, leading to hyperinsulinemia, diabetes mellitus, hyperlipidemia, and perhaps also hypertension [16].

Causal Relationship

For epidemiological data to be considered as proof of a causal relationship several criteria must usually be satisfied. It is of interest to analyse current information on obesity and cardiovascular disease in this regard.

First, the relationship studied should be temporally logical; in other words, in the current situation abdominal obesity should precede cardiovascular disease, and this of course is the case. A dose-response relationship should occur, and this is also the case in both the transsectional and longitudinal data available. The factor analysed should be an independent risk factor, which is the case among women [10] and it seems in more recent studies to also be true in men (Larsson, personal communication, 1986). Finally, a reasonable hypothesis as to the cause-effect relationship should be available, and this is also the case as discussed above. In summary then, it seems that there is sufficient evidence to fulfill the criteria mentioned and to consider that the evidence available strongly suggests a cause-effect relationship between abdominal obesity and cardiovascular disease.

Practical Consequences

In this situation it seems advisable to use the available information for practical purposes. It is clear that we need criteria additional to the conventional measurements to define abdominal obesity, because it seems desirable to diagnose the condition early in order to prevent or diagnose the disorders it may cause. In Scandinavian middle-aged men it seems that when the W:H ratio exceeds 1.0 the risk of various diseases increases steeply. This is a measurement which is so easy that it can be done by anyone, and when the circumference of the waist exceeds that of the hips there is reason for concern. In women this limit is about 0.8. When these values are exceeded further clinical work is needed, including measurements of blood glucose, plasma insulin and lipids, and blood pressure. Treatment is also needed, even if total body weight, BMI or other conventional measurements indicate that general obesity is not present. Conversely, with generalized obesity that is not primarily of the abdominal regions, more excess weight in terms of body weight, BMI, etc., can be tolerated before further testing or treatment is required. In its moderate form generalized obesity seems to be mainly a cosmetic problem.

Conclusions

In conclusion, there is now considerable evidence from several sources, and several kinds of examinations, that only one type of human obesity, namely that localized to the abdominal region, is associated with several of the malignant obesity-related diseases, such as cardiovascular disease. Further research in this area should be fruitful, not least as far as the pathogenesis of the complicating disorders is concerned. For example, the pathogenesis in many cases of noninsulin-dependent diabetes mellitus might be elucidated by this new approach to the problem.

References

1. Blackburn H, Parlin W (1965-1966) Antecedents of disease. Insurance mortality experience. Ann NY Acad Sci 134: 1965-1017
2. Larsson B, Björntorp P, Tibblin G (1981) The health consequences of moderate obesity. Int J Obesity 5: 97-116
3. Hubert HB, Feinlieb M, McNamara PM, Castelli WP (1983) Obesity as an independent risk factor for cardiovascular disease: a 26-year follow-up of participants of the Framingham heart study. Circulation 67: 5
4. Waaler HTh (1984) Height, weight and mortality. The Norwegian experience. Acta Med Scand [Suppl] 67: 1-56
5. Vague J (1956) The degree of masculine differentiation of obesities: a factor determining predisposition to diabetes, atherosclerosis, gout and uric calculus disease. Am J Clin Nutr 4: 20-28
6. Kissebah AH, Vydelingum N, Murray R, Evans D, Hartz A, Kalkhoff R, Adams P (1983) Relation of body fat distribution to metabolic complications of obesity. J Clin Endocrinol Metab 54: 254-260
7. Krotkiewski M, Björntorp P, Sjöström L, Smith U (1983) Impact of obesity on metabolism in men and women - importance of regional adipose tissue distribution. J Clin Invest 72: 1150-1162
8. Kissebah AH, Evans DJ, Peiris A, Wilson CR (1985) Endocrine characteristics in regional obesities: role of sex steroids. In: Vague J, Björntorp P, Guy-Grand B, Rebuffé-Scrive M, Vague Ph (eds) Metabolic complications of human obesities. Excerpta Medica, Amsterdam, pp 115-130 (International congress series 682)
9. Larsson B, Svärdsudd K, Welin L, Wilhelmsen L, Björntorp P, Tibblin G (1984) Abdominal adipose tissue distribution, obesity and risk of cardiovascular disease and death: 13 year follow up of participants in the study of men born 1913. Br Med J 288: 1401-1404
10. Lapidus L, Bengtsson C, Larsson B, Pennert K, Rybo E, Sjöström L (1984) Distribution of adi-

pose tissue and risk of cardiovascular disease and death: a 12 year follow up of participants in the population study of women in Gothenburg, Sweden. Br Med J 289: 1257-1261
11. Ohlsson LO, Larsson B, Svärdsudd K, Welin L, Eriksson H, Wilhelmsen L, Björntorp P, Tibblin G (1985) The influence of body fat distribution on the incidence of diabetes mellitus. 13.5 year follow-up of the participants in the study of men born in 1913. Diabetes 34: 1055-1058
12. Ducimetiere P, Richard J, Cambien F, Avons P, Jacqueson A (1985) Relationships between adiposity measurements and the incidence of coronary heart disease in a middle-aged male population. The Paris prospective study I. In: Vague J, Björntorp P, Guy-Grand B, Rebuffé-Scrive M, Vague Ph (eds) Metabolic complications of human obesities. Excerpta Medica, Amsterdam, pp 31-38 (International congress series 682)
13. Krotkiewski M, Björntorp P (1986) Muscle tissue in obesity with different distribution of adipose tissue. Effects of physical training. Int J Obesity 10: 331-341
14. Evans D, Hoffman RG, Kalkhoff RK, Kissebah AH (1983) Relationship of androgenic activity to body fat topography, fat cell morphology and metabolic abberations in premenopausal women. J Clin Endocrinol Metab 57: 304-310
15. Rebuffé-Scrive M, Enk L, Crona N, Lönnroth P, Abrahamsson L, Smith U, Björntorp P (1985) Fat cell metabolism in different regions in women. J Clin Invest 75: 1973-1976
16. Björntorp P (1985) Regional patterns of fat distribution. Ann Intern Med 103: 994-995

Lipoproteins and Apolipoproteins in the Prediction of Coronary Artery Disease

G. Assmann

Introduction

Atherosclerotic cardiovascular disease is the leading cause of death and also the most frequent cause of early invalidity in most European countries. Clinical conditions such as coronary heart disease (angina pectoris, myocardial infarction, acute cardiac death), cerebrovascular insufficiency (apoplexy), and peripheral arterial occlusive disease (intermittent claudication, gangrene) become manifest following decades of asymptomatic development of atherosclerotic vascular stenosis. In evaluating coronary risk there is a distinction made between primary risk factors (hypercholesterolemia, nicotine abuse, hypertension) and secondary risk factors (diabetes mellitus, obesity, lack of physical activity). The primary risk factors are individually capable of producing clinical complications of atherosclerotic vascular disease. Secondary risk factors, as a general rule, evoke clinical complications only in conjunction with one or more other factors. Individual risk factors should not be viewed as isolated in the course of a disease, since they frequently occur in combination. The incidence of cardiovascular disease increases cumulatively with the presence of multiple risk factors. The concept of a multifactorial basis for the origin of atherosclerotic vascular disease is principally derived from the findings of epidemiological studies. It has been demonstrated quite convincingly in the example of acute cardiac death that risk factors can be identified in the overwhelming majority of cases and that individual risk factors are interrelated.

Without drawing attention from the importance of other risk factors, particular emphasis must be placed on the close correlation between hypercholesterolemia and atherosclerosis. Supported by the results of epidemiological studies as well as clinical findings and the results of animal experiments, there can be no doubt about the role of cholesterol in the pathogenesis of coronary heart disease. The cornerstone of this viewpoint is the dose-response relationship between serum cholesterol level and the risk of coronary heart disease, as determined in various epidemiological studies. Suitable preventive measures and expert diagnosis, i.e., recognition of high-risk patients as well as application of modern treatment procedures, are equally important in order to reduce morbidity and mortality due to coronary heart disease. On all of these aspects there have recently been developments which are referred to below.

Strategies for Primary Prevention of Coronary Heart Disease

Experts in the United States and Europe have worked out recommendations for the primary prevention of coronary heart disease [1, 2]. The unanimnous opinion is that cholesterol values should not exceed 200 mg/dl. These recommendations are founded on the results of various prospective epidemiological surveys [3-6]: in the Multiple Risk Factor Intervention Trial with a sample of approximately 350000 men aged between 35 and 57 years, a linear increase of mortality due to coronary heart disease and the serum cholesterol level was found (Fig. 1) [6]. A cholesterol level between 200 and 260 mg/dl apparently doubles the risk of death due to coronary heart disease! The United States consensus conference has defined cholesterol values which are age dependent and require treatment with moderately raised and high coronary risk (Table 1). Since lowering serum cholesterol can reduce the frequency of coronary heart disease [7, 8], various medical organizations

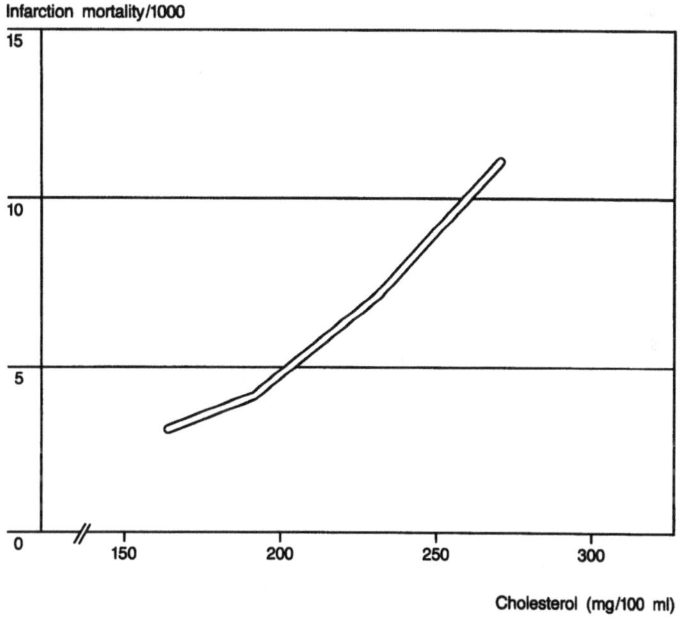

Fig. 1. Myocardial infarction mortality over a 6-year period according to the Multiple Risk Factor Intervention Trial data, 356222 men, aged 35-57 years [6]

Table 1. Cholesterol values requiring treatment according to the recommendations of the USA consensus conference [1]

Age (years)	Moderate risk		High risk	
	mg/dl	(mmol)	mg/dl	(mmol)
20-29	>200	(5.17)	>220	(5.69)
30-39	>220	(5.69)	>240	(6.21)
>40	>240	(6.21)	>260	(6.72)

in the USA have recently taken part in a national campaign, the "National Cholesterol Education Program". The prime aim of this program is to inform the medical profession about new aspects of the diagnosis and treatment of hypercholesterolemia.

The recommendations of the European consensus conference are similar in content, but for the individual risk prognosis and the necessity for treatment greater emphasis has been put on serum triglycerides, HDL cholesterol, and the overall risk (family history, smoking habit, hypertonus, diabetes mellitus, male sex) (Table 2) [2]. In many European countries it is usual to consider cholesterol values above 260 mg/dl as pathological. In contrast to this, the European consensus conference has agreed that in all adult persons cholesterol values above 200 mg/dl require medical attention. For most patients with cholesterol values between 200 and 250 mg/dl nutritional advice and treatment of other risk factors are recommended. In pronounced hypercholesterolemias (250–300 mg/dl) an intensive dietary treatment and, if necessary, application of lipid-lowering drugs with regular checks on effectiveness are recommended. Values above 300 mg/dl require consultation with a specialist to determine the exact diagnosis and for guidelines on therapy. In order to reach the target level of 200 mg/dl cholesterol and hence successfully reduce the frequency and severity of coronary heart disease, the European consensus conference refers to individual and mass strategies. The individual or high-risk strategy aims to identify those persons in the population who run a particularly high risk of coronary infarct (e.g., because of hypercholesterolemia) by employing a variety of clinical and laboratory tests. A combination of selective screening (search for risk factors when the following constellation is found: familial disposition to cardiovascular disease or hyperlipidemia; xanthomas; xanthelasms or arcus corneae, obesity, diabetes mellitus, hypertonus, smoking, gout) and screening as part of preventive medical care (at regular intervals by a general practitioner, as part of occupational medical care, or at the time of taking up employment) can to date be considered to be an optimal strategy in European countries to detect a large number of at-risk patients.

The mass strategy aims to alter habits within the population, where especially a change in eating habits, regular physical activity and cessation of smoking can be expected to lead to a reduced number of infarcts in the population. Nutritional advice recommends an individually adjusted calorie intake to avoid obesity, reduction of fat intake to less than 30% of the daily calorie intake, and that saturated fatty acids should amount to less than 10%. Consumption of monounsaturated and polyunsaturated fatty acids is recommended, as are a reduction of cholesterol intake to less than 300 mg/day and a simultaneous increase in complex carbohydrates (fruit, vegetables and fibrous foods), as well as a restriction of alcohol and salt intake. These preventive measures should be observed by the whole population as well as by patients with cholesterol values of more than 200 mg/dl. The implementation of such nutritional strategies requires the cooperation of doctors, government offices and the food industry. This needs public education programs, suitable labelling of foods, and a nutritionally sound range of foods in restaurants and canteens, as well as political measures through national and international organizations.

Hypercholesterolemia is a widespread problem. Extensive research in the Federal Republic of Germany (Prospective Cardiovascular Münster (PROCAM)

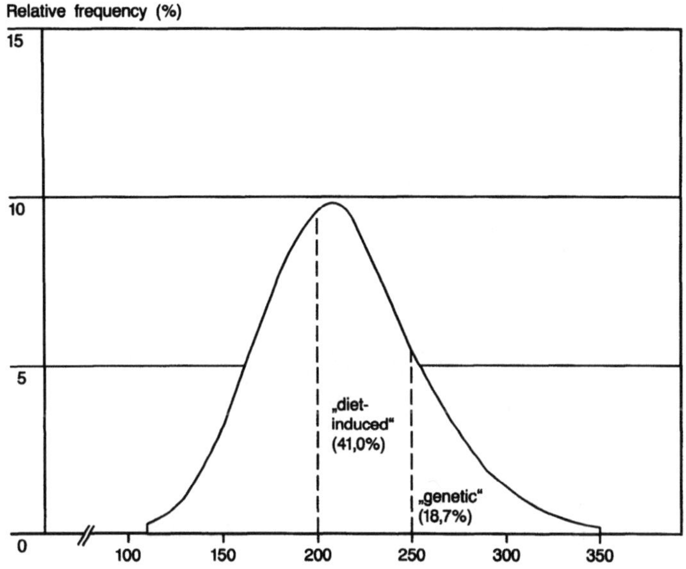

Fig. 2. Frequency distribution of cholesterol values in 20–50 year old men ($n = 11\,091$), from PROCAM data [9]

study) [9] revealed that about 60% of men aged 20–50 years had cholesterol values of above 200 mg/dl (Fig. 2). In most hypercholesterolemics with values between 200 and 250 mg/dl (41%) a reduction of serum cholesterol (low-density lipoprotein (LDL) cholesterol) can be achieved by correcting nutritional habits (reducing dietary cholesterol, saturated fatty acids and calorie intake). The pathologic mechanisms which cause increased LDL cholesterol levels are well understood today (Fig. 3): a cholesterol-rich diet leads to a suppression of hepatocellular LDL receptors, a calorie-rich diet to the overproduction of very low density lipoprotein (VLDL) and hence indirectly to LDL, and saturated fatty acids lead to a reduced catabolism of intermediate density lipoprotein (IDL) and LDL. Hypercholesterolemias with values above 250 mg/dl (18.7%) frequently have a genetic component.

The recognition of high-risk patients is, as a rule, not possible solely from determination of the cholesterol level. Triglyceride and HDL cholesterol levels should also be determined. The European consensus recommends the following evaluation for these two parameters.

In contrast to hypercholesterolemia whose causal role in the pathogenesis of coronary heart disease is undisputed, the evaluation of a hypertriglyceridemia with regard to an associated coronary risk is often difficult. Slightly raised triglyceride values are often related to obesity, alcohol consumption and/or badly adjusted diabetes mellitus. The correction of these factors often leads to a reduction to normal levels. Especially in familial combined hyperlipidemia and type III hyperlipoproteinemia, the hypertriglyceridemia is an expression of a metabolic disorder of triglyceride-rich lipoproteins which is connected with a high coronary risk. Trigly-

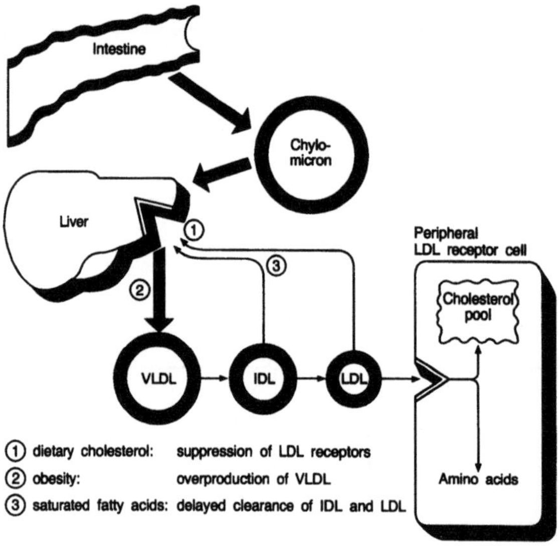

Fig. 3. Pathophysiologic effect of nutritional cholesterol, obesity and saturated fatty acids on the concentration of LDL cholesterol in blood

ceride values of more than 1000 mg/dl are often associated with a risk of pancreatitis and require treatment.

Low HDL cholesterol levels are in many people associated with a high risk of coronary heart disease. The inverse relationship between the HDL cholesterol level and the risk of coronary heart disease has been demonstrated in several epidemiological studies. Low HDL cholesterol levels are often associated with a lack of physical exercise, obesity, cigarette smoking and/or hypertriglyceridemia. A correction of these factors leads, as a rule, to an increase in HDL cholesterol values. Moderate hypercholesterolemias are frequently a result of high HDL cholesterol values. The treatment of the hypercholesterolemia is not indicated in such cases. In daily practice the question of whether intense treatment of hyperlipidemia should be given is significantly influenced by the presence of high or low HDL cholesterol levels.

As a result of the German PROCAM study and taking into account the American and European recommendations for an early identification of 40–65 year old men who are at risk for heart disease, the following practice-orientated strategies have been developed (Fig. 4) [9]:

1. A determination of the cholesterol level as the sole measure for a risk evaluation is considered to be insufficient. Much more satisfactory is the following strategy which is based on the parameters cholesterol, triglyerides and HDL cholesterol. Subjects with cholesterol values of 300 mg/dl and higher (fields 1 and 2) are classified as at risk, those with cholesterol and triglyceride concentrations below 200 mg/dl (field 5) as not at risk or at low risk (Fig. 4 above). The remaining subjects, i.e., those with triglyceride values above 200 mg/dl and cholesterol values below 300 mg/dl (fields 4 and 6) or with triglyceride values below 200 mg/dl and cholesterol values between 200 and 300 mg/dl (field 3), are classified according to their HDL cholesterol values: if the HDL cholesterol value is below 35 mg/dl a high risk is diagnosed, otherwise a low risk. In the "high risk" group identified

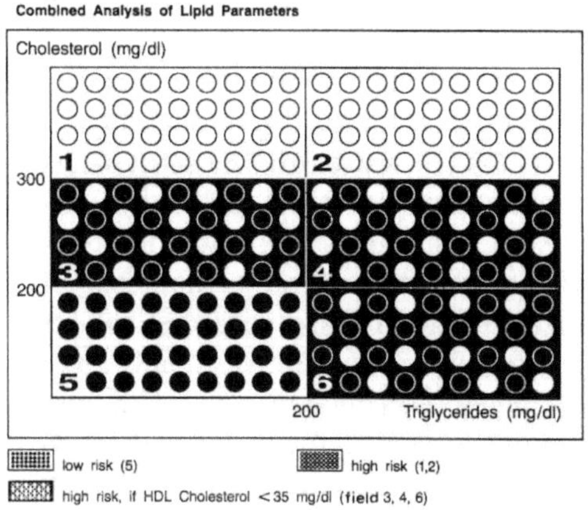

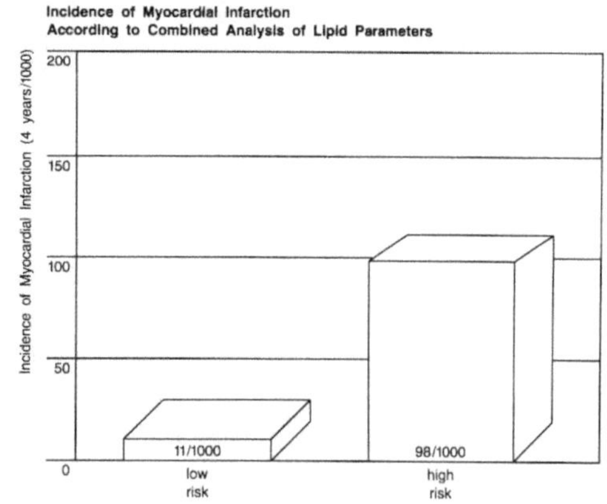

Multiple Logistic Function

- Family history of myocardial infarction
- Diabetes mellitus
- Current cigarette smoker
- Angina pectoris
- Age
- Systolic Blood Pressure
- Cholesterol
- HDL Cholesterol

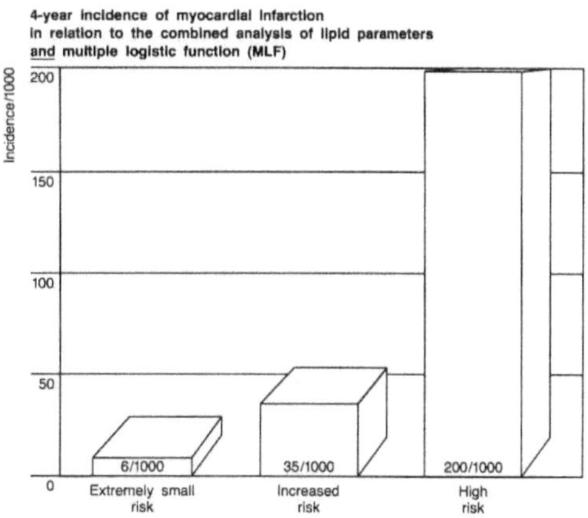

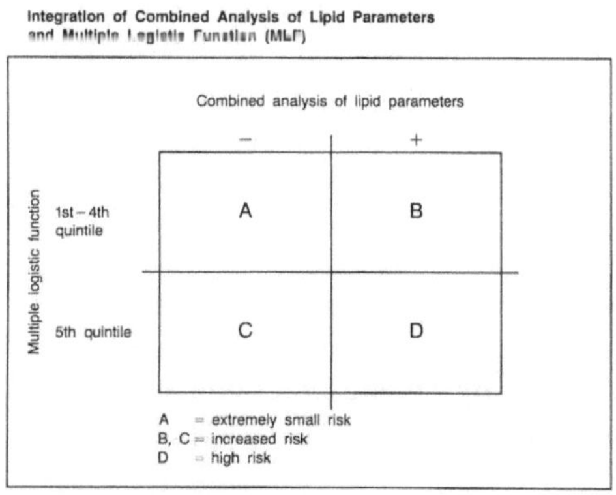

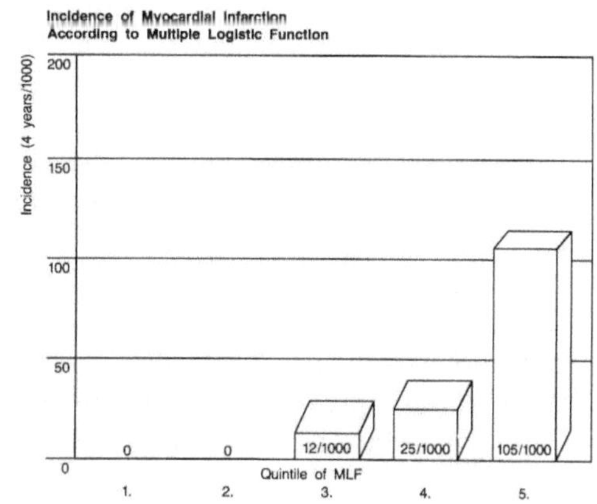

Fig. 4. Strategies for the early recognition of men at risk of a myocardial infarction (40-65 years of age). *Above:* Combined analysis of lipid parameters. *Middle:* Multiple logistic function. *Below:* Integration of combined analysis of lipid parameters and multiple logistic function (MLF)

with this strategy, the incidence rate was almost nine times that of the remaining group.

2. In order to use the information generated by measuring several parameters (the most important risk factors) the mathematical method for the discrimination and classification of the multiple logistic function (MLF) was used. The most clear-cut independent factors (i.e., heart infarct in the family, diabetes mellitus, smoking, angina pectoris, age, systolic blood pressure, total cholesterol, and HDL cholesterol) were taken into account. Depending on the level of these parameters in each individual the risk of each participant developing a myocardial infarct within the next 4 years was calculated. The group was split into five equally large groups (quintiles) in ascending order of calculated risk (Fig. 4 middle). Although in the lower two quintiles no myocardial infarcts occurred, the incidence rose in the third to the fifth quintiles from 12 to 25 to 105 per thousand. Two-thirds of all the infarcts occurred in the uppermost quintile. The risk in these patients was almost twelvefold: one in 10 people in this group suffered from an infarct within a period of 4 years compared with one in 119 in the other 80%.
3. When the methods of combined lipid metabolism diagnosis and multiple logistic function analysis of the risk factors are further integrated in order to optimize predictive statements (Fig. 4 below) people with very low (6/1000), increased (35/1000), and high (200/1000) risk can be differentiated (Fig. 4 below). Of all infarcts 56% occur in the high-risk group (8% of all subjects) but only 16% in the low-risk group (70% of all cases). Therefore, the incidence of myocardial infarcts in the high-risk group is about 30 times higher than in the low-risk group.

The above-mentioned strategies (combined lipid metabolism diagnosis, multiple logistic function) cover ⅔–¾ of all myocardial infarcts and can be applied in screening for early recognition of individuals at risk. With these methods, which can be applied by all general practitioners without great financial involvement, a group at risk of myocardial infarct can be identified with relatively high sensitivity. Lipid parameters alone can be used directly without further aids, but the multiple logistic function analysis requires a certain number of calculations. With a fixed-wire pocket calculator which is fed with the values of the eight parameters and which then automatically calculates a risk factor, the individual risk can be determined. One advantage of this calculation method is that the changes in the individual risk factors during a therapy, which might simultaneously influence several risk factors, can be evaluated objectively. For the calculation of the cost : benefit ratio within the scope of primary prevention this method can be a valuable aid. Also, affected patients can in this way be motivated to alter their lifestyle.

The practice-orientated methods introduced here for the recognition of high-risk patients are suitable to predict the risk of myocardial infarct individually as part of preventive medicine. Application of this procedure by general practitioners and in occupational preventive medicine allows a cost-effective primary prevention aiming to reduce the risk of infarction.

Classification of Lipid Metabolism Disorders

The classification system for hyperlipoproteinemia phenotypes using lipoprotein electrophoresis (types I-V) developed by Fredrickson and his research team has found worldwide acceptance and is today used in numerous laboratories as part of the lipid metabolism diagnosis. The relatively simple classification into types I-V does, however, have significant disadvantages. In routine practice the diagnosis is usually restricted to the determination of the "type", although present knowledge warrants further thoughts and investigations. Therefore, several aspects are listed below which argue against a differentiation into various lipoprotein types as the basis for a precise metabolic diagnosis and which throw doubt on lipoprotein electrophoresis as an additional test, or even make it seem superfluous [10].

1. The quantitative determination of cholesterol and triglycerides as well as the examination of fasting serum ("refrigerator test") permit the determination of the lipoprotein type with great accuracy, as long as some simple rules are observed. Chylomicrons can, for instance, be seen with the unaided eye in serum left overnight in the refrigerator. The precise evaluation and the assignment of the lipoprotein pattern are quite simple without lipoprotein electrophoresis, especially in cases of pronounced hyperlipidemia.
2. In daily practice the physician frequently finds slightly increased levels of cholesterol and/or triglycerides and is required to differentiate phenotypes II b (mixed hyperlipidemia) from IV (isolated hypertriglyceridemia). Without a quantitative determination of cholesterol in the various lipoprotein classes, especially LDL cholesterol and HDL cholesterol, as well as apolipoprotein B (LDL apo B), a correct grouping is usually not possible.
3. The differentiation of hyperlipoproteinemia phenotypes has only a restricted biochemical and genetic value. It is not possible, either by the determination of lipids or by lipoprotein analysis, to establish the genetic form of the hyperlipidemia accurately. The basis for a genetic classification, in addition to consideration of the clinical findings, consists of family studies and specific biochemical tests. Except for familial hyperchylomicronemia (type I), all hereditary hyperlipidemias may exhibit more than one lipoprotein phenotype. This is particularly evident in the case of familial combined hyperlipidemia, in which phenotypes II a, II b, and IV occur with approximately equal frequency in the family of a hyperlipidemic patient. Occasionally, high apo B concentrations (hyperapobetalipoproteinemia) are found with only moderate hyperlipidemia.
4. The informative value of the type I-V classification is limited by the fact that a lipoprotein phenotype is frequently observed to be inconstant in a patient and that the lipoprotein pattern in influenced by the ingestion of medications, reduction of food intake, and in particular by diets and alcohol (leading to a "type change").
5. Certain lipoprotein fractions visible on electrophoresis (double pre-β band, broad β band) do not have any clear-cut diagnostic or therapeutic relevance and may, in fact, lead to an improper interpretation.
6. According to Fredrickson, the classification of lipid metabolism disorders does not take into account the concentration of HDL cholesterol. However, recent epi-

demiological clinical and biochemical findings leave no doubt about the diagnostic value of HDL cholesterol.

In summary, it must be emphasized that not classification, but rather the differentiation of secondary and familial disorders should be the prime concern in the diagnosis of disorders of lipid metabolism. For nearly all patients the classification scheme of the European consensus conference (i.e., the determination of cholesterol, triglycerides, and HDL cholesterol, and evaluation of the fasting serum in addition to the clinical findings) is sufficient to provide the foundation for implementing any therapeutic measures which may be indicated (Table 2).

Special diagnostic procedures are, however, required if one of the following diseases/situations are found: myocardial infarct before the age of 45; myocardial infarct or vessel disease in two or more family members; or cholesterol level over 300 mg/dl and/or triglycerides over 500 mg/dl (group E, Table 2).

Table 2. Guidelines for the management of hyperlipidemia according to the recommendations of the European Consensus Conference [2]

A Total cholesterol 200–250 mg/dl Triglycerides <200 mg/dl Assess overall risk for CHD, taking into account family history of CHD, hypertension, diabetes, male sex, younger age, smoking, low HDL-cholesterol, e.g. <35 mg/dl Restrict food energy if overweight, give nutritional advice and correct other risk factors if present	***B*** Total cholesterol 250–300 mg/dl Triglycerides <200 mg/dl Assess overall risk of CHD as under A Restrict food energy if overweight, prescribe lipid lowering diet and monitor response and compliance. If cholesterol remains high, consider use of lipid-lowering drug
C Total cholesterol <200 mg/dl Triglyceride 200–500 mg/dl Seek underlying causes of hypertriglyceridemia, e.g. obesity, excessive alcohol intake, diuretics, betablockers, exogenous oestrogens, diabetes Restrict dietary energy if overweight, deal with underlying causes if present. Prescribe and monitor lipid-lowering diet. Monitor cholesterol and triglyceride levels	***D*** Total cholesterol 200–300 mg/dl Triglyceride 200–500 mg/dl Assess overall risk of CHD as in A, seek underlying causes of hypertriglyceridemia as in C Restrict dietary energy if overweight, deal with underlying causes of hypertriglyceridemia if present and proceed according to A or B. Prescribe and monitor lipid-lowering diet. If serum lipid response is inadequate and overall CHD risk is high, consider use of lipid lowering drug
E Total cholesterol >300 mg/dl and/or Triglycerides >500 mg/dl Consider referral to a lipid clinic or to specialized physician for investigation and initiation of treatment by diet and, if necessary, drugs	

The following laboratory tests have been particularly useful in the recognition of familial defects which entail a high risk of a myocardial infarct [10-14]:

LDL receptor determination for the recognition of familial hypercholesterolemia. The quantification of the LDL receptors is done on cultivated skin fibroblasts (tissue culture), on circulating lymphocytes by means of monoclonal fluorescence-marked receptor antibodies or by means of complementary DNA (cDNA) hybridization techniques and the determination of restriction fragment length polymorphisms.

Apo B quantification for the recognition of hyperapobetalipoproteinemia. The quantification of total apo B and LDL apo B involves the use of polyclonal, monospecific antibodies and ELISA techniques.

Apo E polymorphisms for the recognition of familial type III hyperlipoproteinemia (apo E_2 homozygosity). Isoelectric focusing of VLDL apolipoproteins permits a differentiation into six apo E phenotypes. Oligonucleotide hybridization techniques permit a genotype characterization. Relatively high LDL cholesterol concentrations are frequently the result of apo E_4 homozygosity (2% of the German population) or apo E_4 heterozygosity (E_4/E_3, 20% of the German population).

Apolipoprotein mutants. Various mutant forms have been described for apolipoproteins A I, A IV, B, C II, C III and E. These are discovered by means of isoelectric focusing of isolated lipoproteins or by means of cDNA hybridization techniques. Particularly in familial hypoalphalipoproteinemia (a group of biochemically and genetically different diseases with low HDL cholesterol) the particular familial defect can be defined with special diagnostic methods.

Restriction fragment length polymorphisms. These are genetic markers which are potentially linked to the changes in regulatory or structural genes important in lipoprotein metabolism. Although molecular diagnostics so far only succeed in some cases to specify the familial aspects of a defect (cosegregation of haplotypes), a rapid development regarding the classification of lipid metabolism disorders can be expected.

LP(a). Occasionally hypercholesterolemia is the result of an increased concentration of this lipoprotein. Quantification is done by ELISA techniques or immunoelectrophoretical quantification.

Most of the above-mentioned special procedures are offered by only a few laboratories. Demand will, without doubt, increase due to the therapeutic implications and laboratories will be adjusting to this situation.

Modern Treatment Procedures

Hypercholesterolemia. According to the European guidelines for the treatment of hypercholesterolemia (Table 2), in moderate (200-250 mg/dl) and pronounced (250-300 mg/dl) hypercholesterolemia nutritional advice and a low-fat diet is indicated before commencing drug therapy. A low-fat diet (< 300 mg/day) can lead to a drastic lowering of serum cholesterol in apo E_3/E_4 homozygotes (20% of the population) and in apo E_4 homozygotes (2% of the population). Reductions of 50–100 mg/dl are frequently observed. Therefore, quite a few patients can with regard to their serum cholesterol values be treated without medication by means of a low-cholesterol, low-fat diet.

There are at present five essential principles for the drug treatment of hypercholesterolemia, the so-called anion exchange resins, the derivatives and analogues of clofibric acid, the nicotinic acid derivates, the thyroxine derivatives and probucol. Since probucol frequently leads to a drastic reduction in HDL cholesterol, the effects of which are at present difficult to comprehend, this should not be the first choice for treatment. There are substances in their first clinical trial phase which selectively reduce the cholesterol synthesis in the organism (so called HMG CoA reductase inhibitors). Further results are pending.

Also in their clinical trial phase are procedures for the selective elimination of LDL from plasma, e.g., LDL apheresis via antibody columns or dextran sulfate columns, LDL precipitation during plasmapheresis, and absorption of LDL by means of the filtration procedure. Since satisfactory adjustment of extreme hypercholesterolemia (>400 mg/dl) is often not possible despite a combination of diet and drug therapy, the development of procedures for selective LDL elimination has a high priority until new drugs are developed. Surgical intervention (ileum bypass, podocaval shunt, liver transplantation) is rather dubious considering the new developments.

Hypertriglyceridemia. According to the recommendations of the European consensus conference, drug treatment of raised triglyceride levels (group D, Table 2) is necessary if dietary measures (weight reduction, alcohol restriction) are not sufficient and the coronary risk of the patient is increased (e.g., HDL cholesterol < 35 mg/dl). The combination of hypertriglyceridemia and low HDL cholesterol is particularly frequent: in this situation the derivatives and analogues of clofibric acid are the first choice.

In extreme hypertriglyceridemias (> 500 mg/dl) a low-fat diet should always be recommended and, if this is not successful, a specialist should be consulted. As a special diagnostic procedure the determination of apo E polymorphism has been successful in the determination of the arterial risk in hyperlipidemics. In all the cases of apo E_2 homozygosity a consequent normalization of the lipid metabolism to avoid myocardial infarct and peripheral artery disease is indicated. Apo B quantification in hypertriglyceridemia can also provide useful information (? hyperapobetalipoproteinemia) as to the necessity of drug therapy.

These examples show clearly that special diagnostic procedures have become an invaluable part in the planning of therapeutic measures. Given the high morbidity and mortality due to coronary heart disease it will be necessary to employ modern procedures for the diagnosis and therapy of metabolic disorders consistently.

References

1. (1985) Lowering blood cholesterol to prevent heart disease. Consensus Conference. JAMA 253: 2080-2086
2. Strategy for the prevention of coronary heart disease. A policy statement of the European Atherosclerosis Society. Eur Heart J (in press)
3. Kannel WB, Gordon T (1976) The Framingham study: an epidemiological investigation of cardiac disease: the results of the Framingham study applied to four other US based epidemiologic studies of cardiovascular disease. Publication (NIH) 76-1083, section 31. US Dept of Health, Education and Welfare
4. Pooling Project Research Group (1978) Relationship of blood pressure, serum cholesterol, smoking habit, relative weight, and ECG abnormality to incidence of major coronary events: final report of the Pooling Project. J Chronic Dis 31: 201-306
5. Multiple Risk Factor Intervention Trial Research Group (1982) Multiple risk factor intervention trial. Risk factor changes and mortality results. JAMA 248: 1465-1477
6. Stammler J, Wentworth D, Neaton JD (1986) Prevalence and prognostic significance of hypercholesterolemia in men with hypertension. Prospective data on the primary screenees of the multiple risk factor intervention trial. Am J Med 80 (suppl 2A): 33-36
7. Lipid Research Clinics Program (1984) The lipid research clinics coronary primary prevention trial results: I. Reduction in incidence of coronary heart disease. JAMA 251: 351-374
8. Lipid Research Clinics Program (1984) The lipid research clinics coronary primary prevention trial results: II. The relationship of reduction in incidence of coronary heart disease to cholesterol lowering. JAMA 251: 365-374
9. Assmann G, Schulte H (1986) Procam-trial. Panscientia, Zürich, 1986
10. Assmann G (1982) Lipidstoffwechsel und Atherosklerose. Schattauer, Stuttgart
11. Assmann G (1983) Apolipoproteinopathien. Klin Wochenschr 61: 169-182
12. Assmann G, Lenzen HJ (1985) Apolipoprotein E-Polymorphismen. Hyperlipidämie und Herzinfarktrisiko. Internist 26: 692-700
13. Schriewer H, Nolte W, Robeneck H, Assmann G (1986) Apolipoprotein B determination in the dissolved precipitate obtained after precipitation of LDL with polyvinylsulphate. An alternative method for the determination of LDL apolipoprotein B without using ultracentrifugation. J Clin Chem Clin Biochem 24: 347-352
14. White R, Leppert M, Bishop DT, Backer D, Berkowitz J, Brown C, Callahan P, Holm T, Jerominski L (1985) Construction of linkage maps with DNA markers for human chromosomes. Nature 313: 101-105
15. Brown MS, Goldstein JL (1981) Lowering plasma cholesterol by raising LDL receptors. N Engl J Med 305: 505-517
16. Grundy SM (1984) Recommendations for the treatment of hyperlipidemia in adults. A joint statement for the nutrition committee and the council on arteriosclerosis of the American Heart Association. Arteriosclerosis 4: 445-468
17. Havel RJ, Kane JP (1982) Therapy of hyperlipidemic state. Annu Rev Med 33: 417-433
18. Heel RC, Brogden RN, Speight TM, Avery GS (1978) Probucol: a review of its pharmacological properties and therapeutic use in patients with hypercholesterolemia. Drugs 15: 409-428
19. Illingworth DR, Sexton GJ (1984) Hypercholesterolemic effects of mevinolin in patients with heterozygous familial hypercholesterolemia. J Clin Invest 74: 1972-1978
20. Levy RI (1985) Primary prevention of coronary heart disease by lowering lipids: results and implications. Am Heart J 110: 1116-1122

Prevalence of Hyperlipidaemia in British Compared with North American Men

G. R. Thompson, D. Robinson, S. L. Allaway, E. A. Bevan, and C. D. Ritchie

Introduction

The distribution of plasma lipid and lipoprotein values within the North American population was determined between 1971-1976 during the Lipid Research Clinics (LRC) Prevalence Study [1, 2]. Fasting plasma cholesterol and triglycerides were measured in over 17000 white men between the ages of 20-64 [1] and low-density lipoprotein (LDL) and high-density lipoprotein (HDL) cholesterol levels were subsequently determined in nearly 2500 of these men [2]. To compare the prevalence of hyperlipidaemia in these North American men with their British counterparts, we have analysed data on over 8000 men of similar age undergoing health screening in London during 1984, making appropriate corrections for differences in methodology. Despite these corrections the range of values obtained in this particular sample of British men differed appreciably from those in the LRC study. This possibly reflects dietary differences and may have some bearing on current mortality from coronary heart disease (CHD) being higher in Britain than in the United States and Canada [3].

Methods

Blood samples were obtained after an overnight fast (12-14 h) from 8836 men aged 20-69 who voluntarily attended the British United Provident Association (BUPA) Medical Centre in London for health screening during 1984. All men answered a standard questionnaire and underwent a clinical examination, which included an electrocardiogram. Most of those attending were white (94%) and resident in Britain. Serum was analysed enzymatically for its content of total cholesterol [4], triglyceride [5] and HDL cholesterol [4], the latter after precipitation of very low-density lipoprotein (VLDL) and LDL by dextran sulphate and magnesium [6]. The enzymatic analyses were undertaken using a Technicon SMAC system. To compensate for interlaboratory differences the system was calibrated against reference standards supplied by the Centers for Disease Control (CDC), Atlanta, which had supervised quality control during the LRC study. By calculating the linear regression of BUPA values for these standards against the CDC values it was possible to correct for analytical variations which exceeded CDC criteria of acceptability. Three different concentrations of reference standards for total cholesterol (TC), triglyceride (TG) and HDL cholesterol (HDL-C) were analysed in sextuplicate, each on three separate occasions. The resultant regression equations were used to correct the computerised results (in mmol/litre) of the BUPA samples, as follows:

$$\text{Corrected TC} = \frac{\text{BUPA value} + 0.31}{1.07}.$$

$$\text{Corrected TG} = \frac{\text{BUPA value} + 0.14}{1.12}.$$

$$\text{Corrected HDL-C} = \frac{\text{BUPA value} + 0.04}{0.93}.$$

Values for LDL cholesterol were then calculated for all BUPA samples with a triglyceride of <4.5 mmol/litre, using the formula of Friedewald et al. [7]. A correction was also made to allow for the fact that serum values are approximately 3% higher than those obtained using plasma [8].

Results

The mean ± SD of uncorrected fasting serum total cholesterol and triglyceride in 8836 BUPA men according to age over the range 20-69 years is shown in Fig. 1. Corresponding values for HDL cholesterol and LDL cholesterol for these men are

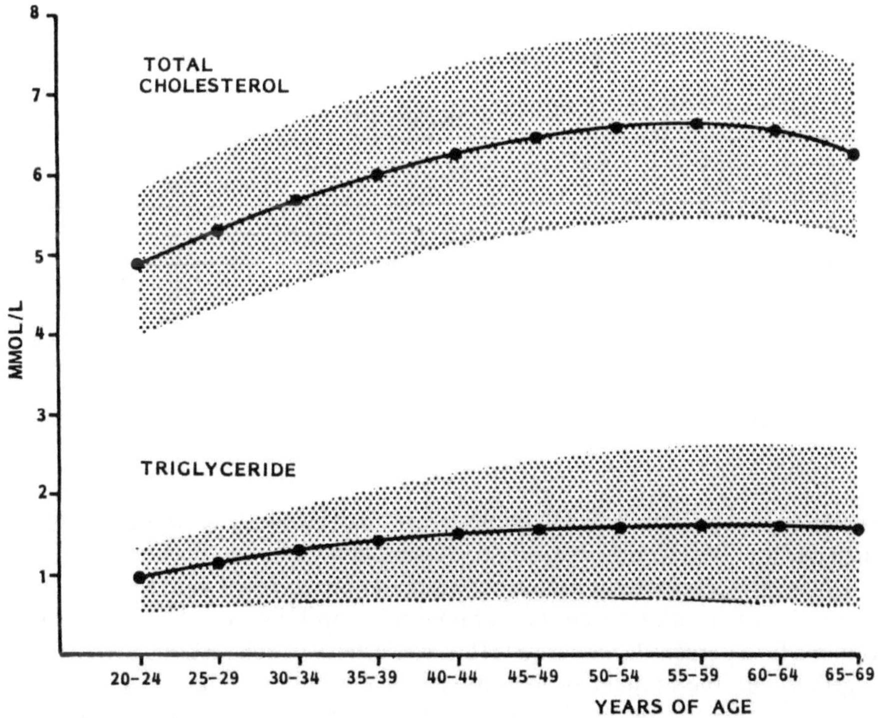

Fig. 1. Mean ± SD of serum lipids in fasted men according to age

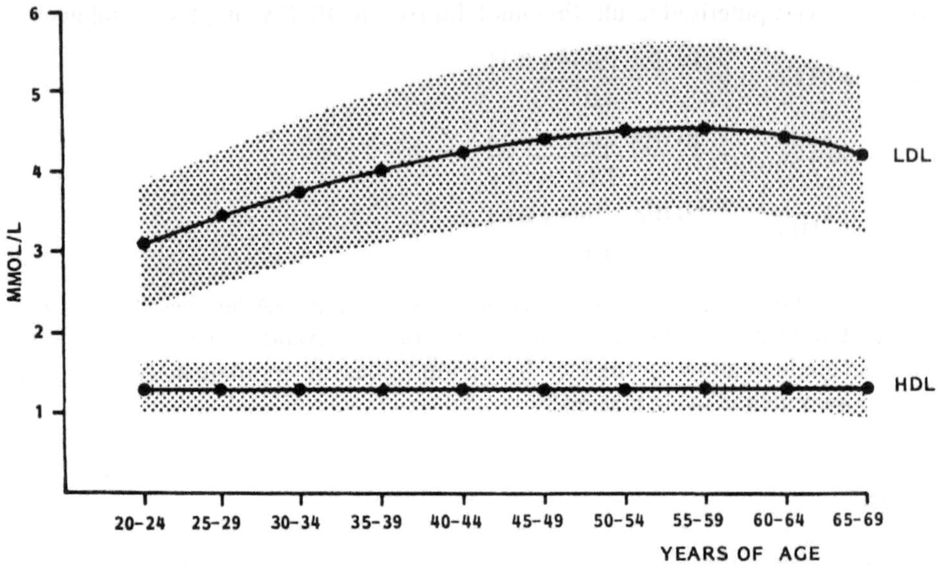

Fig. 2. Mean ± SD of LDL and HDL cholesterol according to age

Table 1. Limits of statistical normality for fasting serum lipids and HDL cholesterol (measured) and for LDL cholesterol (calculated) in men screened at BUPA Medical Centre during 1984

Age	No.	TC	TG	LDL-C[a]	HDL-C	
		95th percentile (mmol/litre)			5th percentile (mmol/litre)	95th percentile
20-24	383	6.4	1.9	4.5	0.9	1.9
25-29	650	7.2	2.3	5.2	0.9	1.9
30-34	1169	7.7	2.6	5.7	0.8	1.9
35-39	1711	8.0	2.9	5.9	0.8	1.9
40-44	1398	8.1	3.1	5.9	0.8	1.9
45-49	1233	8.3	3.1	6.2	0.8	1.9
50-54	1030	8.4	3.1	6.2	0.8	1.9
55-59	680	8.5	3.0	6.4	0.8	1.9
60-64	427	8.5	3.2	6.3	0.8	2.0

[a] $\text{LDL-C} = \text{TC} - (\text{HDL-C} + \frac{\text{TG}}{2.19})$ mmol/litre, excluding the 149 subjects with TG > 4.5 mmol/litre.

shown in Fig. 2. Total and LDL cholesterol values rise with age to peak at 55-59 and then decline. Triglyceride values rise in a similar manner but decline less after 55-59 whereas HDL cholesterol values were remarkably constant between 20-69.

The 95th percentile values for serum lipids and HDL and LDL cholesterol and also the fifth percentile values for HDL cholesterol in 8681 BUPA men aged 20-64, together with the number of men in each age group, are shown in Table 1. These data were then corrected for analytical variation and converted from serum to 'plasma', as shown in Table 2. This resulted in appreciable decreases in the 95th per-

Table 2. Data in Table 1 corrected to conform with CDC standards and converted from serum to 'plasma'

Age	TC	TG	LDL-C	HDL-C	
	95th percentile (mmol/litre)			5th percentile (mmol/litre)	95th percentile
20-24	6.1	1.8	4.1	1.0	2.0
25-29	6.8	2.1	4.8	1.0	2.0
30-34	7.3	2.4	5.2	0.9	2.0
35-39	7.6	2.6	5.4	0.9	2.0
40-44	7.6	2.8	5.5	0.9	2.0
45-49	7.8	2.8	5.7	0.9	2.0
50-54	7.9	2.8	5.6	0.9	2.0
55-59	8.0	2.7	5.8	0.9	2.0
60-64	8.0	2.9	5.8	0.9	2.1

Table 3. Percentage of BUPA men aged 20-59 (n=8254) with corrected 'plasma' values above or below the statistical limits of normality of white North American men of similar age screened during the Lipid Research Clinics Prevalence Study

Total cholesterol	> LRC 95th percentile	13.8%
Triglyceride	> LRC 95th percentile	1.6%
LDL cholesterol	> LRC 95th percentile	11.6%
HDL cholesterol	< LRC 5th percentile	0.75%
	> LRC 95th percentile	17.5%

Table 4. Ratios (mean ± SD) of HDL cholesterol to total cholesterol (HDL-C/TC) and to LDL cholesterol (HDL-C/LDL-C) in 'plasma' of BUPA men aged 20-59 compared with white North American men of similar age, using published data from the LRC Prevalence Study [9]. The t test was used to compare differences

Ratio	BUPA	LRC	p
HDL-C/TC	0.250 ± 0.077 (n=8132)	0.231 ± 0.071 (n=2448)	<0.001
HDL-C/LDL-C	0.406 ± 0.199 (n=8117)	0.364 ± 0.159 (n=2448)	<0.001

centile values for total and LDL cholesterol and triglyceride, and slight increases in the fifth and 95th percentile values for HDL cholesterol.

Table 3 shows the percentage of BUPA men in whom corrected 'plasma' values of total, LDL cholesterol, HDL cholesterol and triglyceride exceeded the 95th percentile values of men of comparable age in the LRC study and also the percentage with an HDL cholesterol below the corresponding fifth percentile [1, 2]. The percentage with total and LDL cholesterol values above the LRC cut-off values was more than doubled whereas the percentage with raised triglycerides or a reduced HDL cholesterol was less than one-third of that of their North American counterparts. The ratios of HDL cholesterol to total cholesterol and HDL cholesterol to LDL cholesterol in BUPA and LRC men aged 20-59 are compared in Table 4. Both ratios were significantly higher in the Britons.

Discussion

Valid comparisons of the prevalence of hyperlipidaemia in different countries are not easily made retrospectively, for obvious reasons. However, we have attempted this by comparing published data from the LRC study in North America with data from men attending the BUPA Medical Centre in London. The LRC values for total cholesterol and triglyceride were based on analysis of fasting plasma samples during 1971-1976 from over 17000 white men aged 20-64 [1] whereas values for LDL and HDL cholesterol were derived from just under 2500 men aged 20-59 [2]. BUPA values for total cholesterol, triglyceride and HDL cholesterol were obtained in over 8000 fasted men, screened during 1984, in whom values of LDL cholesterol were then calculated. Increases in total and LDL cholesterol and triglyceride with age were similar in both surveys, as was the constancy of HDL cholesterol, but the prevalence of hyperlipidaemia differed. Significant hypercholesterolaemia, i.e. a value above the LRC age-related 95th percentile, was present in 13.8% of BUPA men, compared with 5% of LRC men. This was mainly due to an increase in LDL cholesterol, which exceeded the LRC 95th percentile in nearly 12% of BUPA men, but also reflected an increase in HDL cholesterol in that 17.5% had a value above the LRC 95th percentile. In contrast the prevalence of hypertriglyceridaemia was decreased in BUPA men, only 1.6% of whom had a value above the LRC 95th percentile.

Much effort has been made to minimise the effects of experimental variability between the two sets of data. Serum values in BUPA men were converted to plasma values so as to make them comparable with LRC plasma values. Cholesterol and triglyceride were measured non-enzymatically during the LRC study whereas enzymatic methods were used to analyse BUPA samples. To overcome this difference appropriate corrections were applied to BUPA values using regression equations based on analysis of CDC reference standards. Similar corrections were applied to HDL cholesterol values, which were determined after heparin-manganese precipitation [10] in the LRC study compared with dextran sulphate-magnesium precipitation of BUPA samples. The latter method gives values approximately 0.03 mmol/litre lower than the former [6]. Another difference was that LDL cholesterol was calculated in the LRC study by subtracting HDL cholesterol from cholesterol in the $d > 1.006$ fraction of ultracentrifuged plasma [10] whereas the formula of Friedewald et al. [7] was used to calculate LDL cholesterol in BUPA samples. Excellent correlation exists between these two methods with the proviso that samples with a triglyceride concentration of > 4.5 mmol/litre must be excluded from the Friedewald analysis, as was done.

Another source of variation was the manner in which individuals were selected. In the LRC study this was done so as to obtain a representative sample of the entire North American population whereas BUPA men were self-selected. The latter procedure is open to bias with respect both to socio-economic grouping and the possibility that an increased proportion of individuals with hyperlipidaemia opt to undergo screening on account of a positive family history or symptoms of CHD.

The likelihood that the BUPA data were indeed biased by self-selection can be assessed indirectly by examining the results of another survey carried out recently in Britain, which was free from this potential source of error. The Regional Heart Study [11] surveyed a geographically and socio-economically representative sample of almost 8000 men aged 40–59 in the United Kingdom during the period 1978–1980. Mean values of serum cholesterol, triglyceride and HDL cholesterol were 6.30, 2.05 and 1.15 mmol/litre respectively [12] compared with values of 6.34, 1.54 and 1.28 mmol/litre in aged-matched BUPA men. The higher triglycerides in the Regional Heart Study can be explained by the fact that subjects were not fasted whereas their lower HDL cholesterol levels possibly reflected the use of phosphotungstate-magnesium as the precipitating agent, which is known to give lower values than other methods [13, 14]. Alternatively, higher levels of HDL cholesterol in BUPA men could have been a reflection of higher alcohol intake or less cigarette smoking [11] since high HDL cholesterol levels were also evident in an earlier BUPA survey, despite use of the phosphotungstate-magnesium method [15]. The similarity of mean serum total cholesterol levels in the BUPA and Regional Heart Studies is striking, however, suggesting that differences in the method of selection of subjects had no effect on this particular variable.

Assuming that the differences between LRC and BUPA data are real, how best can they be explained? The fact that LRC data were gathered 8–13 years before the BUPA data is unlikely to account for the lower prevalence of hypercholesterolaemia in North America since cholesterol levels appear to have been falling there rather than rising [1]. The finding that an increased proportion of BUPA men had LDL and HDL cholesterol levels above the LRC 95th percentile is compatible with British men having a higher intake of dietary saturated fat and cholesterol and/or, a lower intake of polyunsaturated fat than North Americans [16, 17]. Analysis of the linoleic acid content of adipose tissue samples supports the latter explanation [18]. The lower proportion of BUPA men with hypertriglyceridaemia conceivably reflects differences in the prevalence of obesity and glucose intolerance in the two study populations [19]. Evidence that obesity is less common in at least one country in Europe, Holland, than in the United States has recently been published [20]. A similar trend in Britain could account for the lower triglyceride values of BUPA men since these are positively correlated with obesity [19].

Do these international differences in the prevalence of risk factors have any epidemiological significance? British men not only have higher levels of total and LDL cholesterol, both of which are positively correlated with CHD [21], but also have higher levels of HDL cholesterol. The latter was negatively correlated with CHD in the Framingham Study in the United States [21] but not in the British Regional Heart Study [22]. The ratio of HDL cholesterol to both total and LDL cholesterol was higher in BUPA men than in the LRC study which could be regarded as advantageous in the context of CHD, as could their lower prevalence of hypertriglyceridaemia. However, the significance of hypertriglyceridaemia as a risk factor is debatable [23] and the inverse correlation between the HDL: total cholesterol ratio and CHD mortality [24] has been disputed [25].

Current statistics show that CHD mortality rates in the United States and Canada are now appreciably lower than in the nations which comprise the United Kingdom [3]. The decline in CHD mortality in the United States during the past 15 years has coincided with a decrease in serum total cholesterol [26], but comparable data on HDL cholesterol are lacking. Thus on the basis of the evidence available it would seem reasonable to attempt to lower total and LDL cholesterol levels in Britain to North American levels by dietary means [27]. Future trends in HDL cholesterol levels and CHD mortality need to be carefully monitored since it remains to be established that the two are causally related. Despite this uncertainty, measurement of HDL cholesterol continues to be useful, not only to avoid unnecessary treatment of hyperalphalipoproteinaemia, a benign condition [28], but also because it enables one to calculate LDL cholesterol so conveniently.

Summary

Data on fasting serum lipids obtained from over 8000 men screened at the BUPA Medical Centre during 1984 have been compared with published data from the Lipid Research Clinics Prevalence Study. After correcting for analytical variation the results suggest that BUPA men, who were mainly British, had a higher prevalence of increased levels of total, LDL and HDL cholesterol in plasma than North American men of comparable age and a decreased prevalence of hypertriglyceridaemia. These differences may be of dietary origin and could have a bearing on the current excess mortality from coronary heart disease in Britain compared with North America.

Acknowledgement. We thank the staff of J.S. Pathology Services Ltd. for their cooperation, Dr. A. Hainline for generously providing CDC reference samples and Mrs. E. Manson for typing the manuscript.

References

1. LRC Program Epidemiology Committee (1979) Plasma lipid distributions in selected North American populations: the Lipid Research Clinics Prevalence Study. Circulation 60: 427–439
2. Heiss G, Tamir I, Davis CE, et al. (1980) Lipoprotein-cholesterol distributions in selected North American populations: the Lipid Research Clinics Program Prevalence Study. Circulation 61: 302–315
3. World Health Organization (1984) World Health Statistics Annual. WHO, Geneva
4. Lie RF, Schmitz JM, Pierre KJ, Gochman N (1976) Cholesterol oxidase-based determination, by continuous-flow analysis, of total and free cholesterol in serum. Clin Chem 22: 1627–1630
5. Bucolo G, David H (1973) Quantitative determination of serum triglycerides by the use of enzymes. Clin Chem 19: 476–482
6. Warnick GR, Benderson J, Albers JJ (1982) Dextran sulfate-Mg^{2+} precipitation procedure for quantitation of high density-lipoprotein cholesterol. Clin Chem 28: 1379–1388
7. Friedewald WT, Levy RI, Fredrickson DS (1972) Estimation of the concentration of low-density lipoprotein cholesterol in plasma, without use of the preparative ultracentrifuge. Clin Chem 18: 499–502
8. Laboratory Methods Committee of the Lipid Research Clinics Program of the NHLBI (1977) Cholesterol and triglyceride concentrations in serum/plasma pairs. Clin Chem 23: 60–63

9. Green MS, Heiss G, Rifkind BM, Cooper GR, Williams OD, Tyroler HA (1985) The ratio of plasma high density lipoprotein cholesterol to total and low density lipoprotein cholesterol: age-related changes and race and sex differences in selected North American populations. The Lipid Research Clinics Prevalence Study. Circulation 72: 93-104
10. Rifkind BM, Segal P (1983) Lipid Research Clinics Program. Reference values for hyperlipidemia and hypolipidemia. JAMA 250: 1869-1872
11. Shaper AG, Pocock SJ, Walker M, et al. (1981) British Regional Heart Study: cardiovascular risk factors in middle-aged men in 24 towns. Br Med J 283: 179-186
12. Thelle DS, Shaper AG, Whitehead TP, et al. (1983) Blood lipids in middle-aged British men. Br Heart J 49: 205-213
13. Warnick GR, Cheung MC, Albers JJ (1979) Comparison of current methods for high density lipoprotein cholesterol quantitation. Clin Chem 25: 596-604
14. Durrington PN (1980) A comparison of three methods of measuring serum high density lipoprotein cholesterol in diabetics and non-diabetics. Ann Clin Biochem 17: 199-204
15. Williams P, Robinson D, Bailey A (1979) High-density lipoprotein and coronary risk factors in normal men. Lancet 1: 72-75
16. Schaefer EJ, Levy RI, Ernst MD, et al. (1981) The effects of low cholesterol, high polyunsaturated fat, and low fat diets on plasma lipid and lipoprotein cholesterol levels in normal and hypercholesterolemic subjects. Am J Clin Nutr 34: 1758-1763
17. Schonfeld G, Patsch W, Rudel LL, et al. (1982) Effects of dietary cholesterol and fatty acids on plasma lipoproteins. J Clin Invest 69: 1072-1080
18. Katan MB, Beynen AC (1981) Linoleic acid consumption and coronary heart disease in USA and UK. Lancet 2: 371
19. Cowan LD, Wilcosky T, Criqui MH, et al. (1985) Demographic, behavioural, biochemical and dietary correlates of plasma triglycerides. Lipid Research Clinics Program Prevalence Study. Arteriosclerosis 5: 466-480
20. Rookus MA, Deurenberg P, van Sonsbeek JLA (1986) Obesity in North America and the Netherlands. Lancet 1: 100
21. Kannel WB, Castelli WP, Gordon T (1979) Cholesterol in the prediction of atherosclerotic disease. New perspectives based on the Framingham Study. Ann Intern Med 90: 85-91
22. Shaper AG, Pocock SJ, Walker M, Phillips AN, Whitehead TP, Macfarlane PW (1985) Risk factors for ischaemic heart disease: the prospective phase of the British Regional Heart Study. J Epidemiol Community Health 39: 197-209
23. Hulley SB, Rosenman RH, Bawol RD, Brand RJ (1980) Epidemiology as a guide to clinical decisions. The association between triglyceride and coronary heart disease. N Engl J Med 302: 1383-1389
24. Kannel WB, Castelli WP (1979) Is the serum total cholesterol an anachronism? Lancet 2: 950-951
25. Knuiman JT, West CE (1981) HDL cholesterol in men from thirteen countries. Lancet 2: 367-368
26. Havlik RJ, Feinleib M (eds) (1979) Proceedings of the Conference on the Decline in Coronary Heart Disease Mortality. NIH, Washington, Publication, no 79-1610
27. Committee on Medical Aspects of Food Policy (1984) Diet and cardiovascular disease. HMSO, London (Report on health and social subjects, no 28)
28. Glueck CJ, Fallat RW, Millett FA, Steiner PM (1975) Familial hyperalphalipoproteinemia. Arch Intern Med 135: 1025-1028

Low-Density Lipoprotein: Its Metabolic Determinants and Its Role in Coronary Heart Disease

B. Lewis

The relation between coronary heart disease mortality rate and serum cholesterol is seen both in cross-cultural and in single-population studies. In the largest longitudinal studies of each type, respectively the Seven Country Study [1] and the follow up of MRFIT screenees [2], the relation is direct and continuous, with no indication of a threshold in the range 4–8 mmol/litre. In some studies the slope of the relationship is curvilinear and suggests a greater increment in risk for an increment of serum cholesterol in the high range than for an increment of serum cholesterol in the low range, but this is not seen consistently. All published studies have been based on single measurements of serum cholesterol and therefore, for statistical reasons, they underestimate the steepness of the relationship; that is, the increase of risk in persons with higher cholesterol levels is greater than is suggested by such studies. In normal populations, plasma cholesterol levels reflect levels of low-density lipoprotein (LDL) cholesterol; in a study of five populations we found the correlation between these variables was $r=0.96$ [3].

There is acceptable evidence that the epidemiological relationship reflects cause-and-effect. Peto's overview [4] of 17 randomised controlled trials of cholesterol reduction by diet and drugs (total number of subjects was 36000) provides evidence of a very strong association between cholesterol lowering and reduction in coronary heart disease incidence. La Ville in our laboratory, in collaboration with Woolf, has studied the effect of serum cholesterol reduction using the drug lovastatin in a strain of genetically hyperlipidaemic rabbits in which aortic atherosclerosis is present by the age of 6 months; if cholesterol levels are reduced towards normal from the time of weaning, little or no atherosclerosis develops by this age. In other studies on animals, diet-induced hyperlipidaemia results in aortic and coronary atherosclerosis-like lesions, which show marked partial regression over a period of 12–40 months if cholesterol levels are reduced to normal (see for example [5, 6]). In man, we have measured the net fluxes of LDL and intermediate-density lipoprotein (IDL) from plasma into arterial intima. These rates are directly related to plasma levels of these lipoproteins. As the cholesterol of atherosclerotic lesions is derived from that of plasma, the findings provide evidence for one mechanism by which high plasma levels of cholesterol-rich lipoproteins may accelerate lipid accumulation in the arterial wall.

In view of the evidence that high levels of plasma LDL cholesterol play an aetiological role in coronary heart disease, we have been interested in mechanisms determining levels of this lipoprotein. One basis for the wide variation of LDL cholesterol and, consequently, of total cholesterol levels within single populations is genetic. Inherited, polygenic determinants account for some 30% of variability in serum cholesterol [7]. One such allele codes for the primary structure of apolipoprotein (apo) E which may be present in one of three main polymorphic forms, each in homozygous or heterozygous state. Persons with the common $E_3/_3$ phenotype tend to have intermediate levels of serum cholesterol, while the mean for those with the $E_2/_2$ phenotype is lower, and the mean for those with the $E_4/_4$ is higher [8]. Utermann has discussed the possible metabolic basis for this relationship in terms of the binding affinity of these phenotypes for hepatic apo B100, E receptors; the lower affinity of E_2 for the receptor would lead to reduced uptake of IDL compared with that in persons with E_3 or E_4 phenotypes, and in consequence to up-regulation of these receptors and, in turn, to increased fractional catabolism of LDL. In keeping with this, we have reported that in normolipidaemic and type III hyperlipidaemic persons with the $E_2/_2$ phenotype, the rate of conversion of IDL to LDL is considerably lower than in control subjects [9]. Generally, in severe hypertriglyceridaemic states LDL cholesterol levels tend to be low, and the mechanism maintaining such LDL levels is an increase in fractional catabolic rate [10].

We have described the kinetic bases of primary genetic hyperlipidaemias [11]. Using methods modified from those developed for such kinetic studies, for use in an epidemiological context, we investigated LDL metabolism in normal population samples to obtain an understanding of the mechanisms underlying variation in plasma cholesterol levels within populations and between populations. This international collaborative study involved P.R. Turner, J.A. Rossouw, M. Mancini, Ll. Masana, T.A. Miettinen and their colleagues [12].

We studied five population samples with wide differences in mean serum cholesterol and congruent differences in national mortality rates from coronary heart disease; in decreasing sequence these were Caucasians in the United Kingdom, Finland, Italy and Spain, and Africans in South Africa. We identified 109 healthy persons with LDL cholesterol in the highest, modal and lowest deciles of the distribution for each population and measured LDL apo B production rate and fractional catabolic rate. We also measured the rate of LDL degradation by freshly isolated blood mononuclear cells in vitro. The two catabolism-related variables were, significantly, directly correlated ($r=0.49$, $p<0.01$). The LDL apo B production rate was directly related to LDL cholesterol and LDL apo B concentrations, and LDL apo B fractional catabolism was inversely related to these levels.

The independent effect of differences in production rate was greater than that of fractional catabolic rate, the latter mechanism playing a major role in maintaining levels of LDL cholesterol in the lowest decile. These relationships were consistent within all five population samples.

In seeking metabolic differences between populations, we found that the strikingly low modal concentration of LDL cholesterol in the African population sample was due to comparably low production rates of LDL. Among the European populations the lowest LDL cholesterol levels, in the Spanish sample, were maintained by a relatively low LDL production rate and a high fractional catabolic rate; variation between the remaining three European samples was attributable to differences in fractional catabolism. The relationship between dietary fatty acids and these kinetic variables proved to be of considerable interest. The production rate of LDL apo B was directly related to intake of saturated fatty acids, while the fractional catabolic rate was directly related to intake of monounsaturated fatty acids.

These findings are congruent with the known relationship between serum cholesterol levels and dietary patterns in the five communities studied.

How does LDL interact with cellular and other elements of the arterial intima to accelerate the progression of atherosclerosis? This has been alluded to in an earlier section. LDL undergoes lipid peroxidation when incubated with rabbit endothelial cells. This modified lipoprotein is taken up by mouse macrophages [13].

In more recent work in our laboratory by Masana et al. [14], these interactions have been confirmed using human cells. Lipid peroxidation is involved in the modification of LDL by human endothelial cells derived from umbilical cords, the altered lipoprotein showing increased electrophoretic mobility and avid uptake by human macrophages, by contrast with native LDL. Modified LDL shows more rapid fractional catabolism than native lipoprotein when injected into rabbits. Further studies on patients undergoing vascular surgery confirm that lipoproteins undergo lipid peroxidation in vivo (Shaik et al., in preparation); these observations may contribute to our understanding of the mechanisms involved in conversion of macrophages into foam cells in the developing atherosclerotic plaques.

Since the cholesterol-rich LDL and very low-density lipoprotein (VLDL) remnant particles play a major role in determining the risk of atherosclerotic heart disease, public policy aimed at reducing this risk must be based on a secure knowledge of the prevalence of lipoprotein risk factors. In a population in which this prevalence is low, some emphasis should probably be placed on case finding with a view to individual care of persons at high relative risk, such as those with familial hypercholesterolaemia. Where the prevalence is high, a strategy with the dual goals of reducing the distribution of risk in the entire population and individual care is mandatory. The nationwide Risk Factor Prevalence Study in the United Kingdom is addressing this and related issues [15]. Approximately 13000 men and women aged 25-59 years have been examined up to the present time. One of the successes of the British National Health Service has been the free access of the population to primary medical care. As some 75% of the population see their general practitioners at least once each year, frequent contact between patients and doctors in primary health care provides an outstanding opportunity for health education and for case finding of persons at high risk of cardiovascular disease. Hence our population sample was based on patients registered with urban general practitioners in four major cities.

No less than 63% of this sample proved to have serum cholesterol levels exceeding 5 mmol/litre, i.e. to have levels in the range conferring higher risk of coronary heart disease than persons with levels below this value. Almost one-quarter, 23%, had levels exceeding 6.5 mmol/litre, an unequivocally high value. This underlies the essential role of population measures to combat the very high mortality from coronary heart disease in the United Kingdom. Other findings in the study also have bearing on strategic considerations in the prevention of coronary disease. One has been the opportunity to examine quantitatively the concept of "selective screening", that is, the view that measurement of lipid risk factors be reserved for persons believed, on clinical and anamnestic grounds, to be likely to have abnormal findings. Indeed, persons with a positive family history of cardiovascular disease, those with xanthelasmas, arcus or suspected xanthomas, and those with Body Mass Index exceeding 25 have a substantial frequency of hyperlipidaemia and should undoubtedly undergo screening. However the converse proved to be invalid. From the viewpoint of detection of persons at high risk of coronary heart disease, selective screening proved insensitive and quite inadequate. For example, the presence of a positive family history would necessitate testing 36% of the population, and would lead to the detection of 43% of persons with cholesterol levels exceeding 6.5 mmol/litre. Another aspect of the study was the yield of case finding by two different methods. The proportion of persons coming forward for health examination on the basis of one invitation mailed by their general practitioners was about 55%; on the other hand, an invitation issued verbally by the practitioner in the course of a consultation for an intercurrent medical problem (so-called case finding) was accepted by 90%. This is a rewarding vindication of the doctor-patient relationship as a basis for preventive medicine, and corresponds with the model exemplified and taught by Prof. Gotthard Schettler whose 70th birthday is honoured in this volume.

References

1. Keys A (1981) Seven countries. Harvard University Press, Cambridge
2. Neaton JD, Kuller LH, Wentworth D, Borhani NO (1984) Total and cardiovascular mortality in relation to cigarette smoking, serum cholesterol concentration, and diastolic blood pressure. Am Heart J 108: 759-769
3. Lewis B, Turner PR, Rossouw JE, Masana Ll, Mancini M, Miettinen TA, et al. (in press) Metabolic epidemiology of plasma cholesterol: a study of the mechanisms of variation of cholesterol levels within populations and between populations. In: Nestel PJ (ed) Atherosclerosis VII. Elsevier, Amsterdam
4. Peto R, Yusuf S, Collins R (1985) Cholesterol-lowering trial results in their epidemiologic context. Circulation 72: III-451
5. Weber G, Fabbrini P, Resi L, Jones R, Vesselinovitch D, Wissler RW (1977) Regression of arteriosclerotic lesions in Rhesus monkey aortas after regression diet. Atherosclerosis 26: 535-547
6. Clarkson TB, Lehner NDM, Wagner WD, St Clair RW, Bond MG, Billock BC (1979) A study of atherosclerosis regression in *Macaca Mulatta*. Exp Mol Pathol 30: 360-385
7. Meyer K (1962) Serum cholesterol and heredity. Acta Med Scand 172: 401
8. Utermann G, Pruin N, Steinmetz A (1979) Polymorphism of human apolipoprotein E. III. Effect of a single polymorphic gene locus on plasma lipid levels in man. Clin Genet 15: 63
9. Turner PR, Cortese C, Wootton R, Marenah C, Miller NE, Lewis B (1985) Plasma apolipoprotein B metabolism in familial Type III dysbetalipoproteinaemia. Eur J Clin Invest 15: 100-112
10. Sigurdsson G, Nicoll A, Lewis B (1976) The metabolism of low density lipoproteins in endogenous hypertriglyceridaemia. Eur J Clin Invest 6: 151-158
11. Janus ED, Nicoll AM, Turner PR, Magill P, Lewis B (1980) Kinetic bases of the primary hyperlipidaemias. Studies of apolipoprotein B metabolism in genetically defined subjects. Eur J Clin Invest 10: 161-172
12. International Collaborative Study Group. Metabolic epidemiology of plasma cholesterol. Lancet 1986; ii: 991-996
13. Henrickson B, Mahoney EM, Steinberg D (1982) Interactions of plasma lipoproteins with endothelial cells. Ann NY Acad Sci 401: 102-116
14. Masana Ll, Shaikh M, LaVille A, Lewis B (1986) Lipid peroxidation of low density lipoprotein by human endothelial cells modifies its metabolism in vitro. Rev Esp Fisiol 42: 99-104
15. Guyer BM, Lewis B, Mann JI, Rose LB, Shepherd J, Winder A (in press) Prevalence of risk factors for coronary heart disease in the United Kingdom. In: Nestel PJ (ed) Atherosclerosis VII. Elsevier, Amsterdam

Plasma Levels of Lipoproteins and Apolipoproteins in Octo- and Nonagenarians

P. Avogaro, G. Bittolo-Bon, G. Cazzolato, A. Bottecchia, and R. Brugiolo

Introduction

A great deal of attention has been paid in recent years to high-density lipoproteins (HDL) and to their inverse relationship with the occurrence of ischemic heart disease (IHD). This attention to HDL is not new, as pioneer studies have already emphasized its value as a predictor of "de novo" cases of IHD [1], but it is only recently that a revival of interest in HDL has started, originating from both epidemiological and clinical studies. The seminal paper was by Miller and Miller [2], who stressed the inverse relationship existing between HDL and IHD. At about the same time other papers were published which referred to the existence of families whose members appeared to be protected from IHD by high levels of HDL cholesterol (HDL-C) [3, 4, 5] and/or of apolipoprotein A (apo A). Furthermore, Glueck et al. [6] proposed that high levels of HDL-C or low levels of low-density lipoprotein cholesterol (LDL-C), or a combination of the two parameters, constitute the features of a "longevity syndrome." However, data obtained in two subsequent studies [7, 8] do not agree with the proposed biochemical pattern of longevity, although in neither study was the prevalence of hyper-α-lipoproteinemia recorded nor was it ascertained whether any relationship between the mortality rates and the levels of HDL-C existed [8].

The present paper refers to data obtained from a large number of octo- or nonagenarians associated with a geriatric hospital in Venice. In none of the cases studied was a condition of hyper-α-lipoproteinemia (HDL-C and/or apo A-I) recorded, although low levels of apolipoprotein B (apo B) appeared as a noticeable trait.

Material and Methods

Individuals of both sexes (45 males and 69 females) over 80 years old were randomly selected from a population living in a Venetian senior-citizens residence. Of these, 56 (35 males and 21 females) were octogenarians, 53 (10 males and 43 females) were nonagenarians and 5, all females, were centenarians. Most of the subjects lived in private rooms and were self-sufficient; only 15 patients required extensive nursing care, but these were alert and communicative. All of them followed their usual diet. Alcoholic drinks were taken in moderate quantities by 15% of subjects, but only 4 currently smoked. As a control group 79 septuagenarians (40 males and 39 females) were randomly chosen from the same population. None of the investigated subjects was receiving any treatment known to influence lipid metabolism, and none suffered from major atherosclerosis clinical events (i.e., myocardial infarction, stroke, or gangrenous limbs). Body mass index (BMI) was calculated by dividing body weight (expressed in kg) by the square of body height (expressed in m).

Venous blood samples were collected in test-tubes containing disodium EDTA (1 mg/ml) after an overnight fast. The levels of total cholesterol (TC) and triglyceride (TG) were determined enzymatically using reagents from Menarini (Florence, Italy), and the level of HDL-C in the supernatant was determined after precipitation of apo B-containing lipoproteins by phosphotungstate-$MgCl_2$ [9]. LDL-C values were calculated using the formula TC – (TG/5 – HDL-C) [10]. The two apolipoproteins apo A-I and apo B were quantified in fresh untreated plasma according to the method of Laurell [11], using monospecific immune antisera as reported previously [9]. The prevalence of abnormal phenotypes was tested, as characterized by abnormal levels of LDL and/or HDL (defined as values above the 95th or below the 50th percentile of a middle-aged normal population). The cut-off points chosen are shown in Table 3.

Results

The octo- and nonagenarian males showed values of BMI, TC, TG, HDL-C, apo A-I, and apo B that were significantly lower than those of the septuagenarians of the same sex, but the ratios LDL-C:HDL-C and LDL-C:apo B were significantly higher in the octo- or nonagenarians. No significant differences between males over 80 and septuagenarians were observed for blood pressure, LDL-C, or for the apo A-I:apo B ratio. In females a similar pattern was observed, although in contrast with males, significantly higher values of LDL-C were observed in octo- and nonagenarian females than in septuagenarians; the two groups also showed similar values of TG. The group of females over 80 had a significantly higher mean age than the males. They also had significantly higher systolic blood pressure (SBP), TC, HDL-C, and apo B than males of the same age group, but values of apo A-I and of the ratios apo A-I:apo B and LDL-C:apo B were significantly lower. There were no statistically significant differences between the sexes for BMI, diastolic blood pressure (BDP), TC, LDL-C and the ratio LDL-C:HDL-C (Tables 1, 2). No statistically significant differences were observed between octogenarian and nonagenarian subjects of the same sex (not shown). Table 3 shows the prevalence of lipoprotein and/or apolipoprotein abnormalities in octo- and nonagenarians, according to the criteria stated earlier. In this group there is little prevalence of hyper-LDL-C, with only one female showing values of LDL-C diagnostic for hypo-β-lipoproteinemia; none of the examined subjects showed HDL-C values above the normal limits, but about half of the octo- and nonagenarians had HDL-C values lower than the 5th lower percentile of a middle-aged population.

Table 1. Mean values of age, body mass index (BMI) blood pressure (SBP, systolic; DBP, diastolic), total cholesterol (TC), triglyceride (TG), low-density lipoprotein cholesterol (LDL-C), and high-density lipoprotein cholesterol (HDL-C) in octo- and nonagenarian and septuagenarian males and females (values are expressed as means with one standard deviation)

	Age (years)	BMI	SBP (mmHg)	DBP (mmHg)	TC (mg/dl)	TG (mg/dl)	LDL-C (mg/dl)	HDL-C (mg/dl)
Octo- and nonagenarians Males [45]	86.7 4.5	22.6[d] 2.9	144.3 17.5	79.8 9.5	177.9[d] 32.7	101.2[d] 34.1	127.5 26.4	30.1[d] 6.9
Females [69]	90.7[b] 6.2	21.3[d] 4.3	151.3[a] 19.0	81.7 8.5	190.8[d] 37.6	125.7[a] 67.0	131.3[d] 32.0	34.3[a,d] 9.5
Septuagenarians Males [40]	75.3 2.9	25.1 4.6	140.5 18.8	78.2 7.5	202.9 41.4	121.6 41.2	135.3 37.9	43.3 11.1
Females [39]	75.2 2.7	26.3 3.7	150.3 21.9	83.7 10.5	222.3[a] 43.1	130.2 58.4	151.3[a] 38.5	45.3 9.7

[a] $p < 0.05$. [b] $p < 0.01$ vs males (same decades). [c] $p < 0.05$. [d] $p < 0.01$ vs 8th decade (same sex).

Table 2. Amounts of apoproteins B (apo B) and A-I (apo A-I) and the ratios apo A-I : apo B and LDL-C : apo B in octo- and nonagenarian and septuagenarian males and females (values are expressed as means with standard deviation)

	Apo B (mg/dl)	Apo A-I (mg/dl)	LDL-C: HDL-C	Apo A-I: apo B	LDL-C: apo B
Males 80[c] [45]	74.8[d] 16.2	72.2[d] 17.7	4.40[d] 1.19	1.00 0.29	1.73[d] 0.24
Females 80[c] [69]	83.3[a,d] 18.5	65.6[a,d] 15.1	4.04[d] 1.26	0.81[b] 0.21	1.59[b,d] 0.25
Males 70-79 [40]	103.5 23.3	90.0 18.4	3.39 1.39	0.93 0.25	1.31 0.28
Females 70-79 [39]	114.9[a] 27.0	89.1 14.2	3.34 1.42	0.81[a] 0.22	1.34 0.26

[a] $p < 0.05$. [b] $p < 0.01$ vs males (same decades).
[c] $p < 0.05$. [d] $p < 0.01$ vs 8th decade (same sex).

Table 3. Prevalence of some lipoprotein abnormalities in octo- and nonagenarian males and females

	Males		Females	
	n	%	n	%
Hyper-LDL-C[a]	2	4.3	3	4.4
Hypo-LDL-C[b]	0	0	1	1.4
Hyper-HDL-C[c]	0	0	0	0
Hypo-HDL-C[d]	23	48.9	37	53.6

[a] LDL-C $\geqslant$190 mg/dl.
[b] LDL-C $\leqslant$70 mg/dl.
[c] HDL-C $\geqslant$70 mg/dl.
[d] HDL-C $\leqslant$30 mg/dl for men and $\leqslant$35 mg/dl for women.

Discussion

The "revival" of the idea that HDL is an anti-risk factor is based upon some apparently sound arguments [2-6]. One of the more widely quoted is the belief that increased values of HDL-C and/or apo A-I, or decreased values of LDL-C or apo B, or a combination of the two represent the main features of the "longevity syndrome" [6].

The data referred in this paper do not fit with this hypothesis. In our large sample of elderly people HDL-C was significantly lower in octo- and nonagenarians than in septuagenarians; moreover not a single case of hyper-HDL (HDL-C and/or apo A-I) was recorded. In a previous study of 103 nonagenarians of both sexes [7] hypo-α-lipoproteinemia was the most frequently encountered lipid abnormality but only a few cases of hyper-α-lipoproteinemia and a single case of hypo-β-lipoproteinemia were observed. A recent study [8] has recorded low levels of LDL-C, high levels of HDL_2, and a high ratio of $HDL_2 : HDL_3$. No variation of HDL-C with age or any relationship between mortality rate and plasma level of HDL-C has been observed. The protective role of HDL has recently been questioned; an epidemiological study by a British group did not record a significant relationship between the prevalence of IHD and the level of HDL; they concluded that HDL-C is not a major risk-factor in coronary heart disease in Britain [12].

We do not have any reasonable hypothesis to explain the diverent results obtained in our study and Glueck et al.'s study [6]. However, it is notable that our sample had equal numbers of each sex whereas Glueck et al.'s was mostly females [6]. There are some data which support our findings. HDL increases in athletes or in people performing sustained physical activity [13]; this is surely not the case in aged people. Also, the consumption of alcohol, a substance known for its capacity for increasing HDL [14], usually decreases in the elderly for economic reasons [15]. HDL originates from triglyceride-rich, very low-density lipoproteins through the action of a lipoprotein lipase which is synthetized by adipocytes and skeletal myocytes and then transferred to the capillary endothelium [16-18]. Adrenergic agents, especially epinephrine, increase the synthesis of lipoprotein lipase by adipocytes [19]. Lipoprotein lipase is reduced in the elderly [20], possibly due to a decline in adrenergic activity; moreover, triglycerides also decrease [20] in the elderly, thus explaining the decrease in HDL. This does not mean that the presence of high levels of HDL may not be a prerequisite for a long life. It is possible that old age is mostly reached by people who have normal or high levels of HDL in middle age, although data supporting this view are not available. In our elderly people both of the major apolipoproteins, apo A-I and apo B, decreased without any significant variation in their ratio; in our experience [21] this represents the strongest biochemical discriminator between atherosclerotic patients and controls. Our present data support the view [6] that low levels of apo B represent a major biochemical trait of the elderly, thus confirming its role as an effective discriminator and/or predictor of atherosclerotic events [21]. In the octagenarians a significantly increased value of the ratio LDL-C : apo B was also recorded. This is an interesting finding as, according to Sniderman [22] and ourselves [23], atherosclerotic patients have lower LDL-C : apo B ratios than normal individuals. The reverse of this seems to be a biochemical trait of longevity.

Females over 80 show a biochemical pattern which is more "atherogenic" than males, thus confirming a trend already described for cholesterol, triglycerides, and the main lipoprotein classes [20].

In summary, the most remarkable finding of our study is that HDL does not represent a marker of longevity but that apo B does. These data, as well as those coming from other studies [7, 8, 12], do not properly accord with the role that has been assigned to HDL as an aging factor.

References

1. Gofman JW, Young W, Tandy R (1966) Ischemic heart disease, atherosclerosis and longevity. Circulation 34: 679
2. Miller CJ, Miller NE (1975) Plasma high density lipoprotein concentration and development of ischaemic heart disease. Lancet I: 16
3. Glueck CJ, Fallat RW, Millet F, Steiner PM (1975) Familial hyperalphalipoproteinemia. Arch Int Med 136: 1025
4. Avogaro P, Cazzolato G (1975) Familial hyper-HDL-(α)-cholesterolemia. Atherosclerosis 22: 63
5. Naito HK, Lewis LA, Mac Cormack LJ, Hofstetter G, Amihanovic J (1975) Hyper-alpha-Lipoproteinemia: a case study. Clin Chem 21: 639
6. Glueck CJ, Gartside PS, Steiner PM, Miller M, Todhunter T, Haof J, Pucke M, Terrana M, Fallat RW, Kastryap ML (1977) Hyperalpha and hypobetalipoproteinemia in octogenarian kindreds. Atherosclerosis 27: 387
7. Heckers H, Burkard W, Schmahl FW, Fuhrmann W, Platt D (1982) Hyper-alpha-lipoproteinemia and hypo-beta-lipoproteinemia are not markers for a high life expertancy. Gerontology 28: 176
8. Deutscher S, Bates MW, Caines MJ, La Porte RE, Puntereri A, Taylor FH (1986) Determinants of lipid and lipoprotein level in elderly men. Atherosclerosis 60: 221
9. Kostner GM, Avogaro P, Bittolo Bon G, Cazzolato G, Quinci GB (1979) Determination of high density lipoproteins: screening methods compared. Clin Chem 25: 939
10. Friedewald TW, Levy RI, Fredrickson DS (1972) Estimation of the concentration of low density lipoprotein cholesterol in plasma without use of a preparative ultracentrifuge. Clin Chem 18: 49
11. Laurell CB (1966) Quantitative estimation of proteins by electrophoresis in agarose gel containing antibodies. Anal Biochem 15: 45
12. Pococh SJ, Shaper AG, Phillips AN, Walker M, Whitehead TP (1986) High density lipoprotein cholesterol is not a major risk factor for ischaemic heart disease in British men. Br Med J 292: 515
13. Wood PD, Williams PT, Haskell WL (1984) Physical activity and high-density lipoproteins. In: Miller NE, Miller GJ (eds) Clinical and metabolic aspects of high-density lipoproteins. Elsevier, Amsterdam, pp 133-166
14. Avogaro P, Cazzolato G (1975) Changes in the composition and physico-chemical characteristics of serum lipoproteins during ethanol-induced lipaemia in alcoholic subjects. Metabolism 24: 1231
15. Mishara BL, Kastenbaum R (1980) Alcohol and old age seminars. In: Greenblatt M (ed) Psychiatry. Academic, London
16. Ashby P, Bennet DP, Spencer IM, Robinson DS (1978) Post translational regulation of lipoprotein lipase activity in adipose tissue. Biochem J 176: 865
17. Bragby GJ, Lin MS, Spitzer JA (1977) Lipoprotein Lipase activity in rat heart myocites. Life Sci 21: 467
18. Lithell H, Lindgarde F, Mygaard E, Saltin P (1981) Capillary supply and lipoprotein-lipase activity in skeletal muscle in man. Acta Physiol Scand 111: 383
19. Ashby P, Robinson DS (1980) Effects of insulin glucocorticoids and adrenaline on the activity of rat adipose-tissue lipoprotein lipase. Biochem J 188: 1985
20. Avogaro P, Crepaldi G (1961) Aspetti del metabolismo lipidico nel vecchio. Giorn Gerontol 9: 339

21. Avogaro P, Bittolo Bon G, Cazzolato G, Quinci GB (1979) Are apolipoproteins better discriminators than lipids for atherosclerosis? Lancet I: 901
22. Sniderman AD, Wolfson C, Teng B, Franklin FA, Bachoric PS, Kwiterovich PO (1982) Association of hyperapobetalipoproteinemia with endogenous hypertriglyceridemia and atherosclerosis. Ann Intern Med 97: 833
23. Avogaro P, Bittolo Bon G, Cazzolato G, Quinci GB, Belussi F (1978) Plasma levels of apolipoprotein A-I and apolipoprotein B in human atherosclerosis. Artery 4: 385

Cholesteryl Ester Transfer, Lipoproteins, Hypertriglyceridemia, and Atherosclerosis

S. Eisenberg

Cholesteryl Ester Transfer Proteins

Cholesteryl ester (CE) and triglyceride (TG) transfer reactions in human plasma were first described more than two decades ago by Nichols and Smith [1]. The results of this study differed from earlier reports in two important respects: it showed first, that the lipids that moved between lipoproteins were the hydrophobic core-molecules, TG and CE, and secondly, that the reaction caused enrichment of the TG-rich very low density lipoprotein (VLDL) with CE, whereas the CE-rich low- and high-density lipoproteins (LDL and HDL) acquired TG molecules. The observations, however, remained almost unnoticed for another decade. Renewed interest in the reaction began when Zilversmit et al. reported in 1975 that a protein or proteins present in lipoprotein-deficient rabbit plasma [density (d) >1.25 g/ml] promoted exchange of labeled CE between VLDL and LDL from hypercholesterolemic rabbit plasma [2]. This protein has been named cholesteryl ester transfer protein (CETP) or, more properly, lipid transfer protein (LTP).

The properties of LTP, its distribution among lipoproteins, and its mechanism of action have recently been reviewed [3]. The protein has a molecular weight of approximately 60000–70000 daltons and it facilitates exchange of CE, TG, and PL molecules. Whenever tested, the three lipid transfer activities copurify during the different purification steps and are most probably mediated by the same protein. In plasma, LTP is associated mainly with HDL [4], but after centrifugation distributes equally between HDL and lipoprotein-deficient plasma ($d>1.25$ g/ml). Binding of LTP to VLDL and LDL has been demonstrated, but whereas VLDL- and LDL-LTP complexes rapidly dissociate, HDL-LTP complexes remain stable [5]. Lipid transfer activity is identified in the plasma of some, but not all, animal species [6]. High activities are found in the rabbit, possum, and trout, while low or undetectable activities are found in the rat, sheep, cow, pig, and dog. Humans have intermediate activity.

Lipid transfer reactions cause either an exchange (replacement of a molecule in a lipoprotein by the *same* molecule of another lipoprotein) or a transfer (replacement of a molecule in a lipoprotein by a *different* molecule of another lipoprotein). These two reactions have been termed homoexchange and heteroexchange respectively [5], and appear to be mediated by the same mechanism [7]. In heteroexchange reactions, the core lipid composition of both donor and acceptor lipoproteins changes; TG-rich lipoproteins lose TG molecules and acquire equimolar amounts of CE, while CE-rich lipoproteins lose CE and acquire TG molecules. It is this heteroexchange phenomenon that causes alterations of the structure, composition, and metabolism of the lipoproteins. In a recent study, we investigated the capacities of three VLDL density subfractions (VLDL-I, VLDL-II, VLDL-III) to serve as acceptors of CE from HDL, as compared with LDL [8]. The study demonstrated homoexchange of CE with all four lipoprotein fractions that was proportional to the surface area of the lipoproteins. Heteroexchange (measured by increments of CE content in the VLDL's and LDL), however, was best correlated to the TG:CE ratios of the lipoproteins and accounted for 80% of total CE transfer between HDL and VLDL-I, but only 5%-10% of total CE transfer to LDL; VLDL-II and VLDL-III exhibited intermediate behavior.

Two mechanisms have been proposed for the mode of action of LTP. The first assumes that LTP acts as a carrier of lipid molecules between lipoproteins, i.e., a ping-pong mechanism [9]. However, Ihm et al. provided evidence that LTP facilitates lipid transfer by enhancing formation of a ternary collision complex consisting of LTP, donor lipoprotein, and acceptor lipoprotein [10].

In Vitro Remodelling of Lipoproteins

Many investigators have reported that VLDL actively participates in CE transfer reactions [3]. Back-transfer of TG from VLDL to HDL and LDL has been clearly demonstrated [11, 12]. There are both homo- and heteroexchange processes, and the VLDL-CE mass increases [8]. As mentioned above, mass CE transfer is clearly related to the TG:CE ratio in the acceptor lipoproteins. Tall et al. [14] demonstrated that VLDL lipolysis by bovine milk lipoprotein lipase enhances transfer of CE from HDL to VLDL, and speculated that accumulation of fatty acids in the VLDL (and HDL) increases binding of LTP to the lipoproteins. This, in turn, enhances CE transfer [13, 14]. CE transfer to VLDL and chlomicrons also takes place in vivo. Nestel et al. calculated that the apparent flux of CE from HDL to VLDL is similar to reported values for total cholesterol esterification in human plasma in vivo [15]. Thus, most or even all of the lecithin:cholesterol acyl transferase (LCAT)-derived CE in human plasma is metabolized after being transferred to TG-rich lipoproteins.

Heteroexchange of CE and TG between LDL and VLDL has been studied in depth by us [16-18]. More than half of the CE molecules in LDL are replaced by TG after 18 h incubation of LDL with VLDL and a LTP source [16, 18]. This change of core lipid composition is associated with a change of the surface composition of the LDL, and the LTP-modified LDL (M-LDL) acquires apoprotein (apo) AI, apo C, and apo E from the VLDL and/or the lipoprotein-deficient plasma fraction. Next, we attempted to deplete the M-LDL of transferred TG molecules by adding lipoprotein lipase to the incubation mixture. More than 80% of M-LDL-TG could be hydrolyzed. This resulted in the composition of M-LDL changing towards that of the native CE-rich lipoprotein, with loss of the added apoproteins. However, the postlipolysis M-LDL was significantly smaller than either M-LDL or the native LDL. Thus, the cycle of transfer and lipolysis resulted in net loss of core lipids from the LDL. Two other observations are worth mentioning: first, the artificial TG lipid emulsion, Intralipid, is as active in similar experiments as VLDL [19], indicating that none of the VLDL-specific constituents (e.g., apoproteins) is necessary, and secondly, CE-depleted, TG-enriched LDL is less effective than native LDL in regulating cellular cholesterol synthesis and LDL-receptor activity [18].

Remodeling of HDL particles by varying the amounts of core lipids - predominantly CE - is a process responsible for the regulation of HDL subpopulation (HDL_1, HDL_2, HDL_3, HDL_4) distribution [20, 21]. In this complex cycle, supply of free cholesterol and phospholipid (from lipolysis and cell membranes), together with LCAT, is responsible for conversion of the small, dense HDL_3 to HDL_2 [21, 22], while heteroexchange of CE and TG in HDL_2 followed by hydrolysis of transferred TG causes a reverse conversion of HDL_2 to HDL_3 [20, 21]. The events occurring during the reverse-conversion process were recently reported by us [23]. Using systems similar to those described above for LDL, human HDL_2 was incubated with human VLDL in the presence of LTP sources. As with LDL, HDL_2 lost CE to, and acquired TG from, VLDL. The modified HDL_2 then lost most of the acquired TG molecules after incubation with either hepatic lipase or bovine milk lipoprotein lipase. After repetitive in vitro cycles of incubating HDL_2 with VLDL and LTP followed by M-HDL_2 lipolysis, HDL_2 became more like HDL_3, as judged by the increased density, and decreased CE content (by ⅔) and particle size [23]. Although in these cycles both lipoprotein lipase and the hepatic lipase were active against HDL-TG, in vivo it is the latter enzyme that most probably is responsible for the reverse-conversion process.

In Vivo Effects of Lipid Transfer Reactions

Until recently the metabolic implications of lipid transfer processes, if any, were obscure. Yet, it was clear that transfer of CE and TG molecules between lipoproteins must affect the structure, composition, and metabolism of the particle. For example, addition or deletion of CE molecules is a process that must affect the function of lipoproteins, e.g., their capacity to regulate cellular metabolic pathways. Elucidation of such metabolic consequences of lipid transfer processes, has, surprisingly, begun only in the last few years, when studies of three in vivo models have been initiated: plasma lipoproteins in rats, an animal species devoid of lipid transfer; human patients with abetalipoproteinemia, when acceptors for CE are absent; and patients with hypertriglyceridemia (HTG), a condition with presumed excessive lipid transfer. These data are discussed according to the various lipoproteins investigated.

Very Low Density Lipoproteins. Data on the structure and composition of VLDL that can be related to the LTP reaction are available in rats and in humans with HTG. In rats, VLDL contains only a few CE molecules, 1.5%-2.5% of total lipoprotein mass [24], and the fatty acid pattern of VLDL-CE indicates the hepatic origin of these molecules. The structure and composition of VLDL from subjects with HTG before and after initiation of lipid-lowering therapy (with bezafibrate) was recently reported [25]. As compared with normal VLDL (N-VLDL), VLDL from subjects with HTG (HTG-VLDL) contains less protein, more free and esterified cholesterol and less TG, but no change is found for total phospholipids. These abnormalities are strongly and significantly related to plasma TG levels and revert towards normal when TG-lowering therapy is instituted. In a subsequent study [26], VLDL was fractionated into three populations. Of the three, VLDL-I, the fraction containing the largest and least dense particles, was found to be the most abnormal. HTG-VLDL-III, in contrast, was almost normal, while HTG-VLDL-II was moderately abnormal. It thus appears that abnormalities of the large VLDL particles are responsible for most of the abnormalities of HTG-VLDL. The metabolic processes that are responsible for enrichment of HTG-VLDL with CE are presumably related to an excessive lipid transfer process. Experiments carried out in vitro [8] demonstrated the high capacity of VLDL-I to serve as an acceptor of CE and donor of TG in lipid transfer reactions. VLDL-II had a moderate capacity to participate in the reaction, while VLDL-III had the least. It is therefore possible that in vivo, during their prolonged circulating lives, large VLDL particles become excessively enriched with CE molecules.

Two abnormalities of VLDL metabolism are common to all HTG patients, regardless of disease entity, experimental procedure, or method of analysis [27]. One is a slow delipidation rate, and the other a decreased fractional conversion of VLDL apo B to LDL apo B. The first abnormality reflects most probably the pathogenesis of HTG states; the absolutely, or relatively (to high synthetic rates) decreased rates of VLDL-TG transport. The metabolic basis of the reduced VLDL→LDL conversion is possibly due to the excessive CE content of HTG-VLDL. To test this hypothesis, we determined the structure and composition of "in vitro LDL" produced by nearly complete TG hydrolysis of three VLDL subfractions (I, II, and III) obtained from normal and HTG human subjects [26]. LDL-like particles (by density, diameter, and lipid and protein composition) are produced from all three N-VLDL fractions. By contrast in HTG, LDL-like particles are found only after lipolysis of VLDL-III. Neither VLDL-I nor VLDL-II (especially the former) produce LDL-like particles, in spite of almost complete TG hydrolysis (>95%). Postlipolysis VLDL-I and VLDL-II in such patients is enriched with CE, less dense, and much larger than LDL. These data suggest that the bulk of HTG-VLDL-I and -II cannot form LDL and is degraded independently of the LDL pathway. Hence, in HTG states, only VLDL-III is the source of LDL. We suggest that with therapy, VLDL delipidation rate is accelerated, less CE molecules are transferred to VLDL (especially VLDL-I and VLDL-II), and more VLDL particles complete the VLDL→LDL conversion pathway.

Low-Density Lipoproteins. Abnormalities of LDL in HTG states have been reported by several investigators [25, 28]. In our study [25], LDL from 16 patients with HTG (plasma TG 245–2500 mg/dl) was analyzed before and during TG-lowering therapy. In a zonal ultracentrifugation system, HTG-LDL separates into two or even three populations. The main LDL (corresponding to N-LDL) was further characterized. HTG-LDL is denser than N-LDL, relatively enriched with protein (predominantly apo B) and TG, and contains significantly less free and esterified cholesterol. In addition, HTG-LDL is smaller (by electron microscopy) than N-LDL, and diameters less than 170 nm (normal is 210–220 nm) are found. These six abnormalities are strongly and significantly related to the degree of triglyceridemia, and tend to revert towards normal when plasma TG is reduced. Of the six abnormalities we focused on the cholesterol content of the lipoprotein. On the basis of regression analysis of the change of LDL core-volume and CE: protein (apo B) ratio we were able to demonstrate a reduced content of cholesterol molecules in HTG-LDL that was curvilinearly related to plasma TG levels [29]. We believe that the abnormal density, composition, and size of HTG-LDL are best explained by excessive lipid transfers between a large pool of slowly turning-over, TG-rich lipoproteins in a system with normal, or even low, rates of LDL production.

The compositional analysis predicts that the catabolism of HTG-LDL is abnormal, and that this abnormality reflects the loss of free and esterified cholesterol from the lipoprotein. This is expected even on theoretical grounds alone. As HTG-LDL is a cholesterol-poor lipoprotein, it should down-regulate cellular receptor activity and cholesterol synthesis less efficiently than N-LDL [30]. Recently, we initiated a series of investigations on the ability of HTG-LDL to regulate LDL receptor activity and cholesterol synthesis in cultured human skin fibroblasts [31]. HTG-LDL exhibits a lower affinity for the apo B, E receptor and is a less efficient regulator of cellular sterol synthesis and cellular receptor activity than N-LDL. These abnormalities are strongly and significantly correlated with the cholesterol content of the LDL and revert towards normal when bezafibrate therapy is instituted. More recently, we determined the actual metabolism of HTG-LDL in regulated cells (unpublished observations). The rate of cellular metabolism of HTG-LDL in cells regulated by HTG-LDL is higher than that of N-LDL in cells regulated by N-LDL. It thus appears that cells exposed to HTG-LDL contain more receptors than cells exposed to N-LDL and degrade considerable amounts of LDL, in spite of the reduced affinity of the LDL for the receptor. The molecular basis for the defective affinity of HTG-LDL for the receptor is yet unknown. This phenomenon must reflect reversible conformational changes of the apo B moiety in HTG-LDL, and this was demonstrated by us in experiments using monoclonal antibodies specific for the receptor-binding domain of apo B [32]. The abnormality of HTG-LDL responsible for the change in apo B, however, remains to be elucidated.

High-Density Lipoproteins. Data on the structure and composition of HDL related either to the absence or excess of lipid transfers are available in humans with abetalipoproteinemia [20], in rats [24], and in human subjects with HTG states [25]. Lessons learnt from all three models have established that core-lipid transfer reactions are the principal modulators of the HDL subpopulation distribution [21]. In abetalipoproteinemia, a condition where chylomicrons, VLDL, and LDL are absent, HDL levels are low, but most of the HDL is associated with an abnormally large, light density, and CE-rich HDL_2, the ABL-HDL_2 [52]. ABL-HDL_3 is also CE enriched [20]. All these deviations from normal are compatible with accretion of LCAT-derived CE molecules in the HDL system, and conversion of small particles into larger ones. Rat HDL is composed of two populations, HDL_2 and HDL_1 [24]. The dense, small HDL_3 has not been identified. Again, these findings are best explained by the absence of LTP activity. A converse situation is found in HTG where excessive transfer between an expanded pool of TG-rich lipoproteins and HDL takes place. In our studies we showed dense, TG-rich, and CE-poor HDL_3 in groups of patients with HTG [25, 33]. These abnormalities are strongly related to plasma TG levels and tend to revert towards normal when TG-lowering therapy (with bezafibrate) is instituted. These findings in HTG are best explained by the mechanism discussed above, i.e., heteroexchange of HDL-CE and VLDL-TG, followed by hydrolysis of the transferred TG molecules.

Taking advantage of the absence of LTP activity in the rat, we have determined the in vivo metabolism of rat plasma lipoproteins labeled in their CE moiety. Using [^{3}H]-CE-labeled rat plasma HDL_2, we showed conversion of some HDL_2 particles to HDL_1 [34]. More recently, we used [^{3}H]CE-labeled human HDL_3 in a similar experimental system [35]. Conversions of the HDL_3 first to HDL_2 and then to apo E-HDL_1 were documented. The experiments were then repeated in rats pre-injected with human LTP. LTP had only a minimal effect on $HDL_3 \rightarrow HDL_2$ conversion, probably because of the rapidity (30-60 min) of this process. However, formation of HDL_1 was markedly affected and the amount of HDL_1 formed during 18 h of circulation was reduced to about one-half. Extrapolation of these in vivo investigations in the rat to the human predicts that HDL subpopulation distribution indeed reflects processes of CE enrichment and removal occurring along a size and density gradient.

Cholesteryl Ester Transfer, Lipoprotein Remodeling, and Atherogenesis

The data and concepts described above have dealt predominantly with individual lipoproteins. Plasma lipid transport in lipoproteins, however, must be viewed as one system where each component is part of a whole. In plasma, chylomicrons, VLDL, IDL, LDL, HDL, and their subclasses are all simultaneously exposed to and affected by lipid transfer processes. LTPs facilitate transfer of TG, phospholipid and CE molecules. In human plasma, redistributions of TG and CE begin as soon as the nascent lipoproteins enter the plasma compartment and continue throughout their circulating lives. TG distributions cause mainly structural and compositional alterations of all lipoproteins but may also affect metabolic routes, e.g., LDL metabolism. CE distributions have immediate metabolic implications, that are possibly related to atheroma formation and development of atherosclerotic diseases. The best example is the lipoprotein system in HTG states where excessive TG and CE transfers occur. Figure 1 illustrates the effects of CE redistribution on plasma cholesterol clearance in normal subjects and in patients with HTG. Let us begin with LDL and HDL. In normotriglyceridemic subjects, an amount of cholesterol and CE (estimated to be 1.5-2.5 g/day) is cleared from the plasma, with irreversible degradation of LDL and HDL. In patients with HTG, however, considerably less cholesterol is cleared from the plasma with these two lipoproteins, even if their degradation is accelerated. That is inferred from the consideration that if normal amounts of cholesterol enter cells (with a larger number of HTG-LDL particles), then LDL-receptor activity would be down-regulated to normal level. Hence, even in the face of accelerated LDL catabolism, the equilibrium reached is bound to reflect subnormal clearance of plasma cholesterol with the lipoprotein. The same considerations lead to the conclusion that cholesterol clearance with HDL in subjects with HTG is also subnormal. Therefore, in patients with HTG, an additional pathway for removal of cholesterol from plasma must exist, and the amounts of cholesterol cleared by that pathway must be quite substantial. Our own studies indicate that direct catabolism of cholesterol- and CE-rich VLDL or VLDL remnants in

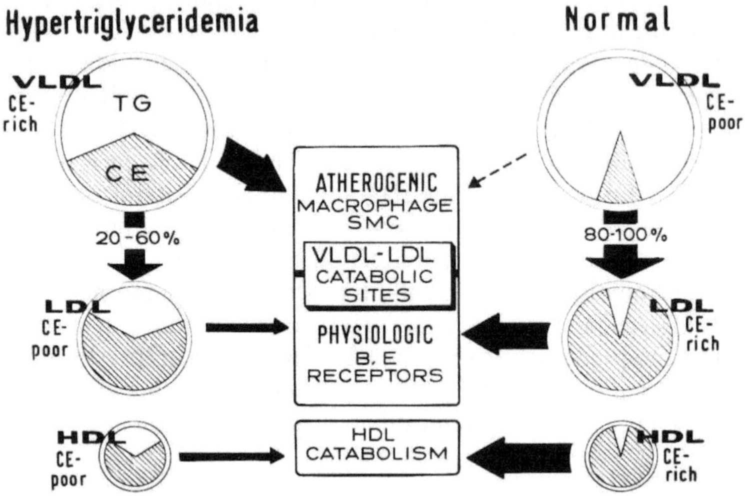

Fig. 1. Effects of cholesterol redistribution on lipoprotein metabolism in normo- and hypertriglyceridemeic states. In the normal state VLDL→LDL conversion is nearly complete, and cholesterol (free and esterified) leaves the plasma mainly with LDL and HDL. It is suggested that the LDL and HDL catabolic routes are nonatherogenic. In HTG, LDL and HDL contain subnormal amounts of cholesterol and do not clear from plasma as much cholesterol as normal lipoproteins. Excess cholesterol (predominantly esterified) is present in VLDL. Such VLDL particles do not complete the VLDL→LDL conversion path and are cleared by alternative routes (macrophages, smooth muscle cell [SMC]) that are potentially atherogenic

HTG provides an "escape" mechanism responsible for the clearance from plasma of cholesterol that is normally catabolyzed with LDL and HDL. Indeed, both fibroblasts and macrophages were shown to degrade large VLDL particles (VLDL-I and VLDL-II) isolated from human subjects with HTG but not from normal subjects [36]. Degradation of β-VLDL-III in macrophages [37] may represent the extreme situation of inefficient VLDL→LDL conversion, and LDL-independent VLDL catabolism. Figure 1 suggests that the pathway is atherogenic although this suggestion remains to be tested.

References

1. Nichols AV, Smith L (1965) J Lipid Res 6: 206-210
2. Zilversmit DB, Hughes LB, Balmer J (1975) Biochim Biophys Acta 409: 393-398
3. Tall AR (1986) J Lipid Res 27: 359-365
4. Pattnaik NM, Zilversmit DB (1979) J Biol Chem 254: 2782-2786
5. Morton RE (1985) J Biol Chem 260: 12593-12599
6. Ha YC, Barter PJ (1982) Comp Biochem Physiol 71 B: 265-269
7. Morton RE, Zilversmit DB (1983) J Biol Chem 258: 11751-11757
8. Eisenberg S (1985) J Lipid Res 26: 487-494
9. Barter PJ, Jones ME (1980) J Lipid Res 21: 238-249
10. Ihm J, Quinn DM, Busch SJ, Chataing B, Harmony JAK (1982) J Lipid Res 23: 1328-1341
11. Hopkins GJ, Barter PJ (1980) Metabolism 29: 546-550
12. Eisenberg S, Perret B (1981) Arteriosclerosis 1: 363a
13. Castro GR, Fielding CJ (1985) J Clin Invest 75: 874-882

14. Tall A, Sammett D, Granot E (1986) J Clin Invest 77: 1163-1172
15. Nestel PJ, Reardon M, Billington T (1979) Biochim Biophys Acta 573: 403-407
16. Deckelbaum RJ, Eisenberg S, Oschry Y, Butbul E, Sharon I, Olivecrona T (1982) J Biol Chem 257: 6509-6517
17. Deckelbaum RJ, Olivecrona T, Eisenberg S (1984) In: Carlson LA, Olsson AG (eds) Treatment of hyperlipoproteinemia. Raven, New York, pp 85-93
18. Chait A, Eisenberg S, Steinmetz A, Albers J, Bierman EL (1984) Biochim Biophys Acta 795: 314-325
19. Granot E, Deckelbaum RJ, Eisenberg S, Oschry Y, Bengtsson-Olivecrona G (1985) Biochim Biophys Acta 833: 308-315
20. Deckelbaum RJ, Eisenberg S, Oschry Y, Cooper M, Blum C (1982) J Lipid Res 23: 1274-1282
21. Eisenberg S (1984) J Lipid Res 25: 1017-1058
22. Patsch JR, Gotto AM, Olivecrona T, Eisenberg S (1978) Proc Natl Acad Sci USA 75: 4519-4523
23. Deckelbaum RJ, Eisenberg S, Oschry Y, Granot E, Sharon I, Bengtsson-Olivecrona G (1986) J Biol Chem 261: 5201-5208
24. Ihm J, Ellsworth JL, Chataing B, Harmony JAK (1982) J Biol Chem 257: 4818-4827
25. Eisenberg S, Gavish D, Oschry Y, Fainaru M, Deckelbaum RJ (1984) J Clin Invest 74: 470-482
26. Oschry Y, Olivecrona T, Deckelbaum RJ, Eisenberg S (1985) J Lipid Res 26: 158-167
27. Eisenberg S (1987) Lipoprotein abnormalities in hypertriglyceridemia: Significance in atherosclerosis. Am Heart 113. January 1987
28. Vakakis N, Redgrave TG, Small DM (1983) Biochim Biophys Acta 751: 280-285
29. Eisenberg S (1985) Adv Exp Med Biol 183: 73-84
30. Brown MS, Goldstein JL (1986) Science 232: 34-47
31. Kleinman Y, Eisenberg S, Oschry Y, Gavish D, Stein O, Stein Y (1985) J Clin Invest 75: 1796-1803
32. Kleinman Y, Schonfeld G, Gavish D, Oschry Y, Eisenberg S (1987) J Lipid Res 27 (in press)
33. Deckelbaum RJ, Granot E, Oschry Y, Rose L, Eisenberg S (1984) Arteriosclerosis 4: 226-231
34. Eisenberg S, Oschry Y, Zimmerman J (1984) J Lipid Res 25: 122-128
35. Gavish D, Oschry Y, Eisenberg S (1987) J Lipid Res 27 (in press)
36. Gianturco SH, Gotto AM Jr, Hwang SLC, Karlin JB, Lin AHY, Prasad SC, Bradley WA (1983) J Biol Chem 258: 4526-4533
37. Fainaru M, Mahley RW, Hamilton RL, Innerarity TL (1982) J Lipid Res 23: 702-714

Importance of Hypertriglyceridemia as an Independent Risk Factor: Investigations with Familial Combined Hyperlipidemia and Familial Hypertriglyceridemia

M. Hanefeld

Introduction

Hypertriglyceridemia (HTG) is one of the most common metabolic abnormalities in adults of industrialized countries with overnutrition and a low level of physical activity. In the Dresden study [10] 10% of the population exhibited triglyceride levels $\geqslant 2.3$ mmol/l. Geographic epidemiology clearly shows a parallel between the prevalence of atherosclerosis and HTG. So far, the epidemiological evidence of the importance of HTG as risk factor is mainly from two types of studies, prospective population-based studies and case-control investigations in high-risk groups.

Population Studies

The association of HTG and coronary heart disease (CHD) is generally accepted. In 11 of 12 large-scale prospective studies reviewed by Lippel et al. [15], univariate analysis showed that elevated TG at entry was a risk factor. Multivariate analysis of these data, however, confirmed HTG as independent risk factor for CHD solely in the Stockholm study [3]. Therefore, the causal hypothesis was rejected by several investigators [11, 17], who requested more evidence before intervention could be recommended. From the geographic point of view, the majority of studies from Scandinavia and central Europe [3, 7, 8] favour an independent role of HTG whereas those from North America [13] do not.

Case-Control Studies

Investigations of survivors of myocardial infarction consistently show that there is a two to five times higher prevalence of HTG among these patients than in controls [7]. This has been confirmed in subjects with coronarogragraphy. Patients with advanced sclerotic lesions exhibit significantly higher triglyceride levels than those with or without mild vascular changes [16, 24]. However, multivariate analysis in this type of study has yielded controversial results [21] with respect to HTG as an independent risk factor.

Type II diabetics with newly manifested ischemic heart disease (IHD) in the diabetes intervention study [20, 9] are characterized by higher TG levels at entry than their counterparts without IHD. This finding is in accordance with most but not all investigations in diabetics concerning the significance of HTG for macroangiopathy [12].

Primary hypertriglyceridemics represent another risk group; HTG is associated with an excessive incidence of myocardial infarction, as shown by a follow-up study of patients with massive hyperlipidemias [8] (Table 1). In this study the correction of elevated TG was associated with a remarkably lower incidence of fatal myocardial infarction and total mortality in comparison with the subset of patients with insufficient control (Table 2).

One explanation for the high incidence of myocardial infarction among the patients with HTG (Table 1) is the fact that the majority represent phenotypic expression of familial combined hyperlipidemia, as described later. The results of our intervention study demonstrate the benefit of substantial triglyceride-lowering treatment. The incidence of myocardial infarction was more than 10 times higher than in the general population of that age range in the GDR [2]. With respect to secondary prevention, drug treatment of HTG in survivors of myocardial infarction (Carlson and Rosenhamer, cited in [24]) resulted in a reduction of coronary death by about 50% in the drug group (32/214) versus diet-treated controls (59/216).

By extrapolation, there are four major difficulties in the evaluation of whether HTG is an independent risk factor or only a marker for CHD. (1) Triglycerides are inextricably connected with at least two other risk factors, high-density lipoprotein

Table 1. Incidence of atherosclerotic vascular diseases per 100 patient years in massive hyperlipoproteinemia (HLP): the Dresden HLP study [8]

	Hyper-cholesterolemia (n=80)	Hyper-triglyceridemia (n=90)	Mixed HLP (n=90)	P
Angina pectoris	2.45	1.19	1.98	NS
Myocardial infarction	0.44	2.57	1.78	0.05
Stroke	0.44	0.60	0.40	NS

Incidence of myocardial infarction for the GDR in the general population 0.18 per 100 person years.

Table 2. Total and myocardial infarction (MI) mortality in massive HLP per 100 patient years in relation to lipid control (average values after 2 years of treatment): the Dresden HLP study [8]

Category of lipid control		Total mortality	Fatal MI
Triglycerides			
perfect	(<2.3 mmol/l)	1.16[b]	0.43[a]
insufficient	(>4.0 mmol/l)	4.36[b]	2.29[a]
Cholesterol			
perfect	(<6.5 mmol/l)	1.73	0.72
insufficient	(>10.3 mmol/l)	3.06	2.29

[a] Significantly different, $P<0.005$.
[b] Significantly different, $P<0.001$.

(HDL) cholesterol and serum insulin. Thus, the use of multivariate logistic regression analysis is problematic since multivariate methods a are based on the assumption that the variables considered are independent from each other. (2) The endpoints used strongly influence the result since definite myocardial infarction and angina pectoris for example differ in their relation to HTG [1]. Thus, studies using myocardial infarction as the reference disease confirm HTG as independent risk factor [4] whereas those which pooled angina pectoris, changes in ECG and myocardial infarction did not [19]. (3) Furthermore, triglyceride concentrations in fasting plasma are strongly influenced by multiple environmental factors resulting in great intraindividual variations. In a follow-up study [14] we found a day-to-day variation of 12%, week-to-week variation of 19%, and variation of 35% after 3.5 years. This is one explanation for the limited relevance of casual triglyceride measurements. Thus, standardized examination conditions and repeated measurements are of particular importance. (4) There is a great heterogeneity of lipoprotein disorders expressing as HTG, with distinct differences not only in the pattern and composition of the lipoprotein fractions but also in their synthesis and catabolism. These will be discussed in chapters by Eisenberg (see pp. 132–139) and Crepaldi/Manzato (see pp. 147–152).

Genetic Hypertriglyceridemias and Atherosclerosis

Investigations of defined types of genetic HTG are a rational approach to evaluate the significance of HTG as a risk marker or causal factor, and to identify forms where preventive measures are indicated. For this purpose we performed family examinations of 116 consecutive index cases with HTG type IV of the Dresden lipid clinic. Selection criteria were two fasting TG values ⩾2.9 mmol/l, cholesterol <7.8 mmol/l and a type IV pattern in lipid electrophoresis (PAGE). Exclusion criteria were secondary HTG and combination with overt diabetes. The distribution of different froms of HTG is shown in Fig. 1. The findings suggest that HTG type IV usually represents the phenotypic expression of familial combined hyperlipidemia (fCHL) and that fCHL and familial HTG (fHTG) are the most common forms of genetic HTG in the patients of the Dresden lipid clinic. We therefore analysed the risk factor profile and IHD prevalence in first-degree relatives (FDR) of index cases with fHTG ($n = 29$) and fCHL ($n = 66$), and normolipidemic spouses ($n = 26$) of FDR of patients with HTG. Cut-off points for HTG in adults were TG ⩾2.3 mmol/l and cholesterol <7.8 mmol/l, and ⩾1.7 mmol/l and cholesterol <6.2 mmol/l for probands below 21 years. The baseline characteristics of the study probands are given in Table 3. Affected FDR in general are significantly older and

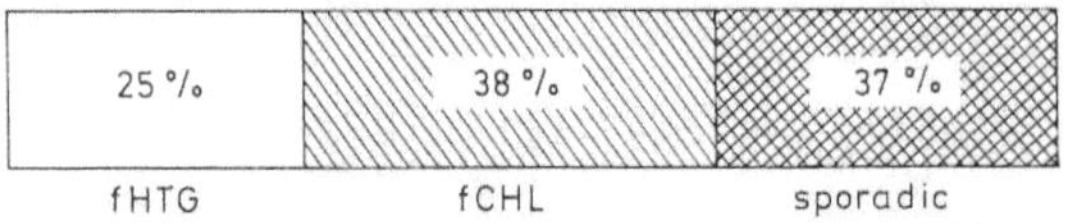

Fig. 1. Distribution of HTG forms among 116 consecutive index cases with HTG (TG ⩾2.3 mmol/l), excluding of type III and V

exhibit a higher weight index and blood pressure than their nonaffected relatives. The distribution of affected FDR fits well with a dominant inheritance of both forms of HTG. The family history with respect to major cardiovascular events reveals a higher incidence of these diseases in patients with fHTG or fCHL in comparison with spouses (Table 4). Presumably because of the high cardiovascular risk, the parents and grandparents of the index cases with HTG have a shorter life expectancy than the general population (Table 5). To reduce bias caused by the improvement of medical care, we excluded deaths before 30 years of age and subjects who

Table 3. Baseline characteristics ($\bar{x}$ ± SEM) of the investigated groups

Subgroup	No. males	No. females	Age (years)	Blood pressure (mmHg)		Ideal weight index
				Systolic	Diastolic	
fHTG						
Affected	19	19	41.6 ± 20.5	140 ± 26[a,b]	84 ± 15	1.22 ± 0.2[a,b]
Normolipidemic	24	25	39.3 ± 20.5	129 ± 17	84 ± 8	1.11 ± 0.19
HTG	20	13	46.7 ± 16.7	146 ± 26	87 ± 10	1.23 ± 0.19
HC	23	38	39.7 ± 18.99	131 ± 18	80 ± 12	1.16 ± 0.18
Mixed HLP	16	13	46.9 ± 15.6	139 ± 22	87 ± 8	1.21 ± 0.16
All fCHL	59	64	43.1 ± 17.9[a]	137 ± 21[a,c]	83 ± 11	1.18 ± 0.18
Normolipidemic	39	56	37.3 ± 18.2	131 ± 19	82 ± 9	1.14 ± 0.19
Spouses	2	24	41.1 ± 6.7	123 ± 17	81 ± 10	1.12 ± 0.18

[a] $P < 0.05$ affected vs. normolipidemic. [b] $P < 0.05$. [c] $P < 0.01$ affected vs. spouses.

Table 4. Major cardiovascular events (%) in the medical history of the family (absolute numbers in parentheses)

	fHTG ($n = 29$)	fCHL ($n = 66$)	Spouses ($n = 33$)
Myocardial infarction	55.2 (16)[a]	37.1 (25)[a]	12.1 (4)
Stroke	37.9 (11)[a]	22.7 (15)[c]	6.1 (2)
Peripheral arterial disease	35.5 (10)	30.1 (20)	18.2 (6)

[a] $P < 0.01$. [b] $P < 0.05$ vs. spouses. [c] $P < 0.01$ vs. fHTG.

Table 5. Average age at death of parents and grandparents of subjects with familial hypertriglyceridemia in comparison with the life expectancy of the GDR population (people older than 30 years, excluding unnatural causes of death)

	Males		Females	
	n	Age (years)	*n*	Age (years)
fHTG	15	67.1	12	71.2
fCHL	37	63.2[a]	29	68.1[a]
Population	94607	72.3	120928	76.7

[a] $P < 0.001$.

had 'unnatural' deaths. Our data for fCHL fit well with calculations from the WHO Health Statistics Report [25] with respect to life shortening by cardiovascular diseases. Of course, more data with larger sample sizes are needed before these findings can be generalized, especially for fHTG. ECG examination has shown a significantly higher percentage of IHD (according to Minnesota classification codes 1.1-1.3, 4.1-4.3, 5.1-5.3, 6.1, 6.2, 7.1, and 8.3) in affected FDR with HTG compared with nonaffected FDR and spouses (Fig. 2). Both forms of HTG seem to be equally affected. The subjects with IHD, however, also were significantly older, had higher systolic blood pressure and higher body weight. Tobacco consumption was not a significant discriminator. To elucidate the importance of HTG as an independent risk factor we looked for statistical 'twins' for FDR with IHD among their counterparts without IHD. For this purpose probands were matched for age, sex, and blood pressure (Table 6).

Matched-pair analysis was used to overcome the problems with multiple-regression analysis caused by the clustering of interrelated risk factors which is typical for both

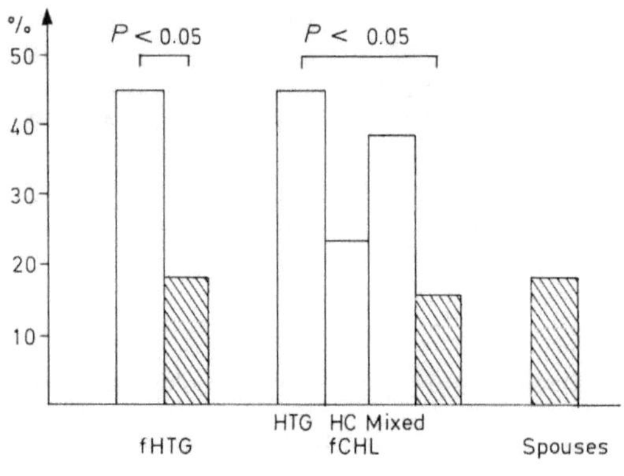

Fig. 2. Prevalence of IHD (Minnesota codes) in first degree relatives of index cases with fHTG or fHCL, and spouses. ▭, Affected; ▨, normolipidemic; *HC*, phenotypic hypercholesterolemia

Table 6. Triglycerides and cholesterol as predictors of IHD prevalence in first-degree relatives of index cases with fHTG and fCHL: matched pairs for age, sex, and hypertension

	fCHL (30 pairs)		fHTG (8 pairs)	
	with IHD	without IHD	with IHD	without IHD
Age (years)	48.1 ± 14.3	47.4 ± 13.9	44.1 ± 16.5	43.3 ± 18.7
Blood pressure (mmHg)				
Systolic	139 ± 21	130 ± 18	138 ± 25	133 ± 15
Diastolic	83 ± 7	81 ± 8	82 ± 13	81 ± 7
Triglycerides (mmol/l)	2.21 ± 1.36[b]	1.64 ± 1.09	3.72 ± 3.66[a]	1.53 ± 0.86
Total cholesterol (mmol/l)	7.89 ± 1.56[c]	6.93 ± 1.55	6.02 ± 1.74	5.63 ± 0.87

[a] $P < 0.1$. [b] $P < 0.05$. [c] $P < 0.01$.

forms of HTG. The results favour of an independent role of HTG as a risk factor for both forms of HTG. In seven out of the eight pairs of the fHTG subset, triglycerides were distinctly higher in FDR with IHD.

Conclusions

Our investigations cannot give a definite answer with respect to a causal role of HTG as coronary risk factor. However, the high prevalence of cardiovascular complications in the family history, the shortened life expectancy in the parental and grandparental generations of index cases, and the higher prevalence of ECG changes in affected FDR in comparison with nonaffected FDR, favour this hypothesis, in particular with respect to HTG as a phenotypic expression of fCHL. Moreover, our data for fCHL, as well as for fHTG, persuasively show that people with HTG are a high-risk group, since HTG, for many reasons, is a sensitive marker of atherogenic disturbances in lipoprotein metabolism [18] of hyperinsulinemia [23], and of coagulation alterations [5] which must be treated. Inclusion of HDL cholesterol and apo lipoprotein B [22] in prospective studies and kinetic investigations [18] could contribute to identifying subgroups of fHTG which actually need no preventive measures. Since no genetic marker exists so far, the epidemiological evidence, including intervention studies, together with the growing recognition [8] that a high percentage of triglyceride-rich lipoproteins in most patients with HTG is catabolised via the scavenger pathway that favors the deposition of cholesterol in the vascular wall, suggests that measures to correct HTG are a rational approach in the prevention of coronary heart disease.

References

1. Aberg H, Lithell H, Selinus J, Hedstrand H (1985) Serum triglycerides are a risk factor for myocardial infarction but not for angina pectoris. Atherosclerosis 54: 89
2. Böthig S, Schneider J, Schaedel H (1972) Herzinfarktregister Berlin, Erfurt, Pasewalk-Konzeption und Zwischenergebnisse. Dtsch Gesundh-Wesen 27: 1501
3. Carlson LA, Böttiger LL, Anfeldt FC (1979) Risk factors in the Stockholm prospective study. Acta Med Scand 206: 351
4. Carlson LA, Böttiger L (1981) Serum triglycerides, to be or not to be a risk factor for ischaemic heart disease? Atherosclerosis 37: 287
5. Cucuianu M (1985) Hyperlipoproteinemia and hemostatic variables. In Haller H, Hanefeld M, Jaross W, Leonhardt W, Dude H (eds) Advances in lipoprotein and atherosclerosis research, diagnostics and treatment. Proceeding of the 5th international, Dresden lipid symposium, p 394
6. Eisenberg S (1986) Physiology and pathophysiology of plasma triglyceride transport: role of lipid exchange reactions. In: Fidge NH, Nestel PJ (eds) Atherosclerosis vol 7. Elsevier, p 209
7. Goldstein J, Schrott HG, Hazzard WR, Bierman E, Motulsky AG (1973) Hyperlipidemia in coronary heart disease II. Genetic analysis of lipid levels in 176 families and delineation of a new inherited disorder combined hyperlipidemia. J Clin Invest 52: 1544
8. Hanefeld M, Hora C, Schulze J, Rothe G, Barthel U, Haller H (1984) Reduced incidence of cardiovascular complications and mortality in hyperlipoproteinemia (HLP) with effective lipid correction Atherosclerosis 53: 47
9. Hanefeld M, Schulze J, Fischer S, Schmechel G, Julius U, Dude H, Vater H, Haller H, the DIS Group (1986) The diabetes interventions study (DIS): a prospective intervention trial in type II diabetes. In Fidge NH, Nestel PJ (eds) Atherosclerosis vol 7. Elsevier, p 557

10. Hanefeld M, Leonhardt W, Haller H, Moser W (1973) Häufigkeit und Interrelationen metabolischer Risikofaktoren: Die Dresdner Studie. Dtsch Gesundh-Wesen 28: 1585
11. Hulley SB, Rosenman R, Bawel R, Brand R (1980) Epidemiology as a guide to decisions. The association between triglyceride and coronary heart disease. N Engl J Med 302: 1383
12. Janka HU, Grünwald P, Waldmann G, Standl E, Mehnert H (1984) Kardiovaskuläre Risikofaktoren bei Typ I und Typ II Diabetikern: Die Schwabinger Studie. Acta Endocrinol 4: 85
13. Kannel WB, Castelli W, Gordon T (1979) Cholesterol in the production of atherosclerotic disease. New perspectives based on the Framingham Study. Ann Intern Med 90: 85
14. Leonhardt W, Hanefeld M (1981) Intraindividuelle Variation der Cholesterol- und Triglyceridkonzentrationen im menschlichen Serum. Dtsch Gesundh-Wesen 36: 618
15. Lippel K, Tyroler H, Eder H, Gotto A, Vahouny G (1981) Relationship of hypertriglyceridemia to atherosclerosis. Arteriosclerosis 1: 406
16. Murray R, Tweddel A, Hird J, Hutton J, Hillis W, Lorimer A, Lawre T (1975) Relation between exent of coronary artery disease and severity of hyperlipoproteinemia. Br Heart J 37: 1205
17. NIH (1984) NIH consensus development summary. Arteriosclerosis 4: 296
18. Oschry Y, Olivecrona T, Deckelbaum R, Eisenberg S (1985) Is hypertriglyceridemic very low density lipoprotein a precursor of normal low density lipoprotein? J Lipid Res 26: 158
19. Rosenman RH, Brand R, Jenkins C, Friedman M, Straus R (1975) Coronary heart disease in the Western Collaborative Group Study. J Am Med Ass 233
20. Schmechel H, Schwanebeck U, Lippold C, Hanefeld M, the DIS Group (1985) Metabolic and clinical findings in newly manifested type II diabetics with myocardial infarction during a four year follow up period. In Haller H, Hanefeld M, Jaross W, Leonhardt W, Dude H (eds) Advances in lipoprotein and atherosclerosis research, diagnostics and treatment. Proceedings of the 5th international Dresden lipid symposium, p 357
21. Schmidt S, Wasserman A, Muesing R, Schlesselman S, Larosa J, Ross A (1985) Lipoprotein and apolipoprotein levels in angiographically defined coronary atherosclerosis. Am J Cardiol 55: 1459
22. Sniderman A, Wolfson C, Teng B, Franklin F, Bachorik P, Kwiterovich P (1982) Association of hyperapobetalipoproteinemia with endogenous hypertriglyceridemia and atherosclerosis. Ann Intern Med 97: 833
23. Steiner G, Vranic M (1982) Hyperinsulinemia and hypertriglyceridemia, a vicious cycle with atherogenic potential. Int J Obesity 6: suppl 1, 117
24. Walldius G (1986) Plasma triglycerides and the development of atherosclerotic disease. In Fidge NH, Nestel PJ (eds) Atherosclerosis, vol 7 Elsevier, p 205
25. World Health Organization (1972) Health statistics report 25. WHO, Geneva

The Plasma Lipoproteins in Hypertriglyceridemia as Risk Factors for Atherosclerosis

G. Crepaldi and E. Manzato

Introduction

A correlation between plasma cholesterol levels and the incidence of atherosclerosis has been clearly demonstrated by several epidemiological and experimental studies. The relationship between plasma cholesterol and atherogenesis is mediated by low-density lipoprotein (LDL). In fact, this class of plasma lipoproteins seems to be directly involved in forming the vascular lesion [1].

Much less data can be collected in the literature about plasma triglyceride levels and atherosclerosis. Several authors have reported elevated plasma triglycerides in patients with coronary artery disease [2, 3], but conflicting epidemiological data about hypertriglyceridemia as an independent risk factor have been published [4]. In particular, a final demonstration that high levels of plasma triglycerides are directly linked to vascular disease is still needed. If this can be proved we would also be able to find out which lipoprotein(s) in hypertriglyceridemia is harmful for the vessel wall.

In this paper we will review some data that we have obtained by analyzing the plasma lipoproteins in patients with severe hypertriglyceridemia and we will attempt a critical evaluation of the lipoprotein modifications produced during treatment of these patients.

Very Low-Density Lipoprotein

The very low-density lipoproteins (VLDL) are a class of lipoproteins containing heterogeneous molecules with variable dimensions, flotation rates (from S_f 400 to 20), and protein-lipid composition. Most of the VLDL triglycerides in normolipidemic subjects are transported by small VLDL with S_f <175 [5]. In patients with hypertriglyceridemia (type IV) the VLDL increase is mainly due to large triglyceride-rich particles with S_f >100 [6]. In type V patients there is an increase in large VLDL and chylomicrons are present in the plasma [7]. On the basis of cholesterol concentration most VLDL in type V patients is of S_f 100–200, although the amounts of S_f >200 (including large VLDL and chylomicrons) and of S_f 20–100 are also increased (Table 1).

Comparing the VLDL subclass distribution in type V with type I patients, it seems that the catabolism of VLDL of S_f 20–100 is less dependent on lipoprotein lipase activity since there is no accumulation of this VLDL class in type I patients [8]. Analysis of the VLDL subclass distribution could be useful to define different

Table 1. Cholesterol concentrations (mg/dl; mean ± SD) in VLDL subclasses in type I patients, in type V patients before (basal) and after 15 (+15) and 30 (+30) days of dietary treatment, and in normal individuals (for serum lipid levels in type V patients see Table 2)

	S_f			
	>200	100–200	60–100	20–60
Type I (*n*=6)	88 ± 36	63 ± 24	19 ± 8	19 ± 9
Type V				
basal (*n*=9)	76 ± 71	137 ± 62	58 ± 17	66 ± 29
+15 (*n*=7)	12 ± 9	40 ± 30	29 ± 15	60 ± 37
+30 (*n*=8)			41 ± 34	
Normals (n = 12)			12 ± 4	

genetic forms of hypertriglyceridemia since the VLDL composition and production rate seem to differ between familial hypertriglyceridemia and familial combined hyperlipidemia [9, 10].

The VLDL distribution and production rate are also important in determining VLDL catabolism. It has been reported that when VLDL apolipoprotein B (apo B) flux is increased VLDL is not transformed into low-density lipoprotein (LDL) [11]. Moreover, in normals and in type IV patients only VLDL of S_f 12–100 is significantly transformed into LDL [12]. Considering these metabolic properties and the absence of vascular lesions in type I patients, it is possible that only small VLDL (S_f < 100) is of importance in atherogenesis.

In some patients with primary hypertriglyceridemia and in some cases of secondary hypertriglyceridemia characterized by a high frequency of atherosclerotic complication (such as hypothyroidism and chronic renal failure) a double pre-β band is often observed in electrophoresis of lipoproteins. The slow pre-β band (which is a VLDL of S_f 20–100) seems to be a remnant of the fast pre-β band (which is a VLDL of S_f 100–230), as demonstrated by us and by others using different techniques [13, 14]. The slow pre-β band is rich in cholesterol and apo E. The apoprotein composition of VLDL could be particularly important in determining the binding and degradation of these lipoproteins, since large VLDL is preferentially degraded by apo E binding to the B, E receptor, while small VLDL is degraded by apo B binding to its receptor [15, 16]. This difference in metabolic behavior might have some significance for the atherogenic role of different VLDL molecules.

Low-Density Lipoprotein

It is well known that VLDL and LDL levels are inversely related [17]. This inverse relationship holds mainly for cholesterol concentrations in these two classes of lipoproteins and is in part due to the triglyceride enrichment of LDL in hypertriglyceridemia [18, 19]. In patients with severe hypertriglyceridemia LDL is rich in triglyceride and depleted of cholesterol; it is also heterogeneous in terms of physical properties. In type V and type I patients we have isolated and characterized three discrete lipoprotein populations in the density range 1.006–1.063 g/ml (Fig. 1):

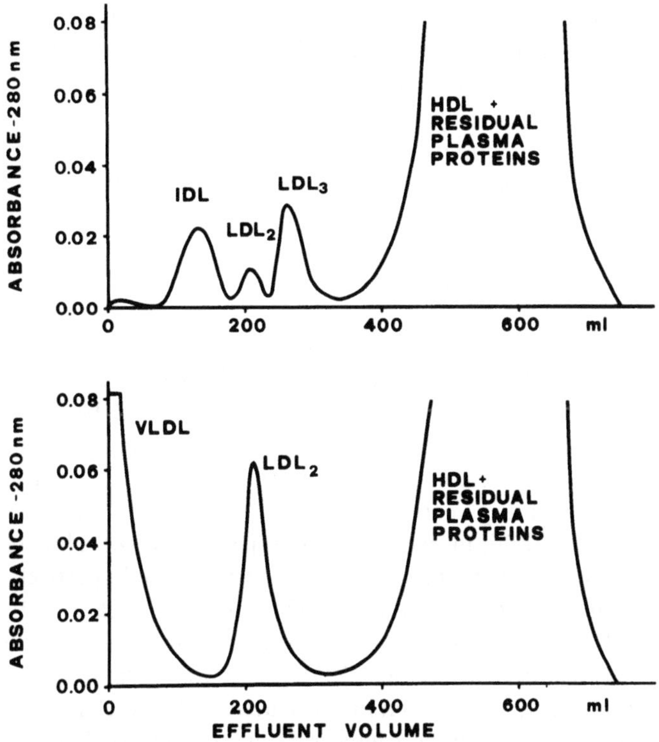

Fig. 1. Absorbance profiles from ultracentrifugation in a zonal rotor of lipoproteins of density >1.006 g/ml from a patient with chylomicronemia *(top)*, and of whole serum from a normolipidemic subject *(bottom)*

Table 2. Lipid levels (mg/dl; mean ± SD) in type V patients before (basal) and after 15 (+15) and 30 (+30) days of dietary treatment

	Serum triglyceride	Cholesterol			
		Serum	IDL	LDL_2	LDL_3
Basal (n=9)	2253 ± 1329	471 ± 129	23 ± 15	16 ± 8	22 ± 11
+15 (n=7)	788 ± 311	317 ± 68	48 ± 22	79 ± 29	
+30 (n=8)	251 ± 151	235 ± 46	16 ± 15	140 ± 47	

intermediate density lipoprotein (IDL; density d = 1.006–1.019 g/ml), LDL_2 (d=1.019–1.045 g/ml), and LDL_3 (d=1.045–1.063 g/ml) [20].

During dietary treatment of type V patients we observed an increase of IDL and LDL_2, while LDL_3 rapidly disappeared when hypertriglyceridemia was only slightly reduced (Table 2). From a metabolic point of view these changes could be due to an activation of the lipolytic cascade of VLDL or to a direct synthesis of IDL. In severe hypertriglyceridemia there is also a stepwise delipidation chain from IDL to LDL_2 and LDL_3 [21].

Familial hypercholesterolemia is characterized by high LDL levels, reduced LDL catabolism, and atherosclerosis, while in hypertriglyceridemia LDL levels are reduced and LDL catabolism is enhanced [22, 23]. In this second situation the low LDL levels and accelerated LDL catabolism could be more atherogenic than normal LDL levels with normal catabolic rate. Moreover, the different protein-lipid composition of hypertriglyceridemic LDL (triglyceride rich and cholesterol depleted) in comparison with normal LDL could be responsible for the abnormal biological properties of hypertriglyceridemic LDL [24].

High-Density Lipoprotein

There is little doubt that high-density lipoprotein (HDL) cholesterol levels are inversely related to the plasma (and VLDL) triglyceride concentration [18, 19, 25]. In hypertriglyceridemia this relationship could be to a large extent due to an exchange of cholesterol for triglyceride between HDL and triglyceride-rich particles. In fact, the composition of HDL in severe hypertriglyceridemia is characterized by high triglyceride and low cholesterol contents [7, 8], probably as a result of the activity of lipid transfer proteins [26]. However, a low HDL concentration seems to be an independent metabolic abnormality in hypertriglyceridemics since in these patients triglyceride reduction often fails to increase HDL [7, 27-29]. The increase of HDL cholesterol observed during treatment in some hypertriglyceridemic patients occurred after the VLDL reduction [30], suggesting that the relationship reported [31, 32] between lipolytic activity and HDL is not a direct one. During dietary treatment of hypertriglyceridemic patients total HDL cholesterol and the HDL subfractions do not seem to be immediately affected by triglyceride reduction, since significant changes to these could not be found using analysis by ultracentrifugation [7].

From these data it seems that the evaluation of HDL in hypertriglyceridemia should be performed by determining HDL constituents other from cholesterol (e.g., phospholipids or apoproteins, in particular apo A-I). Moreover, the in vivo metabolic relationships between HDL and plasma triglycerides should be further studied in order to understand the role of HDL as a factor protecting against atherosclerosis in hypertriglyceridemia.

Conclusions

From the analysis of plasma lipoproteins in hypertriglyceridemia we can conclude that plasma lipoproteins are a complex mixture of heterogeneous macromolecules with different metabolic properties. By studying these functional properties we should be able to obtain a better evaluation of the vascular risk directly linked to hypertriglyceridemia and a more clear definition of the genetic disorders responsible for the elevated triglyceride levels in different patients.

References

1. Grundy SM (1984) Recommendations for the treatment of hyperlipidemia in adults. Circulation 69: 1067 A
2. Goldstein JL, Hazzard WR, Schrott HG, Bierman EL, Motulsky AG (1973) Hyperlipidemia in coronary heart disease. I. Lipid levels in 500 survivors of myocardial infarction. J Clin Invest 52: 1533
3. Carlson LA, Bottiger LE, Ahfeldt PE (1979) Risk factors for myocardial infarction in the Stockholm prospective study. A 14-year follow-up focusing on the role of plasma triglycerides and cholesterol. Acta Med Scand 206: 351
4. Hulley SB, Rosenman RH, Bawol RD, Brand RJ (1980) Epidemiology as a guide to clinical decisions. The association between triglyceride and coronary heart disease. N Engl J Med 302: 1388
5. Kuchinskiene Z, Carlson LA (1982) Composition, concentration, and size of low density lipoproteins and of subfractions of very low density lipoproteins from serum of normal men and women. J Lipid Res 23: 762
6. Packard CJ, Shepherd J, Joerns S, Gotto AM, Taunton OD (1979) Very low density lipoprotein subfraction in type III and type IV hyperlipoproteinemia. Chemical and physical properties. Biochim Biophys Acta 572: 269
7. Manzato E, Marin R, Gasparotto A, Baggio G, Martini S, Gabelli C, Crepaldi G (1986) Lipoprotein modifications during dietary treatment in patients with primary type V hyperlipoproteinaemia. Eur J Clin Invest 16: 149
8. Manzato E, Marin R, Gasparotto A, Baggio G, Fellin R, Crepaldi G (1984) The plasma lipoproteins in familial chylomicronemia. J Lab Clin Med 104: 778
9. Brunzell JD, Albers JJ, Chait A, Grundy SM, Groszek E, McDonald GB (1983) Plasma lipoproteins in familial combined hyperlipidemia and monogenic familial hypertriglyceridemia. J Lipid Res 24: 147
10. Chait A, Albers JJ, Brunzell JD (1983) Very low density lipoprotein overproduction in genetic forms of hypertriglyceridaemia. Eur J Clin Invest 10: 17
11. Reardon MF, Fidge NH, Nestel PJ (1978) Catabolism of very low density lipoprotein B apoprotein in man. J Clin Invest 61: 850
12. Packard CJ, Munro A, Lorimer AR, Gotto AM, Shepherd J (1984) Metabolism of apolipoprotein B in large triglyceride-rich very low density lipoproteins of normal and hypertriglyceridemic subjects. J Clin Invest 74: 2178
13. Manzato E, Pagnan A, Ziron L, Gasparotto A, Braggion M (1984) Double pre-beta lipoprotein. Isolation and characterization of the two populations of very low density lipoproteins by zonal ultracentrifugation. Arteriosclerosis 4: 598
14. Nestel P, Billington T, Tada N, Nugent P, Fidge N (1983) Heterogeneity of very-low-density lipoprotein metabolism in hyperlipidemic subjects. Metabolism 32: 810
15. Gianturco SH, Gotto AM, Hwang SL, Karlin JB, Lin AHY, Prasad SC, Bradley WA (1983) Apolipoprotein E mediates uptake of Sf 100–400 hypertriglyceridemic very low density lipoproteins by the low density lipoprotein receptor pathway in normal human fibroblasts. J Biol Chem 258: 4526
16. Krul ES, Tikkanen MJ, Cole TG, Davie JM, Schonfeld G (1985) Roles of apolipoproteins B and E in the cellular binding of very low density lipoproteins. J Clin Invest 75: 361
17. Wilson DE, Lees RS (1972) Metabolic relationships among the plasma lipoproteins. Reciprocal changes in the concentrations of very low and low density lipoproteins in man. J Clin Invest 51: 1051
18. Hutt VV, Klor HU, Wechsler JG, Ditschuneit H (1984) Composition of VLDL, LDL and HDL lipoprotein fractions in type II a, II b, III, IV and V hyperlipaemic patients and in normal individuals. J Clin Chem Clin Biochem 22: 141
19. Deckelbaum RJ, Granot E, Oschry Y, Rose L, Eisenberg S (1984) Plasma triglyceride determines structure-composition in low and high density lipoproteins. Arteriosclerosis 4: 225
20. Manzato E, Gasparotto A, Marin R, Baggio G, Baldo G, Crepaldi G (1984) Characterization with zonal ultracentrifugation of low-density lipoproteins in type V hyperlipoproteinemia. Biochim Biophys Acta 793: 365

21. Fisher WR, Zech LA, Bardalaye P, Warmke G, Berman M (1980) The metabolism of apolipoprotein B in subjects with hypertriglyceridemia and polidisperse LDL. J Lipid Res 21: 760
22. Sigurdsson G, Nicoll A, Lewis B (1976) The metabolism of low density lipoprotein in endogenous hypertriglyceridemia. Eur J Clin Invest 6: 151
23. Ginsberg HN, Le NA, Gibson J (1985) Regulation of the production and catabolism of plasma low density lipoproteins in hypertriglyceridemic subjects. Effect of weight loss. J Clin Invest 75: 614
24. Kleinman Y, Eisenberg S, Oschry Y, Gavish D, Stein O, Stein Y (1985) Defective metabolism of hypertriglyceridemic low density lipoprotein in cultured human skin fibroblasts. J Clin Invest 75: 1796
25. Schaefer EJ, Levy RI, Anderson DW, Danner RN, Brewer HB, Blackwelder WC (1978) Plasma triglycerides in regulation of HDL cholesterol levels. Lancet II: 391
26. Tall AR (1986) Plasma lipid transfer proteins. J Lipid Res 27: 361
27. Glueck CJ, Stein EA, Kashyap ML (1979) Persistent hypoalpha-lipoproteinemia during therapy of familial type 5 hyperlipoproteinemia. Artery 5: 463
28. Falko JM, Witztum JL, Schonfeld G, Bateman J (1979) Dietary treatment of type V hyperlipoproteinemia fails to normalize low levels of high-density lipoprotein cholesterol. Ann Intern Med 91: 750
29. Witztum JL, Dillingham MA, Giese W, Bateman J, Diekman C, Blaufuss EK, Weidman S, Schonfeld G (1980) Normalization of triglycerides in type IV hyperlipoproteinemia fails to correct low levels of high-density-lipoprotein cholesterol. N Engl J Med 303: 907
30. Carlson LA, Olsson AG, Ballantyne D (1977) On the rise in low density and high density lipoproteins in response to the treatment of hypertriglyceridaemia in type IV and type V hyperlipoproteinaemias. Atherosclerosis 26: 603
31. Kekki M (1980) Lipoprotein-lipase action determining plasma high density lipoprotein cholesterol level in adult normolipaemics. Atherosclerosis 37: 143
32. Magill P, Rao SN, Miller NE, Nicoll A, Brunzell J, St. Hilaire J, Lewis B (1982) Relationships between the metabolism of high-density and very-low-density lipoproteins in man: studies of apolipoprotein kinetics and adipose tissue lipoprotein lipase activity. Eur J Clin Invest 12: 113

Myocardial Infarction in Women on Oral Contraceptives: Risk Factors and Mechanism

V. Beaumont and J. L. Beaumont

Introduction

It is known from epidemiological studies [1-3] that there is a direct relationship between myocardial infarction (M.I.) and the use of oral contraceptives (O.C.). The risk of coronary thrombosis has been estimated as 3 to 4 times greater in O.C. users than in women who have never used them. Little is known as yet about the mechanism that promotes thrombosis of the coronary arteries in women using O.C., but as information has accumulated the responsibility of an atherosclerotic process in this kind of ischemic disease has become questionable. However, determination of the mechanism is of importance since up to now the detection of women predisposed to coronary thrombosis relied on the presence or absence of factors known to be associated with the development of atherosclerosis.

Implications of Factors Increasing the Risk of Atherosclerosis for O. C. Vascular Complications

Numerous retrospective and prospective studies have provided evidence of a strong correlation between ischemic diseases due to atherosclerosis and a number of conditions considered as risk factors. These include hypertension, diabetes, increased serum cholesterol, triglyceride and low-density lipoprotein (LDL) levels, decreased high-density lipoprotein (HDL) levels, and cigarette smoking.

Age and sex are also factors determining the development of atherosclerosis. Until the last 15 years, M.I. was regarded as an uncommon disease in women, especially in those under the age of 50. Recently, however, epidemiological studies have brought to light an increase in M.I. in young women, and a new risk factor had to be taken into account when the evidence of a correlation between O.C. use and M.I. was found [1-4]. However, from the many reports now available it is not always clear whether the risk associated with O.C. is concentrated in women at risk for other reasons, or is a risk per se.

Statistical studies have shown that O.C. induce a discrete elevation of blood pressure in most women, estimated as 1-2 mmHg for diastolic and 5 mmHg for systolic blood pressure [5]. Occasionally, true hypertension may occur, which seems to be related to familial susceptibility, the amount of progestogen in the O.C. [6], and the duration of its use [7]. The risk increases with age. However, hypertension above 150/90 mmHg was estimated as occurring in no more than 5% of the overall group of O.C. users [7] and 10% of the group with thrombosis [8, 9]. O.C. were also found to decrease glucose tolerance in most women. Once more, the effect was small. It was shown to depend upon the estrogen content and the type of progestogen of the different combined O.C. formulations [10]. The glucogenic effect is temporary, and the presence of diabetes is rarely mentioned in O.C. users with vascular complications.

The role of estrogens in lipid metabolism has been extensively studied over the last 30 years. They were shown to decrease serum LDL and cholesterol levels, to increase serum very low-density lipoprotein (VLDL) and triglyceride, and more recently [11] to increase HDL, especially the HDL_2 subfraction. Consequently, estrogens were considered useful to treat hypercholesterolemic patients and prevent atherosclerotic complications. Paradoxically, it was later found that estrogen-treated patients were at increased risk to thrombotic complications [12]. When combined with progestogens, the effects on lipoproteins are different. Progestogens act roughly in a manner opposing that of the estrogens; they decrease VLDL levels, increase LDL and decrease HDL [13]. The net effects of combined O.C. were not always similarly appreciated and conflicting results were reported. Recent studies have provided some evidence that not only the relative content of estrogens and progestogens but also the type of the progestogen influences the lipid and lipoprotein levels. O.C. with a medium or low estrogen content induce little or no modification in serum cholesterol (a lipid fraction highly correlated with coronary heart disease), and usually moderate increase in triglycerides, the participation of which in the disease is more speculative [2, 8, 10, 14, 15]. The effects on HDL are not always concordant. It seems that a decrease in HDL is observed only when the O.C. contain norethindrone and norgestrel, two types of progestogen with strong anti-estrogenic effects [11].

Nevertheless, proof of a correlation between the modifications in the lipoprotein profile and the vascular complications of O.C. is lacking. In nearly all epidemiological studies serum lipoproteins were compared in O.C. users vs. nonusers, and not in healthy users vs. users with thrombosis. When young women with M.I. were studied, hyperlipidemia was shown to be an infrequent finding [8, 9]. However, it cannot be excluded that a moderate but sustained hyperlipidemia may enhance the risk of developing M.I. in older women using O.C. in the long term. In fact, when it is claimed that the risk of M.I. in O.C. users is concentrated in women with other risk factors, those are essentially age and cigarette smoking.

According to the study of the Royal College of General Practitioners [3], the risk of M.I. increases with age. The relative risk in O.C. users compared with nonusers is 2.7 between 30 and 39 years, and 5.7 between 40 and 49 years. These figures are independent of the duration of use.

Cigarette smoking is also known to increase the risk of ischaemic heart disease in men and women. Oliver [16] found that 47% of women with M.I. were smokers, compared with 26% of the general population. The potentiating effects of cigarette smoking and O.C. have been emphasized in many epidemiological studies [1-3, 8, 17, 18]. Shapiro [17] showed that the risk of M.I. increased 4-fold in O.C. users, and increased up to 40-fold in those O.C. users who smoked 25 or more cigarettes per day. Stadel [19], reviewing data from several studies, showed the cumulative effects of both age and cigarette smoking in O.C. users, the risk of M.I. increasing with age, and also, within each age group, with the number of cigarettes smoked. However, it must also be emphasized that M. I. can occur in very young women [20] without any obvious risk factor [9, 20] and after only short-term use of O. C.

Angiographic and Pathological Findings in O. C. Vascular Complications

Although only epidemiologists can give a good appreciation of the frequency of M. I. in O. C. users, practitioners and pathologists can provide different insights into this coronary heart disease.

In women using O. C., coronary heart disease occurs suddenly and results in M. I. Angina pectoris is unusual. Angiographic findings reveal either completely normal vessels or isolated obstruction in otherwise normal, nonatherosclerotic arteries [9], particularly in the youngest women. The absence of a collateral blood supply also suggests a rapid onset of the disease [21].

Histological studies usually confirm the absence of atherosclerotic lesions. The hypothesis that thrombosis may occur on microscopical vascular lesions of a different type is suggested by the autopsy findings of Irey et al. [22]. They showed that the lesions displayed by O. C. users were disseminated along the vascular tree. Some of them essentially consisted of an endothelial and intimal hyperplasia, with more or less narrowing of the vessels; some were associated with an occlusive thrombus. These lesions are not specific and resemble those found in many autoimmune diseases (sclerodermia, periarteritis nodosa, giant cell arteritis). A giant cell thromboangeitis, suggestive of an immunological process, was also described by one of us [23] in a women using O. C. with bilateral carotid thrombosis.

O. C. Thrombosis: An Immunological Disease?

The possibility that an immunological mechanism might be responsible for the vascular thrombosis related to O. C. use was first suggested in 1976, when a monoclonal IgG with anti-ethinylestradiol activity was found in the serum of a 36-year-old woman with pulmonary embolism using O. C. [24]. After this, further studies provided evidence that O. C. may induce antibodies to the synthetic hormones they contain, especially ethinylestradiol. A simple detection of circulating immune complexes by serum precipitation in ammonium sulfate at 25% saturation showed that about 25% of O. C. users were immunoreactive [25, 26]. This simple, but unspecific, method was later changed for a specific radioimmunoassay using radiolabeled ethinylestradiol. This method [27] confirmed that no ethinylestradiol-specific antibodies (anti-EE) could be detected in women who had never used O. C., that about 25%-30% of O. C. users develop anti-EE, and that in O. C. users with a vascular complication, anti-EE could be demonstrated in nearly 90% of cases (Fig. 1). They were not related to the duration of use or to the dose of estrogen. The presence of anti-EE was shown to represent, with cigarette smoking, the main risk factor observed in 50 women who had experienced thrombosis while using O. C., and the sole factor in 44% of them [8]. Furthermore, except for minor differences in age and

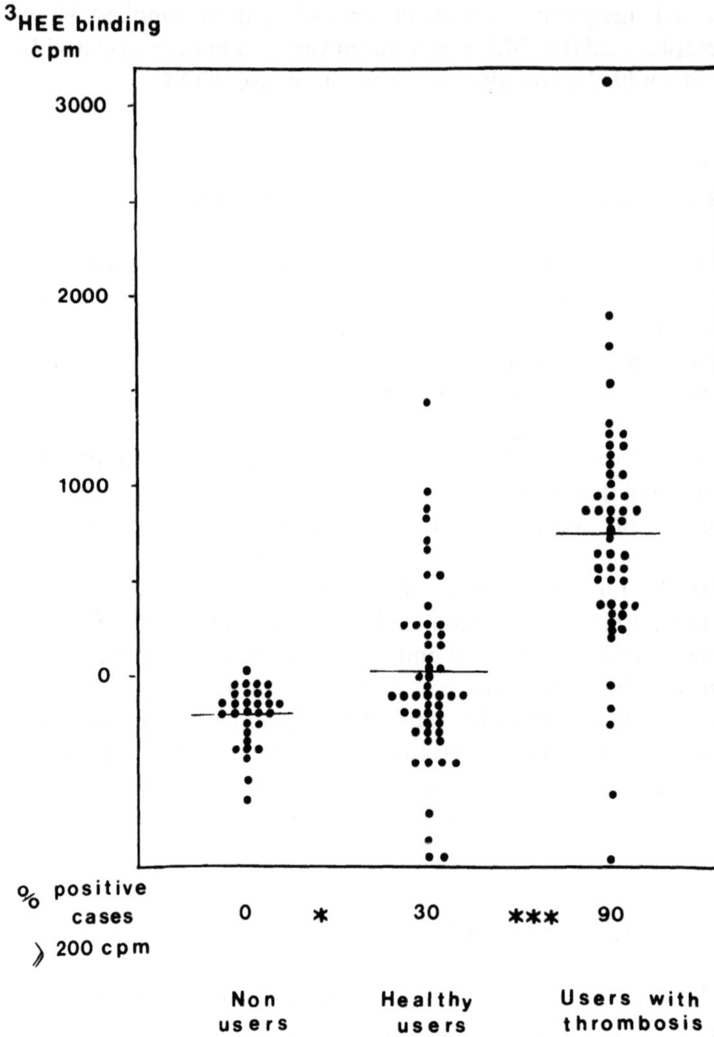

Fig. 1. Binding of tritiated ethinylestradiol (^{3}HEE) in O.C. users and non-users

triglyceride levels, those two factors were the only ones to distinguish O.C. users with thrombosis from healthy users (Fig. 2).

Anti-EE and Cigarette Smoking in O. C.-Related M. I.

Anti-EE were found with a similar frequency in cases of M. I. (95%), cerebrovascular thrombosis (84%), and venous thrombosis (88%). However, the percentage of women who smoked was greater for M. I. (85%) than for the other two diseases (47% and 41% respectively; $P < 0.01$; Table 1). This study seems to indicate that cigarette smoking per se is not a strong risk factor, but is when associated with the presence of anti-EE (Table 2).

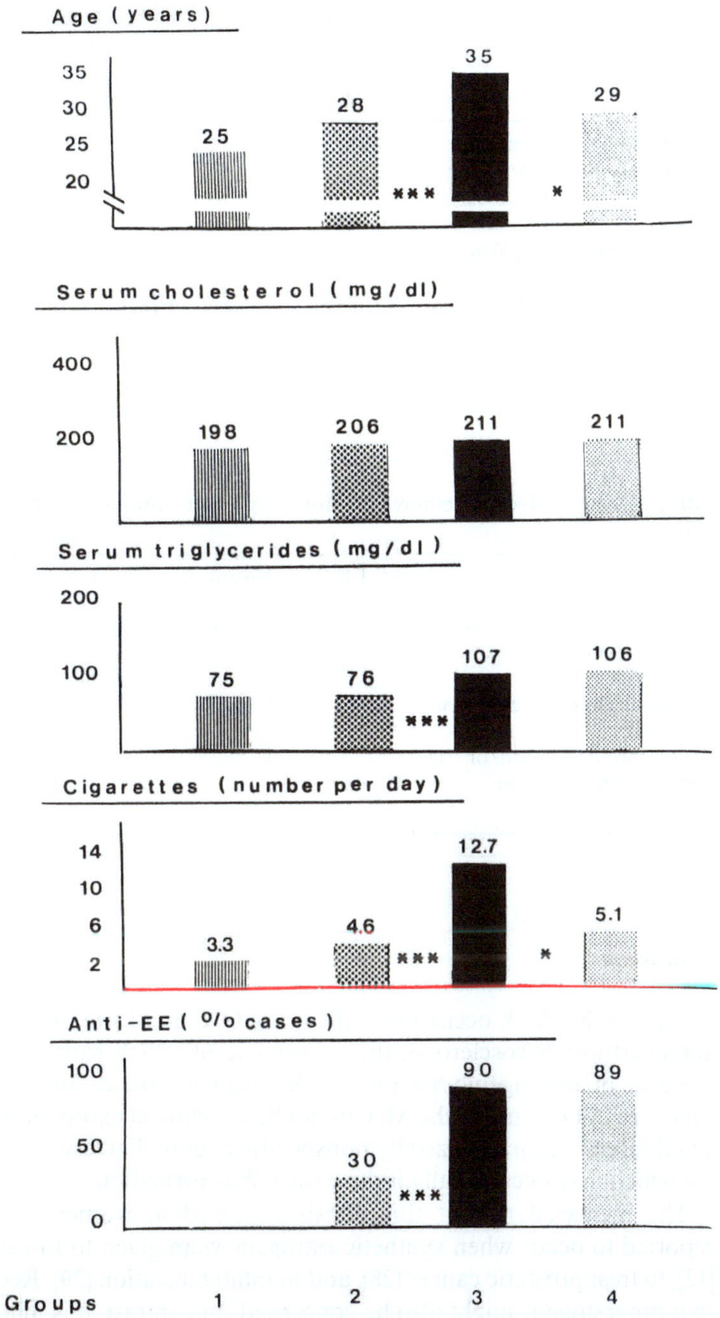

Fig. 2. Risk factors in women according to O.C. use. Group 1, never-users; group 2, healthy users; group 3, users with arterial thrombosis; group 4, users with venous thrombosis. * $P < 0.05$, *** $P < 0.001$

Table 1. Risk factors in O.C. users with thrombosis of different sites

	Myocardial infarction (n=20)	Cerebrovascular thrombosis (n=19)	Venous thrombosis and/or pulmonary embolism (n=17)
Age (mean ± SD, years)	34±6	33±8	28±7
Blood pressure >160/90 mmHg [n (%)]	2 (10)	1 (5)	0
Diabetes	0	0	0
Serum cholesterol >250 mg/dl [n (%)]	2 (10)	5 (26)	3 (18)
cigarettes smoked >10 per day [n (%)]	17 (85)[a]	9 (47)	7 (41)
Anti-EE [n (%)]	19 (95)	16 (84)	15 (88)

[a] P <0.01 between M.I. and the two other groups.

Table 2. Synergic effects of ethinylestradiol-specific antibodies (anti-EE) and cigarette smoking (CS)

	No anti-EE/no CS	No anti-EE/CS	Anti-EE/no CS	Anti-EE/CS
Cerebrovascular diseases (n=19)	2	1	8	8
Ischemic heart diseases (n=20)	0	1	3	16
Venous thrombosis and/or pulmonary embolism (n=17)	1	1	9	6

Conclusion

It appears that M.I. occurring while using O.C. is a form of ischemic heart disease unrelated to atherosclerosis, the occurrence of which cannot be predicted by the presence of atherogenic risk factors. According to the changes observed in the vascular tree of O.C. users, the M.I. might be the clinical expression of a more disseminated disease, characterized by nonspecific endothelial lesions and intimal thickening which may occasionally induce thrombus formation.

The increased risk of thrombosis observed in women using O.C. was also reported to occur when synthetic estrogens were given to lower serum cholesterol [12], to treat prostatic cancer [28], and to inhibit lactation [29]. Recent reports suggest that progestogens might also be concerned. In contrast, it is interesting that, except for one study [30], a significant negative association has been found between coronary heart disease or mortality, and natural estrogen treatments [31, 32, 33].

We have shown that a number of women developed antibodies against the synthetic hormones contained in O.C. These antibodies were the main risk factor in the group with vascular complications. Furthermore, natural estrogens or progestogens, which are not associated with an increased vascular risk, do not induce the formation of antibodies. The possible thrombogenic effect of the antibodies remains to be explained. They have been shown to form circulating immune complexes [26, 27] which might damage the vascular endothelium, promote intimal proliferation, and interfere with coagulation factors, especially platelet aggregation. Cigarette smoking might in turn increase the vascular permeability, facilitate the penetration of complexes, and enhance the coagulation processes.

Thrombosis represents the main risk for users of oral contraception. Determination of antibodies to synthetic sex hormones should be a valuable test to detect oral contraceptive users at risk from vascular complications.

References

1. Mann JI, Vessey MC, Thorogood M, Doll R (1975) Myocardial infarction in young women with special reference to oral contraceptive practice. Br Med J 2: 241-245
2. Mann JI, Inman WHW (1975) Oral contraceptives and death from myocardial infarction. Br Med J 2: 245-248
3. Royal College of General Practitioner's Oral Contraception Study (1981) Further analysis of mortality in oral contraceptive users. Lancet I: 541-546
4. Stamler J, Berkson DM, Lindberg MA (1972) Risk factors: their role in the etiology and pathogenesis of the atherosclerotic diseases. In: Wissler PW, Geer JC (eds) The pathogenesis of atherosclerosis, vol 1. Williams and Wilkins, Baltimore, pp 67-72
5. Ramcharan S, Pellegrin FA, Hoag EJ (1976) The occurence and course of hypertensive disease in users and non-users of oral contraceptive drugs. In: Ramcharan S (ed) The walnut creek contraceptive drug study: a prospective study of the side effects of oral contraceptives, vol 2. Government Printing Office, Washington DC, pp 1-16
6. Royal College of General Practioners' Oral Contraception Study (1977) Effects on hypertension and benign breast disease of progestogen component in combined oral contraceptives. Lancet I: 624
7. Lekieffre J (1979) Arterial hypertension and oral contraceptives. Ann Cardiol Angeiol 28: 35-39
8. Beaumont V, Lemort N, Beaumont JL (1983) Evaluation of risk factors associated with vascular thrombosis in women on oral contraceptives. Possible role of anti-sex steroid hormone antibodies. Artery 11: 331-344
9. Engel HJ, Engel E, Lichtlen PR (1983) Coronary atherosclerosis and myocardial infarction in young women. Role of oral contraceptives. Eur Heart J 4: 1-18
10. Wynn W, Adams PW, Godsland I, Melrose J, Nithyananthan R, Oakley NN, See DH (1979) Comparison of effects of different combined oral contraceptive formulations on carbohydrate and lipid metabolism. Lancet I: 1045-1049
11. Bradley DB, Wingerd J, Petiti DB, Kraus RM, Ramcharan S (1978) Serum high density lipoprotein cholesterol in women using oral contraceptives, estrogens and progestins. N Engl J Med 299: 17-80
12. The Coronary Drug Project Research Group (1973) Findings leading to discontinuation of the 2.5 mg/day estrogen group. JAMA 222: 652-657
13. Baggett B, Nash HA (1980) Effects of contraceptive steroids on serum lipoproteins and cardiovascular disease scrutinized at workshop in Bethesda. Contraception 21: 115-120
14. Wallace RB, Hoover J, Sandler D, Rifkind BM, Tyroler HA (1977) Altered plasma lipids associated with oral contraceptives or estrogen consumption. Lancet II: 11-14
15. Wahl P, Walden C, Knopp R, Hoover J, Wallace R, Heiss G, Rifkind BM (1983) Effect of estrogen/progestin potency on lipid/lipoprotein cholesterol. N Engl J Med 308: 862-867
16. Radford DJ, Oliver MF (1973) Oral contraceptives and myocardial infarction. Br Med J 3: 428-430
17. Shapiro S, Slone D, Rosenberg L, Kaufman DW, Stoley PD, Miettinen OS (1979) Oral contraceptive use in relation to myocardial infarction. Lancet I: 743-747

18. Jick H, Dinan B, Rothman KJ (1978) Oral contraceptives and non fatal myocardial infarction. JAMA 239: 1403-1406
19. Stadel BV (1981) Oral contraceptives and cardiovascular disease. N Engl J Med 305: 672-677
20. Beaumont V, Beaumont JL (1986) Oral contraception and thrombosis. Implication of anti-sex steroid hormone antibodies. In: Oliver MF, Vedin A (ed) Myocardial infarction in young women, vol 1. Churchill-Livingstone London, pp 190-199
21. Dear HD, Jones WB (1971) Myocardial infarction associated with the use of oral contraceptives. Ann Intern Med 74: 236-239
22. Irey NS, Manion WC, Taylor HB (1970) Vascular lesions in women taking oral contraceptives. Arch Pathol 89: 1-8
23. Bakouche P, Vedrenne C, Beaumont V, Chaouat D (1980) Thromboangéite à cellules géantes au cours d'une contraception orale. Etude anatomo-clinique et immunologique. Rev Neurol 136: 509-519
24. Beaumont JL, Lemort N (1976) Oral contraceptives, pulmonary artery thrombosis and anti-ethinylestradiol IgG. Clin Exp Immunol 24: 455-463
25. Beaumont V, Lemort N, Lorenzelli L, Mosser A, Beaumont JL (1978) Hormones contraceptives, risque vasculaire et précipitabilité anormale des gamma-globulines sériques. Pathol Biol 26: 531-537
26. Beaumont V, Delplanque B, Lemort N, Beaumont JL (1982) Blood changes in sex steroid hormone users: I. circulating immune complexes induced by estrogens and progestogens. Incidence in vascular thrombosis. Atherosclerosis 44: 343-353
27. Beaumont V, Lemort N, Beaumont JL (1982) Oral contraception, circulating immune complexes, antiethinylestradiol antibodies and thrombosis. Am J Reproduct Immunol 2: 8-12
28. Byar DP (1972) Treatment of prostatic cancer. Studies by the Veterans Administration Cooperative Urological Research Group. Bull NY Acad Med 48: 751-766
29. Jeffcoate TNA, Miller J, Rooq RF, Tindall VR (1968) Puerperal thromboembolism in relation to the inhibition of lactation by estrogen therapy. Br Med J 4: 19-25
30. Jick H, Dinan B, Rothman KJ (1978) Non-contraceptive estrogens and non fatal myocardial infarction. JAMA 239: 1407-1408
31. Stampfer MJ, Willet WC, Colditz GA, Rosner B, Speizer FE, Hennekens CH (1985) A prospective study of postmenopausal estrogen therapy and coronary heart disease. N Engl J Med 313: 1044-1049
32. Bush TL, Cowan LD, Barret-Connor E, Criqui MH, Karon JM, Wallace RB, Tyroler H, Rifkind BM (1983) Estrogen use and all-cause mortality. JAMA 249: 903-906
33. Rosenberg L, Slone D, Shapiro S, Kaufman D, Stolley PD, Miettinen OS (1980) Non contraceptive estrogens and myocardial infarction in young women. JAMA 244: 339-342

Combined Oral Contraceptives: From Risk to Benefit?

L. W. Hessel

About 25 years ago the first reports of adverse cardiovascular side effects of oral contraceptives (o.c.) began to appear. These included mainly venous thrombosis, pulmonary embolism, and stroke, with risk ratios varying between 2 and 8. Studies reporting increased risk of myocardial infarction were published somewhat later and risk ratios were, as a rule, lower than those for the venous complications.

As time went on and more studies appeared, calculated relative risk figures tended to decrease. This decrease was related to a gradual reduction in hormonal dosage of the contraceptives and was also, at least partly, due to more sophistication in the elimination of bias and other statistical errors. Both earlier and later studies have been challenged in a number of papers, culminating in a comprehensive critical review of all the studies published up to 1984 [21]. After a systematic consideration of the methodologies employed and the many types of bias that are likely to have crept in, it was concluded that, although an association between current use of o.c. and the incidence of venous thromboembolism has consistently been observed, the proposition that o.c. cause cardiovascular disease has not been scientifically proved. Most recent data confirm the view that with modern o.c. there is a slight increase in risk of venous thromboembolism, mainly restricted to older women and to smokers, and no extra risk of myocardial infarction and stroke [20].

As the alarm about deleterious side effects tended to subside reports appeared that showed that o.c. also have distinct health benefits. These include protection against iron-deficiency anemia, endometrial and ovarian cancers, benign breast disease, and perhaps against rheumatoid arthritis. Papers about these advantages have appeared from 1974 onwards; reviews were published in 1982 [18] and in 1986 [7].

Conspicuous by their absence from most epidemiologic studies are data on the composition of o.c. in relation to their positive or negative side effects. One of the aspects to which some attention has been paid is the coincidence of the shift to o.c. with an estrogen content below 100 µg and the drop in the number of adverse reactions. The statistical soundness of these studies has, however, been questioned [14]. We are aware of only one report in which the relation of estrogen content to clinical effects has been studied for o.c. with 50 µg or less estrogen [17]. The data in this report show an advantage for the formulations with 30 µg estrogen; however, the figures are difficult to interpret, as they have not been corrected for differences in progestogen.

With regard to type and quantity of the progestogen component in relation to side effects, available data are almost as scarce as for the estrogen component, especially for the low-dose o.c. A recent summary of the findings in the Royal College of General Practitioners' Oral Contraception Study shows an impressive correlation between doses of the two progestogens norethisterone acetate and levonorgestrel, and the occurrence of arterial disease. Again, the data refer mainly to the older types of o. c. that contain 250 μg or more of the various progestogens [12].

Because of the very low level of total risk and the near impossibility of setting up a randomized trial of sufficient size, it is difficult to prove directly that different brands of modern o. c. carry significantly different levels of risk of, or perhaps protection against, cardiovascular disease. Studies of metabolic effects may, however, be carried out in randomized trials of two or more types of o. c. under carefully controlled conditions. By documenting changes in the various biochemical parameters that are either known or suspected risk factors for cardiovascular disease, an indirect measure of relative safety or benefit may be obtained. In studies of this type differences in effects on risk factors have been identified, especially in the areas of lipid metabolism and hemostasis. Possibly beneficial effects in these areas include increases of levels of high density lipoprotein (HDL) cholesterol and HDL apoproteins, and increases in circulating components of the fibrinolytic system. Elevated levels of HDL and its apoproteins are usually considered as anti-atherogenic. The activity of the fibrinolytic system is a major defense of the body against thrombosis [9].

A first report on the effects of different o. c. of specified composition on HDL cholesterol levels in a large number of women in the United States of America appeared in 1978. It was shown that elevations of HDL cholesterol above the level observed in nonusers was associated with the use of o. c. containing 80 μg or more ethinyl estradiol (EE) or mestranol [2]. In a study carried out in Leiden, The Netherlands, similar results were obtained with respect to HDL cholesterol and apolipoprotein AI (apo AI). Moreover, it appeared that within the class of o. c. with 50 μg EE or less, effects on HDL cholesterol and apo AI could be very different, and that elevations of these HDL constituents were associated with some o. c. of this low-estrogen type [8].

In a later, randomized trial carried out in our laboratory, an o. c. containing 37.5 μg EE and 750 μg lynestrenol was compared with one containing 30 μg EE and 150 μg levonorgestrel. The lynestrenol-containing o. c. increased the level of apo AI and both increased the level of apo AII [4].

Studies on lipoproteins of o. c. of specified composition published up to 1984 have been summarized recently [3]. From this review it can be seen that, of all the low-estrogen o. c., formulations that contain 30 μg EE and 150 μg of the new progestogen desogestrel are unique in increasing not only apo AI but also HDL cholesterol levels. This combination also caused an increase in the ratio of apo AI : apo B. Similar results were reported in a paper in which the same desogestrel-containing preparation was compared with a triphasic levonorgestrel/EE combination. In this report it was suggested that changes seen with both formulations represent beneficial rather than deleterious side effects [16].

As far as protective effects of HDL and its apoproteins are related to cholesterol metabolism, it should be pointed out that the HDL_3 subfraction rather than the HDL_2 subfraction is increased by the triphasic levonorgestrel-containing and the desogestrel-containing preparations [16], whereas it is the HDL_2 subfraction that is said to protect against atherosclerosis ([6], but see also [22]). However, in a recent study carried out in our laboratory, it was shown that there are positive correlations of HDL to parameters of cardiac function that are independent of the degree of coronary atherosclerosis, and that these correlations are stronger for the HDL apoproteins and the HDL_3 subfraction than for HDL cholesterol and the HDL_2 subfraction [13]. Yet, so long as it has not been established that HDL cholesterol levels or apo AI and apo AII levels are causally related to cardiovascular disease or to cardiac function, a protective effect of artificially achieved changes in these levels may not be taken for granted.

A review of the effects of o.c. on coagulation factors and on components of the fibrinolytic system showed increases of fibrinogen, factor VII, and factor X for all preparations that were described. Antithrombin III and plasminogen activators were usually decreased [1]. These changes may be described as procoagulant and this would seem to be in accordance with the observed increase in risk of thrombotic disorders. However, as pointed out by Mammen [15], there is no evidence that links increased clotting factor activities in vitro with hypercoagulability in vivo. Attempts to predict the occurrence of thrombosis must take into account the coagulatory as well as the fibrinolytic arm of the hemostatic balance, and as both of these systems consist of a number of interacting components, rather extensive studies are required. To the extent that these have been carried out with the modern preparations, they have pointed to increases in several profibrinolytic components. In general, o.c. increase concentrations of circulating plasminogen [1], and some low-dose o.c. cause decreases in "histidine-rich glycoprotein" [10], which further increases the activity of free plasminogen. Several other fibrinolytic components are also increased, including activators of the extrinsic as well as the intrinsic system [11].

In a detailed study on two o.c., both of which were of the "sub 50" estrogen type, we found procoagulant as well as profibrinolytic effects and there were considerable differences between the two preparations, especially with respect to tissue-type plasminogen activator, but only minor decreases in antithrombin III [5].

In general it may be assumed that in women taking the low-dose o.c., the increases in coagulation activity are counterbalanced by an increase in fibrinolytic activity; only in a small subgroup of women, where this counterbalance is insufficient, may thrombotic episodes occur. At the same time, there may exist other subgroups, with a non-negligible base line risk of vascular disorder, that may actually benefit from the use of o.c., provided a suitable preparation is prescribed. One such group may consist of nonsmoking women between the ages of 35 and 45. Although data obtained from the use of a variety of formulations lumped together indicate a clear increase in risk in this group, with some o.c. the overall shift in the hemostatic balance (as judged from circulating components) is clearly in the direction of fibrinolysis rather than of coagulation [19].

References

1. Beller FK, Ebert C (1985) Effects of oral contraceptives on blood coagulation. A review. Obstet Gynecol Surv 40: 425
2. Bradley DD, Wingerd J, Petitti DB, Krauss RM, Ramcharan S (1978) Serum high-density-lipoprotein cholesterol in women using oral contraceptives, estrogens and progestins. N Engl J Med 299: 17
3. Fotherby K (1985) Oral contraceptives, lipids and cardiovascular disease. Contraception 31: 367

4. Gevers Leuven JA, Havekes L, van der Kooij-Pontier HA, Starmans RJH, Jansen H, Bouwhuis-Hoogerwerf ML, de Pagter HATh, Hessel LW (1984) Effect of low-dose oral contraceptives on lipoproteins and lipolytic enzymes: differences between two commonly used preparations. Metabolism 33: 1039
5. Gevers Leuven JA, Kluft C, Bertina RM, Hessel LW (1987) Effects of two low-dose oral contraceptives on circulating components of the coagulation and fibrinolytic systems. J Lab Clin Med (in press)
6. Godsland IF, Wynn V (1984) Does the new progestagen desogestrel have metabolic advantages? Lancet ii: 359
7. Grimes DA (1986) Reversible contraception for the 1980s. J Am Med Assoc 255: 69
8. Havekes L, van Gent CM, Stegerhoek CI, Arntzenius AC, Hessel LW (1981) High density lipoprotein cholesterol and apolipoprotein A-I levels in 32-33-year-old women on steroid contraceptives - differences between two frequently used low-estrogen pills. Clin Chim Acta 116: 223
9. Hessel LW, Kluft C (1986) Advances in clinical fibrinolysis. Clin Haematol 15: 443
10. Jespersen J, Kluft C (1982) Decreased levels of histidine-rich glycoprotein (HRG) and increased levels of free plasminogen in women on oral contraceptives low in estrogen. Thromb Haemostas 48: 283
11. Jespersen J, Kluft C (1985) Increased euglobulin fibrinolytic potential in women on oral contraceptives low in oestrogen - levels of extrinsic and intrinsic plasminogen activators, prekallikrein, factor XII, and Cl-inactivator. Thromb Haemostas 54: 454
12. Kay CR (1984) The Royal college of general practitioners' oral contraception study: some recent observations. Clin Obstet Gynecol 11: 759
13. Kempen HJ, van Gent CM, Buytenhek R, Buis R (1987) Association of cholesterol concentrations in LDL, HDL and HDL-subfractions and of apolipoproteins AI and AII, with coronary stenosis and left ventricular function. J Lab Clin Med (in press)
14. Kierkegaard A (1985) Deep vein thrombosis and the oestrogen content in oral contraceptives - an epidemiological analysis. Contraception 31: 29
15. Mammen EF (1982) Oral contraceptives and blood coagulation: a critical review. Am J Obstet Gynecol 142: 781
16. März W, Gross W, Gahn G, Romberg G, Taubert HD, Kuhl H (1985) A randomized crossover comparison of two low-dose contraceptives: effects on serum lipids and lipoproteins. Am J Obstet Gynecol 153: 287
17. Meade TW, Greenberg G, Thompson SG (1980) Progestogens and cardiovascular reactions associated with oral contraceptives and a comparison of the safety of 50- and 30-μg oestrogen preparations. Br Med J i: 1157
18. Mishell DR Jr (1982) Noncontraceptive health benefits of oral steroidal contraceptives. Am J Obstet Gynecol 142: 809
19. Notelovitz M, Levenson I, McKenzie L, Lane D, Kitchens CS (1985) The effects of low-dose oral contraceptives on coagulation and fibrinolysis in two high-risk populations: young female smokers and older premenopausal women. Am J Obstet Gynecol 152: 995
20. Porter JB, Hunter JR, Jick H, Stergachis A (1985) Oral contraceptives and nonfatal vascular disease. Obstet Gynecol 66: 1
21. Realini JP, Goldzieher JW (1985) Oral contraceptives and cardiovascular disease: a critique of the epidemiologic studies. Am J Obstet Gynecol 152: 729
22. Wallentin L, Sundin B (1985) HDL_2 and HDL_3 lipid levels in coronary artery disease. Atherosclerosis 59: 131

Bile Acids, Lipoproteins, and Atherosclerosis

B. Angelin

Introduction

Bile acids represent the major elimination product of cholesterol in humans. These amphiphilic molecules, which are synthesized exclusively in the liver, interact with the metabolism of cholesterol and lipoproteins in several ways (for reviews see [1-4]). Sufficient bile acids are needed in the upper small intestine to ensure adequate absorption of fat and cholesterol. The biliary secretion of bile acids is the major driving force for hepatic bile formation and for the secretion of cholesterol and phospholipids into bile. The rate of degradation of cholesterol to bile acids is regulated by the amount of bile acids returning to the liver in the portal vein. It is thus evident that disturbances of bile acid metabolism may have profound effects on the whole-body cholesterol balance and on lipoprotein turnover. The aim of this paper is to review briefly some recent studies on bile acid metabolism in relation to lipoprotein turnover, and to propose some questions for future research in this field of possible relevance to the development of atherosclerosis.

Bile Acid Enterohepatic Circulation and Cholesterol Metabolism

The quantitatively most important bile acids found in human bile are cholic acid, chenodeoxycholic acid, and deoxycholic acid. The first two are formed from cholesterol in the liver (primary bile acids) via a series of hydroxylation reactions as well as cleavage of the side chain [5]. The initial and rate-limiting step in bile acid formation is the 7α-hydroxylation of cholesterol, a reaction catalyzed by the microsomal enzyme cholesterol 7α-hydroxylase. This enzyme has recently been characterized in human liver [6], and its activity has been demonstrated to be sensitive to feedback inhibition by the amount of bile acids returning to the liver in the portal vein. Under steady-state conditions, the amount of bile acids being synthesized by the liver - about 0.5-1.5 mmol/day (200-600 mg/day) - corresponds to the fecal excretion of bile acids. Normally, about twice as much cholic acid as chenodeoxycholic acid is produced. The pool of bile acids, about 4-10 mmol (1.5-4 g), circulates between 5 and 10 times each day in the enterohepatic circulation [1, 3]. During this enterohepatic circulation, secondary bile acids such as deoxycholic acid are formed by bacterial modifications of the bile acid structure. As a consequence of the efficient intestinal uptake of bile acids, both by active and passive transport mechanisms, a substantial secretion of bile acids can occur with only moderate losses of steroid each day.

Compared with most other species, humans have a relatively limited capacity to synthesize bile acids [2]. Accordingly, a relatively large amount of the net excretion of cholesterol occurs as secretion of free cholesterol into the bile. This explains the relatively high saturation of human bile with cholesterol and the consequent high propensity for formation of cholesterol gallstones that is evident in man.

Cholesterol in the intestinal lumen is derived from dietary as well as from endogenous sources. The latter may generally predominate, and consist of biliary secretion and shedding of cells from the intestinal wall. The high secretion of biliary cholesterol in man could hypothetically be of importance as an atherogenic factor, as it makes a relatively large load of endogenous cholesterol available for absorption. Between 30% and 70% of cholesterol is absorbed after micellar solubilization, in which bile acids are essential [3]. This cholesterol is then transported into the lymph as chylomicrons, which are converted to chylomicron remnants in the peripheral circulation. These particles, which are actively taken up via specific receptors recognizing the E apolipoprotein (apo E) ensure that most of the dietary (and biliary) cholesterol that is absorbed ends up in the liver. Up to now, no clear metabolic regulation of the apo E (or remnant) receptor has been observed under physiological conditions [7-9].

The major endogenous lipoprotein is very-low-density lipoprotein (VLDL) which is secreted from the liver and converted to intermediate- (IDL) and low-density lipoprotein (LDL) in the circulation. Specific receptors recognizing apo B as well as apo E exist in most tissues, but those in the liver and small intestine predominate. The hepatic apo B,E (or LDL) receptors have been shown to be efficiently regulated by the hepatic demand for cholesterol in several species, including man [7-9]. However, the major mechanism for responding to changes in the requirement for cholesterol appears to be the modulation of the activity of the rate-limiting step in cholesterol biosynthesis, the microsomal enzyme hydroxymethyl glutaryl coenzyme A (HMG CoA) reductase [10].

Bile Acid Metabolism in Diseases of Lipoprotein Metabolism

The importance of the liver in the metabolism of cholesterol and lipoproteins is evident from the previous section. Variation in the inflow of cholesterol to the liver should theoretically influence the amount of precursor cholesterol available for bile acid production, and it is of interest to consider the effects of various lipoprotein abnormalities on bile acid production in vivo.

Reduced LDL Receptor Activity. Heterozygous familial hypercholesterolemia (with a reduced expression of LDL receptors) is not associated with any quantitative or qualitative abnormality of bile acid biosynthesis [11]. Patients with a total lack of LDL receptor activity (homozygous, receptor-negative) produce normal amounts of bile acids, and can even increase their synthesis rate in response to interruption of the enterohepatic circulation [12]. Hypothyroidism, which is linked to a reduced hepatic LDL receptor-mediated uptake [13], is not associated with a reduced synthesis of bile acids [14]. In addition, patients lacking VLDL and LDL as the consequence of abetalipoproteinemia still produce normal amounts of bile acids [15].

Thus, the availability of LDL to the liver does not appear to be critical in determining the production rate of bile acids in man.

HDL Deficiency States. HDL has been suggested as a major donor of precursor cholesterol for bile acid synthesis in man [16]. However, in two conditions with heavily reduced HDL levels (fish eye disease and apo AI/CIII deficiency) the production rate of bile acids has been reported to be quantitatively normal [17, 18]. Interestingly, the normal ratio (about 2:1) between the synthesis rates of cholic acid and chenodeoxycholic acid was reversed in both conditions. Thus, HDL deficiency may be associated with a disturbed equilibrium within the precursor pools thought to exist for the two primary bile acids [5, 19].

Reduced Inflow of Chylomicron Remnants. In type III hyperlipoproteinemia, the presence of the variant E-2 isoform of apo E results in defective recognition of chylomicron remnants by the hepatic lipoprotein receptors [20]. In such patients the synthesis of bile acids is increased [21, 22]. This is probably due to the reduced inflow of dietary cholesterol to the liver, resulting in a reduced feedback inhibition of cholesterol synthesis and a consequent increase in bile acid production. Similarly, in situations with cholesterol malabsorption, such as abetalipoproteinemia, coeliac disease, or treatment with β-sitosterol, the synthesis of bile acids is also increased or normal [15, 23, 24].

To summarize, in these various situations of defective lipoprotein uptake by the liver there is no evidence of a reduced capacity to keep a normal bile acid synthesis rate. This reflects the presence of compensatory mechanisms by which the liver may produce precursor cholesterol and retain a normal level of bile acid production. However, further studies on the synthesis of the individual bile acids and the ratio between them in conditions with defective hepatic lipoprotein uptake may be helpful for our further understanding of the compartmentation of hepatic cholesterol in humans.

Disorders of Lipoprotein Metabolism Associated with Disturbances of Bile Acid Turnover

Two situations exist where a primary defect in bile acid metabolism may be considered to be of importance for the development of hyperlipoproteinemia, familial hypertriglyceridemia and polygenic hypercholesterolemia [4].

Familial Hypertriglyceridemia. Endogenous hypertriglyceridemia (type IV lipoprotein pattern) may result from at least two genetic conditions, familial hypertriglyceridemia and familial combined hyperlipidemia. In the first situation, all affected individuals express pure hypertriglyceridemia, i.e., type IV or type V lipoprotein pattern. In familial combined hyperlipidemia, the affected individuals may carry the type IIA, type IIB, or type IV lipoprotein pattern, and the phenotype may also vary within the same individual when studied over prolonged periods of time. Detailed studies of bile acid metabolism in patients with these different forms of genetic hypertriglyceridemia have revealed that patients with familial hypertriglyceridemia, but not those with familial combined hyperlipidemia, have an increased rate of production of bile acids [25]. Also, the fractional catabolic rates of cholic and chenodeoxycholic acids are increased, and the postprandial concentration of serum bile acids is diminished, indicating a reduced capacity for intestinal conservation of the bile acid pool. Mechanistically, it is interesting to consider the corresponding situation in patients treated with cholestyramine; this treatment results in an increased production rate of VLDL triglycerides, and frequently a transient hypertriglyceridemia [26, 27]. As discussed elsewhere [4], the linkage between defective bile acid enterohepatic circulation and VLDL triglyceride overproduction is undefined, but further studies on the regulation of bile acid metabolism in familial hypertriglyceridemia should be performed.

Polygenic Hypercholesterolemia. As discussed above, patients with familial hypercholesterolemia do not have an abnormal bile acid metabolism. In several studies, patients with hypercholesterolemia have been reported to have a reduced bile acid biosynthesis, particularly of cholic acid [28, 29]. Most of the patients mentioned in these reports probably suffered from polygenic hypercholesterolemia or familial combined hyperlipidemia. A recent detailed analysis of cholic acid production rate in relation to serum cholesterol levels in patients with moderate hypercholesterolemia (serum cholesterol 7.5-10 mmol/l) revealed that a reduced fraction of cholic acid synthesis frequently occurs [4]. It is tempting to speculate that this reduced capacity for bile acid synthesis results in a decreased uptake of LDL, and that this is the reason for hypercholesterolemia.

It is of particular relevance to discuss the recent finding of a reduced bile acid biosynthesis with increasing age [30]. It is well known that LDL levels increase with age [31, 32], and recent studies from our laboratory have clearly demonstrated a reduced LDL catabolism with advancing age [33]. Normalization of this situation may be induced by cholestyramine, again strengthening the importance of the relationship between bile acid synthesis and LDL catabolism.

Effects of Perturbations of Bile Acid Metabolism on Lipoprotein Kinetics

LDL Metabolism. A considerable capacity for regulation of hepatic apo B,E receptors in the liver has been demonstrated in several species, whereas the chylomicron remnants (apo E) receptors appear to be refractory to regulation [7-9]. There is generally a reciprocal correlation between plasma LDL level on the one hand and hepatic lipoprotein receptor activity and clearance rates on the other [7]. At least two clinical conditions with increased bile acid production are known to display low LDL levels, type III hyperlipoproteinemia [20] and cerebrotendinous xanthomatosis [34]. Whether this is the result of an increased fractional catabolic rate of plasma LDL has not been established as yet. Also the possibility that the low LDL levels frequently seen in hypertriglyceridemia are related to an enhanced bile acid production rate needs to be investigated.

Feeding with bile acids, particularly chenodeoxycholic acid, reduces bile acid formation [1-3]. Animal studies have indicated that suppression of bile acid production down-regulates LDL receptor binding activity in the liver [35]. Accordingly, LDL levels increase somewhat during treatment with chenodeoxycholic acid but not during treatment with ursodeoxycholic acid [4]; the latter bile acid does not suppress bile acid biosynthesis [36]. Preliminary studies (unpublished) indicate reduced LDL receptor binding in human liver during therapy with chenodeoxycholic acid, as well as reduced catabolism of plasma LDL in vivo.

Thus, whereas abnormalities of LDL receptors and LDL uptake have relatively minor effects on bile acid biosynthesis, the production rate of bile acids appears to be relatively important for the expression of hepatic LDL receptors. Also, the effect of age on bile acid metabolism mentioned above would fit into this scheme. Another intriguing observation is the fact that treatment with disulfiram, which inhibits cholesterol 7α-hydroxylase in animals [37], has been shown to increase LDL levels in treated patients [38].

VLDL Metabolism. Interruption of bile acid enterohepatic circulation results in an increased rate of VLDL triglyceride production [26, 39]. On the other hand, suppression of bile acid biosynthesis by chenodeoxycholic acid reduces VLDL triglyceride formation and decreases the corresponding levels somewhat [26, 40]. Although these effects are generally counterbalanced by reversed changes in the fractional catabolic rate of VLDL particles, the flux of VLDL triglycerides is clearly affected by interference with bile acid metabolism. Possible mechanisms for this relationship have been discussed in detail elsewhere [4], and further studies should clearly be performed in order to characterize it.

HDL Metabolism. Information is very sparse on the effect on HDL metabolism of interference with the enterohepatic circulation of bile acids [41]. Although a considerable proportion of bile acids may be transported through plasma in HDL [42], data on HDL metabolism during bile acid feeding is very limited. The complexity of HDL metabolism makes conclusive studies difficult to perform, but more detailed information on the possible influence of bile acid metabolism on HDL kinetics should be of considerable interest.

Conclusions and Some Questions for the Future

Several important metabolic connections exist between bile acid, cholesterol, and lipoprotein metabolism. Because of the large capacity of the liver to increase its synthesis of cholesterol, deficient uptake of lipoprotein cholesterol by the liver does not result in disturbances of bile acid production. On the other hand, influencing the hepatic demand for cholesterol aimed for bile acid synthesis by interference with enterohepatic circulation appears to affect the expression of LDL (apo B,E) receptors. However, in most situations regulation of cholesterol synthesis appears to be more active. As the liver is by far the most important organ for net excretion of cholesterol from the body, a more detailed knowledge of the concordant regulation of LDL receptors and HMG CoA reductase in human liver will be of utmost importance. By blocking some compensatory mechanisms (as occurs during treatment with the cholesterol synthesis inhibitors mevinolin or compactin), drastic shunting of lipoprotein cholesterol into bile acids may occur.

Although most of our knowledge in this field has been gained during the past 10 years, several very pertinent questions concerning the possible importance of bile acids in the atherosclerotic process still remain to be addressed:

- Can serum levels of bile acids influence lipoprotein composition and, by inducing conformational changes, affect lipoprotein interaction with various receptors and enzymes?
- What is the relationship between HDL and bile acid synthesis?
- Can a reduced bile acid production result in elevated LDL levels, and is such a mechanism responsible for the increase in LDL levels with age?
- Which genetic factors regulate the level of bile acid synthesis?
- Could polygenic hypercholesterolemia result from a low bile acid production?
- What are the effects of sex steroids on bile acid metabolism?
- Can the atherogenic β-VLDL be induced by feeding bile acids as a result of increased cholesterol absorption as well as hepatic lipoprotein receptor down-regulation?
- Does apo E phenotype influence the response to bile acid feeding?
- Can "priming" of bile acid synthetic capacity in early childhood act as a protective factor against atherosclerosis in subsequent years?
- What is the molecular link between bile acid synthesis and VLDL triglyceride production rate?

Although answering these questions will need development of both clinical and biochemical methodology, several will probably be answered within the next 5 years. Due to the importance of the bile acid/bile cholesterol pathways to the net excretion of cholesterol from the body, such knowledge should also have considerable impact on our understanding of some of the mechanisms behind the development of atherosclerosis.

Acknowledgements. The skillful secretarial assistance of Mrs. Lena Ericsson is gratefully acknowledged. The authors' work is supported by the Swedish Medical Research Council (03X-4793 and 03X-7137) and the King Gustaf V and Queen Victoria Foundation.

References

1. Hofmann AF (1976) The enterohepatic circulation of bile acids in man. Adv Intern Med 21: 501-534
2. Grundy SM (1978) Cholesterol metabolism in man. West J Med 128: 13-25
3. Carey MC (1982) The enterohepatic circulation. In: Arias I, Popper H, Schachter D, Shafritz DA (eds) The liver: biology and pathology. Raven, New York, pp 429-465
4. Angelin B, Einarsson K (1986) Bile acids and lipoprotein metabolism. In: Grundy SM (ed) Bile acids and atherosclerosis. Raven, New York, pp 41-66
5. Björkhem I (1985) Mechanism of bile acid biosynthesis in mammalian liver. In: Danielsson H, Sjövall J (eds) New comprehensive biochemistry. Elsevier, Amsterdam, pp 231-278
6. Einarsson K, Angelin B, Ewerth S, Nilsell K, Björkhem I (1986) Bile acid synthesis in man: assay of hepatic microsomal cholesterol 7α-hydroxylase activity by isotope dilution - mass spectrometry. J Lipid Res 27: 82-88
7. Brown MS, Goldstein JL (1983) Lipoprotein receptors in the liver: control signals for plasma cholesterol traffic. J Clin Invest 72: 743-747

8. Mahley RW, Innerarity TL (1983) Lipoprotein receptors and cholesterol homeostasis. Biochim Biophys Acta 737: 197-222
9. Angelin B (1984) Regulation of hepatic lipoprotein receptor expression. In: Calandra S, Carulli N, Salvioli G (eds) Liver and lipid metabolism. Elsevier, Amsterdam, pp 187-201
10. Angelin B, Reihnér E, Rudling M, Ewerth S, Björkhem I, Einarsson K (1987) In vitro studies of lipid metabolism in human liver. Am Heart J (in press)
11. Angelin B (1987) Bile acid metabolism in heterozygous familial hypercholesterolemia: a study comparing affected and unaffected siblings of four kindreds (to be published)
12. Deckelbaum RJ, Lees RS, Small DM, Hedberg SE, Grundy SM (1977) Failure of complete biliary diversion and oral bile acid therapy in the treatment of homozygous familial hypercholesterolemia. N Engl J Med 296: 465-470
13. Thompson GR, Soutar AK, Spengel FA, Jadhav A, Gavigan SJP, Myant NB (1981) Defects of receptor-mediated low density lipoprotein catabolism in homozygous familial hypercholesterolemia and hypothyroidism in vivo. Proc Natl Acad Sci USA 78: 2591-2595
14. Angelin B, Einarsson K, Leijd B (1983) Bile acid metabolism in hypothyroid subjects: response to substitution therapy. Eur J Clin Invest 13: 99-106
15. Illingworth DR, Connor WE, Lin DS, Diliberti J (1980) Lipid metabolism in abetalipoproteinemia: a study of cholesterol absorption and sterol balance in two patients. Gastroenterology 78: 68-75
16. Halloran LG, Schwartz CC, Vlahcevic ZR, Gregory DM, Swell L (1978) Evidence for high-density lipoprotein-free cholesterol as the primary precursor for bile acid synthesis in man. Surgery 84: 1-7
17. Angelin B, Carlson LA (1986) Bile acids and plasma high density lipoproteins: biliary lipid metabolism in fish eye disease. Eur J Clin Invest 16: 157-162
18. Beher WT, Gabbard A, Norum RA, Stradnieks S (1983) Effect of blood high density lipoprotein cholesterol concentration on fecal steroid excretion in humans. Life Sci 32: 2933-2937
19. Einarsson K, Ahlberg J, Angelin B, Holmström B (1979) Evidence for the presence of different cholesterol precursor pools in man. In: Preisig R, Bircher J (eds) The liver. Editio Cantor, Aulendorf, pp 233-238
20. Mahley RW, Angelin B (1984) Type III hyperlipoproteinemia: recent insights into the genetic defect of familial dysbetalipoproteinemia. Adv Intern Med 29: 385-411
21. Andersén E (1980) On the metabolism of cholesterol and bile acids in normo- and hyperlipoproteinemic subjects. Acta Med Scand (Suppl) 643: 1-35
22. Angelin B, Einarsson K, Holmquist L, Leijd B (1987) Bile acid metabolism in primary dysbetalipoproteinemia (to be published)
23. Vuoristo M, Tarpila S, Miettinen TA (1980) Serum lipids and fecal steroids in patients with celiac disease: effects of gluten-free diet and cholestyramine. Gastroenterology 78: 1518-1525
24. Begemann F, Bandomer G, Herget HJ (1978) The influence of β-sitosterol on biliary cholesterol and bile acid kinetics in man. Scand J Gastroenterol 13: 57-63
25. Angelin B, Hershon KS, Brunzell JD (1987) Bile acid metabolism in hereditary forms of hypertriglyceridemia: evidence for an increased synthesis rate in monogenic familial hypertriglyceridemia (to be published)
26. Angelin B, Einarsson K, Leijd B (1978) Effects of cholestyramine and chenodeoxycholic acid on the metabolism of endogenous triglyceride in hyperlipoproteinemia. J Lipid Res 19: 1017-1024
27. Witztum JL, Schonfeld G, Weidman SW (1976) The effects of colestipol on the metabolism of very-low-density lipoproteins in man. J Lab Clin Med 88: 1008-1018
28. Hellström K, Einarsson K (1977) Bile acid metabolism in hyperlipoproteinaemia. Clin Gastroenterol 6: 103-128
29. Miettinen TA (1982) Effects of hypolipidemic drugs on bile acid metabolism. Adv Lipid Res 18: 65-97
30. Einarsson K, Nilsell K, Leijd B, Angelin B (1985) Influence of age on secretion of cholesterol and synthesis of bile acids by the liver. N Engl J Med 313: 277-282
31. Heiss G, Tamir I, Davis GE, Tyroler HA, Rifkind BM, Schonfeld G, Jacobs D, Frantz I (1980) Lipoprotein-cholesterol distribution in selected North American populations: the Lipid Research Clinics Program Prevalence Study. Circulation 61: 302-315

32. Miller NE (1984) Why does plasma low density lipoprotein concentration in adults increase with age? Lancet I: 263-267
33. Ericsson S, Eriksson M, Einarsson K, Berglund L, Angelin B (1987) Reduction of fractional catabolic rate of plasma low density lipoproteins with increasing age (to be published)
34. Schaefer EJ, Levy RI (1985) Pathogenesis and management of lipoprotein disorders. N Engl J Med 312: 1300-1310
35. Angelin B, Raviola CA, Innerarity TL, Mahley RW (1983) Regulation of hepatic lipoprotein receptors in the dog: rapid regulation of apolipoprotein B,E receptors, but not of apolipoprotein E receptors, by intestinal lipoproteins and bile acids. J Clin Invest 71: 816-831
36. Nilsell K, Angelin B, Leijd B, Einarsson K (1983) Comparative effects of ursodeoxycholic acid and chenodeoxycholic acid on bile acid kinetics and biliary lipid secretion in humans: evidence for different modes of action on bile acid synthesis. Gastroenterology 85: 1248-1256
37. Andersson S, Boström H (1984) Effects of disulfiram on rat liver cholesterol 7α-hydroxylase. Biochem Pharmacol 33: 2930-2932
38. Major LF, Goyer PF (1978) Effect of disulfiram and pyridoxine on serum cholesterol. Ann Intern Med 88: 53-56
39. Nestel PJ, Grundy SM (1976) Changes in plasma triglyceride metabolism during withdrawal of bile. Metabolism 25: 1591-1599
40. Begemann F (1978) Influence of chenodeoxycholic acid on the kinetics of endogenous triglyceride transport in man. Eur J Clin Invest 8: 283-288
41. Packard CJ, Shepherd J (1982) The hepatobiliary axis and lipoprotein metabolism: effect of bile acid sequestrants and ileal bypass surgery. J Lipid Res 23: 1081-1098
42. Abberger H, Bickel U, Buscher H-P, Fuchte K, Gerok W, Kramer W, Kurz G (1981) Transport of bile acids: lipoproteins, membrane polypeptides and cytosolic proteins as carriers. In: Paumgartner G, Stiehl A, Gerok W (eds) Bile acids and lipids. MTP Press, Lancaster, pp 233-246

Metabolic Abnormalities in Cerebral and Peripheral Arteriosclerosis

R. Fellin and G. Valerio

Introduction

Numerous clinical and epidemiological studies have shown that various arterial districts (coronary arteries, cerebral arteries, and arteries of the lower limbs) may be simultaneously affected by sclerotic processes in the same patient, confirming that the pathogenetic mechanisms are similar regardless of site. The International Atherosclerosis Project [1], implemented in 19 different geographic areas throughout the world, found a very strong correlation between coronary and aortic lesions. In the Tecumseh study [2] coronary heart disease and absence of peripheral pulses were found to be associated. More recently, the Framingham study [3] showed that claudicatio intermittens was four times more frequent in patients of either sex affected by coronary heart disease (CHD) than in controls. Patients with peripheral artery disease (PAD) were likewise more frequently affected by CHD. Moreover, certain clinical manifestations of CHD, such as angina pectoris and myocardial infarction, seemed to increase the risk of stroke by a factor of 2–4. The Basel prospective study [4] confirmed this reciprocal association between coronary and extracoronary arteriosclerosis, showing that males with PAD presented CHD twice as frequently as controls, and that those with CHD were twice as likely as controls to present PAD. This study also confirmed the findings reported in the Framingham [5] and Seven County studies [6] that arterial hypertension, low-density lipoprotein cholesterol (LDL-C), cigarette smoking, and diabetes mellitus are all risk factors for both CHD and PAD. The most important metabolic risk factors recognized for PAD and cerebrovascular disease (CVD) are reduction of high-density lipoprotein cholesterol (HDL-C), hyperlipidemia, diabetes, and overweight.

Dyslipidemia

In view of the similar etiology of arteriosclerosis at the various arterial sites, the major risk factors for this diseases may correctly be considered as part of the general cardiovascular risk profile. However, numerous authors have reported characteristics peculiar to the site involved, particularly in relation to the lipoprotein factors. High levels of total cholesterol (TC) and/or LDL-C are two of the main risk factors for CHD and PAD, but are not always associated with the clinical manifestations of CVD; numerous studies have in fact shown that TC levels are frequently similar, and sometimes lower, in patients with CVD than in controls.

Hypertriglyceridemia is often encountered in patients with CHD, PAD, and

CVD. However, there is no confirmation that the triglycerides (TG) play any independent role in the absence of concomitant modifications to HDL-C and LDL-C levels. According to Gordon et al. [7], TG determination seems to add little information about the risk of cardiovascular disease to that elicited from HDL-C and LDL-C and other known risk factors. Hypertriglyceridemia is in fact frequently associated with other metabolic and behavioral anomalies, such as obesity, overeating, diabetes, and reduced HDL levels, which all imply a greater risk of arteriosclerosis than high TG levels alone. The significance of apoprotein levels (apo AI, AII, B) in whole serum or in the individual lipoprotein fractions is still under discussion, as it is not yet known whether they are more predictive of arteriosclerosis than the lipid components. According to Pilger et al. [8], a high apo B level is the most reliable individual indicator of risk for PAD, followed by TC, TG and LDL-apo B. In the same patients, apo AI and AII levels were irrelevant, while apo AI : apo B and apo AII : apo B ratios were strongly indicative of the presence/absence of arteriosclerosis. However, Kostner et al. [9] found that low apo AI and AII levels were highly indicative in patients with CVD and, paradoxically, that apo B and LDL-apo B levels were also lower in patients than in controls and hence do not have predictive value. In patients with PAD [10], increased very low density lipoprotein (VLDL-) apo B levels have also been described as a parameter independent of other lipid or lipoprotein components.

High-Density Lipoproteins

A study in Graz [8, 9] found that HDL-C is predictive of both PAD and CVD. For the former it was strongly predictive only as a ratio with LDL-C, but for the latter it proved to be an independent factor. Numerous other observations have shown that low HDL-C levels are the metabolic alteration most frequently encountered in patients with CVD. In a study of 41 male and 19 female stroke survivors, Taggart et al. [11] found that HDL-C levels were significantly lower (−19%) and TG levels significantly higher (+20%) in patients without other alterations of lipid metabolism than in controls. In 61 patients with CVD, Rossner et al. [12] found only a significant reduction in HDL-C. Sirtori et al. [13] and Murai et al. [14], in patients affected by transient ischemia attacks (TIA) or stroke, confirmed the importance of low HDL-C levels in patients affected by TIA and patients affected by TIA or stroke, respectively.

Diabetes Mellitus

Macrovascular complications remain the major causes, in both sexes, of morbidity and mortality in diabetes today. The findings of an international study organized by the World Health Organization [15] clearly suggest that both PAD and CVD correlate strongly with the duration of the disease and fasting glycemia but not with plasma TG, although this is often increased in the presence of reduced HDL-C levels. Diabetes is often associated with other risk factors such as hyperlipidemia, arterial hypertension, and obesity. However, multivariate analysis in the Framingham study [16] showed that diabetes also has an independent role as a risk factor; total mortality from cardiovascular causes was triple in male and double in female diabetics compared with controls. The higher risk of arteriosclerosis linked with diabetes derives from complex modifications caused by the disease in factors both extrinsic (insulin lipoproteins, platelets, etc.) and intrinsic (smooth muscle cells, wall macrophages, etc.) to the arterial wall [17].

Hyperinsulinemia, secondary to the insulin resistance in noninsulin-dependent diabetes mellitus and to exogenous administration in insulin-dependent diabetes mellitus, stimulates the proliferation of smooth muscle cells in the artery wall, hastening the process of artherogenesis. Diabetics have been shown to have increased platelet consumption and reduced platelet survival rates; the platelets become hyperaggregable in correlation with plasma glycemia, and total cholesterol and TG levels, mediated, in part, by an increased thromboxane production. Modifications of the lipid and apoprotein components of the individual lipoprotein fractions have been shown to be sufficient to give rise to significant alterations in their metabolism. For reasons that remain to be demonstrated, VLDLs in diabetics with hypertriglyceridemia are more readily captured by macrophages, giving rise to a rapid increase in foam cells. LDLs, which are abnormally rich in TG and poor in cholesterol, are captured and degraded more slowly by specific receptors; this provokes an excessive accumulation of cholesterol in the plasma and insufficient control of its cellular synthesis. In diabetes, VLDL and LDL become cytotoxic to the cells of the arterial wall as a result of anomalous oxidation processes in the lipid components. The apoproteins of VLDL, LDL, and HDL are subject to nonenzymatic glycosylation and carbamylation; the modified VLDLs and LDLs acquire imumogene properties and the resulting immunocomplexes are potentially damaging to the endothelial cells. The glycosylated HDLs, unlike the LDLs, degrade very rapidly. The increase in the free cholesterol:phospholipid ratio occurring in the VLDLs and LDLs of diabetics facilitates the direct passage of cholesterol to HDL, reducing the removal of tissue cholesterol.

Obesity

The analysis of excess weight as a risk factor in arteriosclerosis is complicated by its frequent association with other known risk factors. The overweight subject frequently has a hypercaloric, hyperlipidic diet and leads a sedentary life. Carbohydrate tolerance deteriorates in direct proportion with the magnitude and duration of excess weight; baseline insulinemia and insulin secretion after stimulation are correlated with development of adipose tissue, so the obese subject is simultaneously hyperinsulinemic and insulin resistant as a result of down-regulation on the specific receptor function. Hyperinsulinemia provokes an increase in the hepatic synthesis of VLDL and cholesterol, while HDL is inversely correlated to TG (VLDL) levels and the body mass index. This complex interdependence of metabolic processes is further complicated by the frequent association of obesity with arterial hypertension. In the light of these considerations, we may well understand the difficulties encountered in the Framingham study [18] (26 years of observation of a general population) in the identification of an independent role of obesity as a risk factor for arteriosclerosis.

Personal Contribution

Low HDL-C levels are one of the few risk factors common to both coronary (CHD) and extra-coronary (PAD, CVD) arteriosclerosis. HDL_2 (density *(d)*= 1.063-1.125 g/ml) and HDL_3 (*d*=1.125-1.21 g/ml) are the two most important subfractions constituting the high-density lipoproteins, and seem to have different predictive values for CHD. According to Anderson et al. [19], plasma HDL_2 cholesterol (HDL_2-C) levels define the coronary risk profile with a 50% better precision than total HDL-C levels. Unlike HDL_3, HDL_2 plasma levels cover a wide range, mainly contributing to influence the concentrations of total HDL. Low HDL_2 levels are associated with several conditions, such as a sedentary lifestyle, obesity, hypertriglyceridemia, carbohydrate-rich diet, and the male sex. High levels are associated with females and physically active individuals. Studies on the formation of HDL_2 and HDL_3 suggest that their plasma concentrations are reciprocally regulated by the activity of lipoprotein lipase. The data are compatible with a concept proposing conversion of HDL_3 to HDL_2 through assimilation of cholesterol, phospholipids, and apoproteins from TG-rich lipoproteins during their degradation by lipoprotein lipase. In particular, the concentration of HDL_2 seems closely related to the rate of intravascular lipolysis. Gidez et al. [20] have proposed a simple and precise method for HDL_2 and HDL_3 subfractionation by polyanion precipitation. Recently, Fellin et al. [21] evaluated the clinical relevance of TC, TG, HDL-C, and the HDL_2 and HDL_3 subfractions in 69 patients affected by PAD and CVD. TC levels were significantly higher in patients (both males and females) than in controls; TG levels were also higher, but the difference was significant only in females. HDL-C levels, on the other hand, were significantly lower in both male (−21.8%) and female (−20.5%) patients. This decrease was more prevalent in HDL_2-C (−32.7% and −32.5% in males and females respectively) than in HDL_3-C (Table 1). The lowest values of HDL-C, HDL_2-C, and HDL_3-C were observed in patients with CVD (Table 2). The TC: HDL-C ratio was significantly higher in both male and female patients as a whole (Table 3). Statistically significant negative correlations between TG and HDL-C and between TG and HDL_2-C were present only in controls. No significant correlation between TG and HDL_3-C was observed (Table 4).

In agreement with other workers, we found a significant reduction in HDL-C

Table 1. Mean values (mg/dl; mean ± SD) of plasma cholesterol, TG, HDL-C, HDL_2-C, and HDL_3-C in patients and controls, and percentage decrease (in parentheses) of HDL-C, HDL_2-C, and HDL_3-C in patients

	Sex	No.	Cholesterol	TG	HDL-C	HDL_2-C	HDL_3-C
Patients	M	55	223.4 ± 47.2[a]	131 ± 54.8	36.2 ± 9.9[c] (21.8%)	10.6 ± 5.6[c] (32.7%)	25.6 ± 6.5[c] (16.5%)
Controls	M	47	205.7 ± 35.4	117 ± 43.8	46.3 ± 10.7	15.7 ± 7.1	30.7 ± 6.2
Patients	F	14	239.0 ± 53[a]	130.9 ± 56.4[b]	43.6 ± 10.5[b] (20.5%)	13.1 ± 6[a] (32.5%)	30.5 ± 6.8[a] (14.2%)
Controls	F	32	212.7 ± 31.5	87.3 ± 32.6	54.8 ± 13.3	19.41 ± 9.2	35.6 ± 6.9

[a] $P<0.05$. [b] $P<0.01$. [c] $P<0.001$.

Table 2. Mean values (mg/dl; mean ± SD) of serum cholesterol, TG, HDL-C, HDL_2-C and HDL_3-C in patients subdivided according to the lesion distribution and in controls

	No.	Sex	Cholesterol	TG	HDL-C	HDL_2-C	HDL_3-C
PAD	31	M	225.4 ± 47.7[a]	125.4 ± 49.3	37.8 ± 8.9[d]	11.1 ± 5.6[c]	26.6 ± 6.1[b]
	8	F	269.4 ± 48.2[d]	157.1 ± 52.7[d]	46.6 ± 9.9	14.9 ± 6.6	33.0 ± 4.8
CVD	11	M	225.8 ± 46.5	147.2 ± 54.1	31.0 ± 10.8[d]	8.3 ± 6.0[c]	22.7 ± 6.4[d]
	6	F	198.5 ± 24.8	96.0 ± 42.6	39.5 ± 10.8[a]	10.7 ± 4.6[a]	27.2 ± 7.9[a]
Both	13	M	216.6 ± 50.0	130.8 ± 68.3	37.1 ± 10.8[b]	11.4 ± 4.9[a]	25.7 ± 7.4[b]
Controls	47	M	205.7 ± 35.4	117.0 ± 43.8	46.3 ± 10.7	15.7 ± 7.1	30.7 ± 6.2
	32	F	212.7 ± 31.5	87.3 ± 32.6	54.8 ± 13.3	19.4 ± 9.2	35.6 ± 6.9

[a] $P < 0.05$. [b] $P < 0.01$. [c] $P < 0.005$. [d] $P < 0.001$.

Table 3. Mean values (mean ± SD) of TC:HDL-C and HDL_2-C:HDL_3-C ratios in patients and controls

	Sex	No.	TC:HDL-C	HDL_2-C:HDL_3-C
Patients	M	55	6.54 ± 1.96[c]	0.43 ± 0.23[a]
Controls		47	4.68 ± 1.37	0.53 ± 0.24
Patients	F	14	5.76 ± 1.82	0.44 ± 0.20
Controls		32	4.06 ± 1.03	0.55 ± 0.23
Patients	M + F	69	6.38 ± 1.94[c]	0.43 ± 0.23[b]
Controls		79	4.43 ± 1.27	0.54 ± 0.23

[a] $P < 0.05$. [b] $P < 0.01$. [c] $P < 0.001$.

Table 4. Correlations *(r)* between the concentration of TG and HDL-C, HDL_2-C, and HDL_3-C values in patients and controls

	TG/HDL-C	TG/HDL_2-C	TG/HDL_3-C
Patients ($n = 69$)	−0.21	−0.24	−0.08
Controls ($n = 79$)	−0.38[a]	−0.43[a]	−0.18

[a] $P < 0.001$.

associated with a slight increase in plasma TC and TG levels, and a significant increase in the TC:HDL-C ratio in patients with PAD and CVD. The HDL reduction was due to a fall in both HDL_2-C and HDL_3-C; nonetheless, an analysis of the HDL_2-C:HDL_3-C ratio disclosed that HDL_2-C was the most reduced. Referring specifically to extracoronary arteriosclerosis, Bradby et al. [22] reported a significant reduction in apo AI (the main HDL_2 apoprotein) in individuals with PAD. Considered in the light of other studies [9, 19, 22], our results tend to suggest that HDL_2 may be the major anti-atherogenic component of the two HDL subfractions. The statistically significant negative correlations between TG and HDL-C and HDL_2-C, but not between TG and HDL_3-C, demonstrated in controls, fits the above-cited hypothesis that HDL_2 formation is regulated by lipoprotein lipase. The absence of a significant correlation between these parameters in patients suggests a possible alteration of this metabolic process.

In conclusion, these preliminary results in patients with PAD and CVD show that the reduction in HDL-C is due to a reduction in both HDL_2-C and HDL_3-C, although the decrease is greater in the former. Since HDL-C is a parameter in the definition of the arteriosclerosis risk profile, we feel that cholesterol determination in the HDL subfractions is advisable.

References

1. International Atherosclerosis Project (1968) The geographic pathology of atherosclerosis. Lab Invest 18: 5-180
2. Johnson BC, Epstein FH (1966) Absence of peripheral pulse in relation to other arterial disease in a community study. Am J Public Health 56: 1482-1492
3. Kannel WB, Shurtleff D (1971) The natural history of arteriosclerosis obliterans. In: Brest, Gifford (eds) Peripheral vascular disease, vol 3. Davis, Philadelphia, pp 38-52
4. Widmer LK, Stahelin HB, Nissen C, Da Silva A (eds) (1981) Venen, Arterien, Krankheiten, Koronare Herzkrankheit bei Berufstätigen. Huber, Bern
5. Kannel WB, McGee FD, Gordon T (1976) A general cardiovascular risk profile: the Framingham study. Am J Cardiol 38: 46-51
6. Menotti A, Giampaoli S (1986) Epidemiology and prediction of cerebral and peripheral vascular diseases. Monogr Atheroscler 14: 11-14
7. Gordon T, Kannel WB, Castelli WP, Dawber TR (1981) Lipoproteins, cardiovascular disease and death. The Framingham study. Arch Intern Med 141: 1128-1131
8. Pilger E, Pristautz H, Pfeiffer KP, Kostner G (1983) Retrospective evaluation of risk factors for peripheral atherosclerosis by stepwise discriminant analysis. Arteriosclerosis 3: 57-63
9. Kostner GM, Marth E, Pfeiffer KH, Wege H (1986) Laboratory parameters as discriminators for peripheral atherosclerosis and stroke. Monogr Atheroscler 14: 119-123
10. Franceschini G, Bondioli A, Matero M, Sirtori M, Tattoni G, Biasi G, Sirtori RC (1982) Increased apoprotein B in very low density lipoproteins of patients with peripheral vascular disease. Arteriosclerosis 2: 74-80
11. Taggart H, Stout RW (1979) Reduced high density lipoprotein in stroke: relationship with elevated triglyceride and hypertension. Eur J Clin Invest 9: 219-221
12. Rossner S, Kjellin KG, Mettinger KL, Siden A (1978) Normal serum cholesterol but low HDL-cholesterol in young patients with ischaemic cerebrovascular disease. Lancet I: 577-579
13. Sirtori CR, Gianfranceschi G, Gritti I, Nappi G, Brambilla G, Paoletti P (1979) Decreased high density lipoprotein cholesterol levels in male patients with transient ischaemic attacks. Atherosclerosis 32: 205-211
14. Murai A, Tomoji T, Myahara T (1981) Lipoprotein abnormalities in the pathogenesis of cerebral infarction and transient ischaemic attack. Stroke 12: 167-172
15. West KM, Ahuja MM, Bennet PH, Czyzyk A, Matco de Acosta O, Fuller JH, Grab B, Grabauskas V, Jarrett J, Kosaka K, Keen H, Krolewski AS, Miki E, Schliack V, Teuscher A, Watkins PJ, Stober JA (1983) The role of circulating glucose and triglyceride concentrations and their interactions with other "risk factors" as determinants of arterial disease in nine diabetic population samples from the WHO multinational study. Diabetes Care 6: 361-369
16. Kannel WB, McGee FD (1979) Diabetes and cardiovascular risk factors: The Framingham study. Circulation 59: 8-13
17. Chait A, Bierman EL, Brunzell JD (1985) Diabetic macroangiopathy. In: Alberti KG, Krall LP (eds) The diabetes annual, vol 1. Elsevier, Amsterdam, pp 323-348
18. Hubert HB, Feinleib M, McNamara PM, Castelli WP (1983) Obesity as an indipendent risk fac-

tor for cardiovascular disease: a 26 year follow-up of participants in the Framingham Heart Study. Circulation 67: 968-977

19. Anderson DW, Nichols AV, Brewer HB Jr (1979) Ultracentrifugal characterization of the human plasma high density lipoprotein distribution. In: Lippel K (ed) Report of the High Density Lipoprotein Methodology Workshop. NIH publication 79, 1661, pp 290-300
20. Gidez LI, Miller GJ, Burstein M, Seagle S, Eder HA (1982) Separation and quantitation of subclasses of human plasma high density lipoproteins by a simple precipitation procedure. J Lipid Res 23: 1206-1223
21. Fellin R, Baroni L, Baiocchi MR, Baldo Enzi G, Grego F, Valerio G (1985) Selective determination of cholesterol in high density lipoprotein subfractions (HDL2 and HDL3) in patients with cerebral and peripheral arteriosclerosis. Clin Chim Acta 147: 233-240
22. Bradby GVH, Valente AJ, Walton KW (1978) Serum high density lipoproteins in peripheral vascular disease. Lancet II: 1271-1274

Elastase-Type Enzymes and Their Relation to Blood Lipids and Atherosclerosis

M. Bihari-Varga and L. Keller

Introduction

The causes and detailed mechanisms of the process leading to the development of the well-known morphological appearance of atherosclerosis are not yet clearly understood. Degradation of the elastic fibers of the arterial wall seems to be an important step in the chain of the complex and multifactorial events of atherogenesis. Although progressive splitting, fragmentation, and lysis of elastic lamellae can be observed in smaller amounts in the course of maturation and aging, the degradation of the elastic fibers is significantly accelerated in atherosclerosis and some other pathological conditions such as pulmonary emphysema, diabetes, arthritis, and several skin diseases.

Few details of the process resulting in the lysis of elastic fibers are known. The elastic fibers contain two distinct ultrastructural components, a microfibrillar component formed by cross-striated fibrotubules and an amorphous one, elastin. From the earliest phase of atherogenesis plasma low-density lipoproteins (LDL) enter the arterial wall and interact with connective tissue macromolecules such as glycosaminoglycans, collagen, and elastin; this selective interaction is considered to be one of the mechanisms of lipid accumulation in atherosclerotic lesions [1-7], although the precise mode of interaction of these components is still not completely understood. The findings of Srinivasan et al. [8] indicated that certain regions of plaque elastin may have affinity for apolipoprotein B (apo B)-containing lipoproteins. According to Kramsch et al. [3, 9, 10], with the permeation of LDL into arterial elastin a change in the protein composition of arterial elastin takes place in localized areas; the result of this process will be further deposition of lipids attracted by the focally altered elastin surface. Accumulated lipids are successively phagocytosed by macrophages, which, after having been destroyed, release their lipid content into the intercellular space, causing damage to both the external and internal elastic membranes of the media.

Atherosclerotic lesions seem to remain focal until the integrity of the elastic structure of the media is maintained, and may become extensive due to a more pronounced fragmentation of the elastic lamellae [11-13]. Noma et al. [14, 15] presented evidence of the in vitro formation of a stable complex between LDL and delipidated arterial elastin, and the inhibition of the LDL binding to elastin in the presence of high-density lipoprotein (HDL); the inhibition proved to be significantly higher with HDL_3 than with HDL_2 [16].

The regulation of elastin metabolism both under physiological and pathological conditions is attributed to humoral and tissue elastases and their inhibitors, and possibly other substances. Disturbances in the equilibrium of elastases and inhibitors might lead to elastic tissue destruction [13, 17].

Elastases, a group of proteolytic enzymes, are endopeptidases capable of solubilizing and degrading insoluble elastin fibers. Baló and Banga [18] were the first to report that elastase extracted from pancreas had a degrading effect on elastin. Elastinolytic enzymes can belong to any of the four classes of proteinases (aspartic-, cysteine-, serine- and metalloproteases). They have been isolated from various sources, and their structures, properties, and specificities have been partially characterized [11-13]. There are data indicating that elastases inhibit the progress of experimental atherosclerosis and enhance lipoprotein lipase activity [19-23]. According to Katsunuma et al. [23] the mechanism of action of elastase consists of the selective degradation of lipid-bound elastin, by which elastase promotes the biosynthesis of newly formed elastin. Hornebeck et al. [24] could not find statistically significant differences between elastase levels in the sera of atherosclerotic and of control subjects. In the circulation the activity of elastases can be modified by high amounts of elastase inhibitors, e.g. α_1-proteinase inhibitor and α_2-macroglobulin [24, 25]. The presence of elastase inhibitors in human aorta has also been reported; it has been suggested that the increase in elastinolytic activity may represent a decrease in the level of inhibitors in the tissue [26]. The local inactivation of α_1-proteinase inhibitor may lead to extensive elastin degradation, as was observed in the lungs of rats in cigarette-smoke inhalation experiments [27].

The aim of our investigation was to gain further insight into the humoral alterations in atherosclerotic vascular disease. Based on the suggestion that changes of elastin metabolism may be reflected in changes of elastase-like activity and of elastase inhibitory capacity of the serum, we have undertaken a series of studies on the behavior of these parameters and their relationship to blood lipids in atherosclerotic patients. It seemed to be of interest to subdivide the atherosclerotic patients according to the localization of the disease, as the factors influencing the anatomical manifestation of the illness have still not been elucidated. As myocardial infarction is the most important acute clinical manifestation of atherosclerosis, investigations were also performed on the dynamics of elastase-like activity, inhibitory capacity, and lipids in the course of myocardial infarction.

Methods

A total of 154 patients between the ages of 40 and 80 years, 130 suffering from advanced ischaemic vascular disease (IVD) of varying localization (coronary, cerebral, peripheral) and 24 with acute myocardial infarction, were studied. The patients were chosen so that the age distribution within each age group was similar. Selection criteria for inclusion were: (1) for patients with ischaemic heart disease (IHD), myocardial infarction at least 6 months prior to the investigation or typical anginal pains and ECG signs of myocardial ischaemia; (2) for patients with cerebrovascular disease (CVD), acute cerebrovascular accident with focal neurological signs in the case history at least 6 months prior to the investigation; (3) for patients with peripheral vascular disease (PVD), intermittent or rest pain with oscillometric and Doppler signs of stenotic or occlusive arterial disease in the lower extremities;

(4) for patients with acute myocardial infarction (AMI), the fulfillment of the criteria for myocardial infarction set by the World Health Organization [28]. As controls 60 age-matched subjects were selected from individuals without histories, symptoms, or findings of IVD. Patients with diabetes mellitus, chronic renal or hepatic disease, endocrine disorders, primary hyperlipidemias, and those treated with drugs affecting lipid metabolism were excluded from the study.

Venous blood was obtained after an overnight fast. Elastase-type protease activity and pancreas elastase inhibitory capacity was measured according to Bieth et al. [29]. Triglyceride, total cholesterol, HDL, HDL_2, HDL_3, LDL, apo A, and apo B contents were determined using Boehringer's Peridochrom and CHOD-PAP test and Sebia's Apofilm plates. Serum glutamic oxaloacetic transaminase (SGOT), lactate dehydrogenase (LDH), and LDH_1 were measured using General Diagnostics' Trans-Ac and Lac-Dehystrate tests. For statistical evaluation conventional t and χ^2 tests were used.

Results and Discussion

Chronic Vascular Disease. Average values of serum elastase activity and pancreatic elastase inhibitory capacity are given in Table 1. Elastase-type enzyme activity was found to be higher in females than in males, probably due to endocrine factors. The mean activity was lower in all three groups of male patients with different localization of IVD than in the controls, while in all three groups of females with IVD elevated elastase activity was measured. Variation with the age of the individuals was not significant. Elastase inhibitory capacity was significantly elevated in all three groups of patients. In healthy individuals of both sexes there exists a significant

Table 1. Elastase activity and pancreas elastase inhibitory capacity (means ± SD) of the sera of patients with IHD, CVD, PVD, and of matched controls

Vascular diagnosis	Sex	Number of patients	Elastase activity (ng ml^{-1} 24 h^{-1})	Inhibitory capacity (ng ml^{-1} 24 h^{-1})
IHD	M+F	54	8.1 ± 4.3	40.8 ± 10.7[a]
	M	30	5.0 ± 2.5[a]	40.2 ± 13.2
	F	24	12.0 ± 6.7[c]	41.6 ± 7.6
CVD	M+F	38	9.5 ± 6.9	40.0 ± 8.4[a]
	M	24	8.9 ± 6.2	39.5 ± 10.3
	F	14	11.0 ± 8.3	43.7 ± 4.9
PVD	M+F	38	10.3 ± 5.8	39.0 ± 8.9[a]
	M	20	7.9 ± 4.8[b]	38.8 ± 10.0
	F	18	12.6 ± 7.0[d]	39.4 ± 7.3
Control	M+F	60	9.3 ± 3.9	31.5 ± 10.4
	M	33	9.3 ± 3.5	30.3 ± 10.1
	F	27	9.2 ± 4.1	33.1 ± 10.8

Significance vs control: [a] $P<0.001$, [b] $P<0.01$.
Significance of M vs F: [c] $P<0.001$, [d] $P<0.01$.

positive correlation ($P < 0.001$) between the elastase-type enzyme activity of sera and their elastase inhibitory capacity; this correlation could not be established in the sera of patients suffering from IVD. This phenomenon points to the possibility that in healthy individuals variation of elastase-type activity is counterbalanced by its inhibitors; the lack of proportionality within the pathological population may well be related to the atherosclerotic process.

From among the serum lipid and lipoprotein parameters, only HDL cholesterol and apo A content showed significant alterations; they were found to be decreased in all three types of IVD compared with matched controls [30, 31]. HDL cholesterol and apo A concentrations showed significant negative correlations with elastase inhibitory capacity (Table 2). This finding may be related to the fact that an elastase-type enzyme could be isolated and characterized in close association with apo A of human HDL preparations [32].

Acute Myocardial Infarction. In our studies significantly increased elastase-type activity was measured in the serum of the patients on the 7th day after AMI (Fig. 1). This might be considered as a part of the response reaction of the organism to the

Table 2. Significance of the correlation between elastase inhibitory capacity of the serum and its HDL cholesterol and apo A contents

Group of patients	Sex	Number of patients	HDL cholesterol		Apo-A	
			t	*P*	*t*	*P*
Arteriosclerotic	M+F	130	4.272	<0.001	3.322	<0.01
	M	74	4.617	<0.001	2.170	<0.05
	F	56	2.813	<0.01	2.100	<0.05
Control	M+F	60	2.926	<0.01	3.000	<0.01
	M	33	5.668	<0.001	2.923	<0.01
	F	27	6.454	<0.001	2.113	<0.05

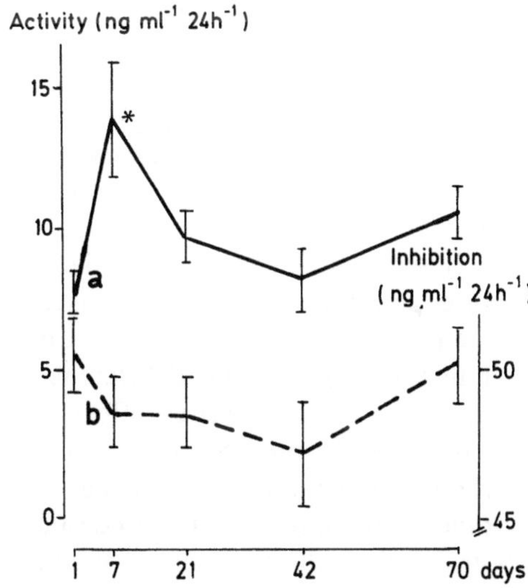

Fig. 1 a, b. Variation of serum elastase-type enzyme activity *(a)* and pancreas elastase inhibitory capacity *(b)* as functions of time following acute myocardial infarction. Mean ± SD; * $P < 0.1$ vs 24 h value

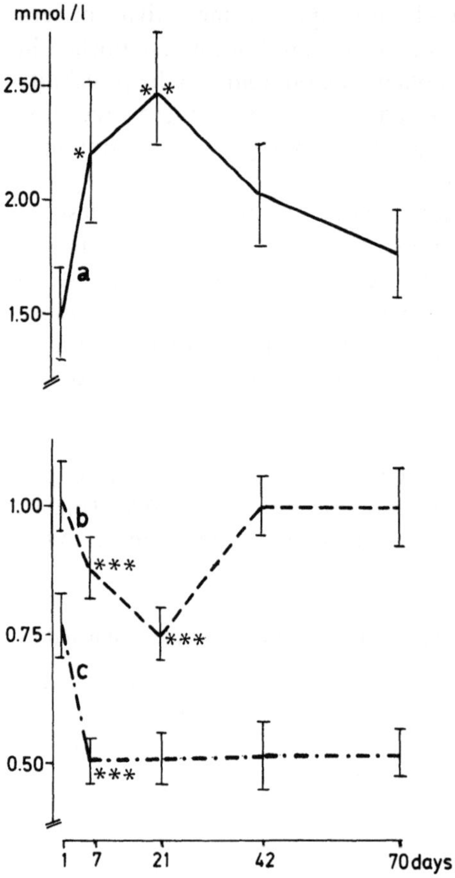

Fig. 2a–c. Variation of serum triglyceride *(a)*, HDL *(b)*, and HDL_2 *(c)* concentration as functions of time following acute myocardial infarction. Mean ± SD; * $P<0.1$ vs 24 h value, ** $P<0.05$ vs 24 h value, *** $P<0.01$ vs 24 h value

injury. Elastase inhibitory capacity was slightly, though not significantly, decreased during the entire observation period. A role for elastase in the repair process seems highly likely, because all elastases have catalytic activity against protein and peptide substrates other than elastin [33], and consequently might also participate in thrombolysis.

Our study confirms reports [34–36] that concentrations of total plasma cholesterol, LDL, and HDL_3 did not vary significantly within the first 70 days after AMI. Triglyceride levels increased significantly, and HDL and HDL_2 fell significantly during the first 1–3 weeks and then gradually tended to return to the initial values (Fig. 2), in accordance with other data in the literature [37, 38]. Other studies have reported decreased [39, 40] or increased [41] total cholesterol, and unchanged triglyceride [38, 41] or HDL [34] levels. Contradictions between the results of various investigators might be due to differences in the severity of the myocardial incidence and in the consequential stress effect, to differences in the selection of patients, or to differences in the protocol of investigation and treatment.

The possible relationship between elastase activity and some acute and chronic risk factors has also been analyzed (Table 3). In the group of patients with elevated elastase activity there was also a significant elevation of SGOT and LDH_1 activity.

Table 3. Acute and chronic risk factors in two groups of patients with acute myocardial infarction

	Group 1[a] (n=11)	Group 2[b] (n=12)	Significance (2 vs1)	
			t/χ^2	P
SGOT (U 1^{-1}; mean ± SD)	54.0 ± 38.6	92.7 ± 47.2	2.10	< 0.05
LDH (U 1^{-1}; mean ± SD)	173.7 ± 46.8	232.9 ± 89.4	1.96	> 0.05
LDH_1 (U 1^{-1}; mean ± SD)	101.9 ± 41.7	158.1 ± 60.2	2.60	< 0.01
Transmural infarction (no. of cases)	6	11	4.10	< 0.001
Hypertension (no. of cases)	4	2	1.20	> 0.1
Smokers (no. of cases)	7	8	0.02	> 0.1

[a] Variation of elastase activity < ±30% during the first 7 days after AMI.
[b] Elevation of elastase activity > ±30% during the first 7 days after AMI.

In these patients the occurrance of transmural infarction was significantly more frequent. These findings suggest that increased elastase-type enzyme activity might be one of the indicators of the severity of a myocardial infarction.

References

1. Kao VCY, Wissler RW (1965) A study of immunohistochemical localization of serum lipoproteins and other plasma proteins in human atherosclerotic lesions. Exp Mol Pathol 4: 465
2. Walton KW, Williamson N (1968) Histological and immunofluorescent studies on the evolution of the human atheromatous plaque. Atherosclerosis 8: 559
3. Kramsch DM, Franzblau C, Hollander W (1971) The protein and lipid composition of arterial elastin and its relationship to lipid accumulation in the atherosclerotic plaque. J Clin Invest 50: 1666
4. Hoff HF, Jackson RL, Mao JT, Gotto AM (1974) Localization of low density lipoproteins in arterial lesions from normolipidemics. Biochim Biophys Acta 351: 407
5. Smith EB (1974) The relation between plasma and tissue lipids in human atherosclerosis. Adv Lipid Res 12: 1
6. Noma A, Takahashi T, Yamada K, Wada T (1979) Elastin-lipid interaction in the arterial wall 1. Atherosclerosis 33: 29
7. Srinivasan SR, Yost C, Radhakrishnamurthy B, Dalferes ER, Berenson GS (1980) Lipoprotein-hyaluronate associations in human aorta fibrous plaque lesions. Atherosclerosis 36: 25
8. Srinivasan SR, Yost C, Radhakrishnamurthy ER, Dalferes B, Berenson GS (1981) Lipoprotein-elastin interactions in human aorta fibrous plaque lesions. Atherosclerosis 38: 137
9. Kramsch DM, Hollander W (1973) The interaction of serum and arterial lipoproteins with elastin of the arterial intima. J Clin Invest 53: 236
10. Kramsch DM, Franzblau C, Hollander W (1974) Components of the protein-lipid complex of arterial elastin. Adv Exp Med Biol 43: 193
11. Balo J, Banga I (1963) Connective tissue changes in atherosclerosis. In: Hall DA (ed) Review of connective tissue research, vol 1. Academic, New York, pp 241-306
12. Robert L, Robert AM (1980) Elastin, elastase and atherosclerosis. In: Robert L (ed) Frontiers of matrix biology. Karger, Basel, pp 130-173
13. Hornebeck W, Bellon G, Brechemier D, Godeau G, Robert L (1981) Control of elastic tissue destruction by elastase inhibitors. In: Deyl Z, Adams A (eds) Connective tissue research. Liss, New York, pp 233-246
14. Noma T, Takahashi T, Wada T (1981) Elastin-lipid interaction in the arterial wall 2. Atherosclerosis 38: 373

15. Noma A, Hirayama T, Yachi A (1983) Studies on the binding of plasma low density lipoproteins to arterial elastin. Connect Tissue Res 11: 123
16. Noma A, Hirayama T, Yachi A (1983) Inhibitory effect of high density lipoprotein subfractions on the in vitro binding of low density lipoproteins to arterial elastin. Atherosclerosis 49: 171
17. Robert L, Bellon G, Hornebeck W (1980) Characterization of different elastases. Bull Eur Physiopathol Res 16: 199
18. Balo J, Banga I (1949) Elastase and elastase inhibitor. Nature 164: 491
19. Butturini U, Pretolani E, Gnudi A (1959) The action of elastase and glucagon on cholesterolemia. Boll Soc Ital Biol Sper 35: 27
20. Osawa A (1970) Antiarteriosclerotic action of elastase. J Jpn Soc Intern Med 59: 230
21. Nakamura H, Ishikawa M (1971) Effect of elastase on cholesterol metabolism. Jpn J Geriatr 8: 225
22. Tono T (1975) Elastase therapy for arteriosclerotic disease. Jpn J Clin Exp Med 53: 1798
23. Katsunuma H, Shimizu K, Ebihara T, Iwamoto T, Kiyokawa M (1983) Anti-atherosclerotic action of elastase. Age Ageing 12: 183
24. Hornebeck W, Potazman JP, De Cremoux H, Bellon G, Robert L (1983) Elastase-type activity of human serum. Clin Physiol Biochem 1: 285
25. Heimburger N, Haupt H (1966) Zur Spezifizität der Antiproteinasen des Humanplasmas für Elastase. Klin Wochenschr 44: 1196
26. Hornebeck W, Brechemier D, Bellon G, Adnet JJ, Robert L (1980) Biological significance of elastase-like enzymes in arteriosclerosis and human breast cancer. In: Sträuli P (ed) Proteinases and tumor invasion. Raven, New York, pp 117-141
27. Janoff A, Carp H, Lee DK, Drew RT (1979) Cigarette smoke inhalation decreases alpha 1-antitrypsin activity in rat lung. Science 206: 1313
28. Ischaemic Heart Disease Registers (1971) Report of the fifth working group. WHO, Copenhagen
29. Bieth J (1978) Elastases. In: Robert L (ed) Frontiers of matrix biology. Karger, Basel, pp 1-8
30. Keller L, Bihari-Varga M, Landi A (1983) A szérum elasztinolitikus aktivitása, elasztáz-gátló kapacitása és néhány lipoprotein konstituense atherosclerotikus betegekben. Magy Belorv Arch 36: 313
31. Bihari-Varga M, Keller L, Landi A, Robert L (1984) Elastease-type activity, elastase inhibitory capacity, lipids and lipoproteins in the sera of patients with ischaemic vascular disease. Atherosclerosis 50: 273
32. Jacob MP, Bellon G, Robert L, Hornebeck W (1981) Elastase-type activity associated with high density lipoproteins in human serum. Biochem Biophys Res Commun 103: 311
33. Werb Z, Barda MJ, McKerrow H, Sandhouse RA (1978) Elastases and elastin degradation. J Invest Dermatol 79: 154
34. Heldenburg D, Rubenstein A, Levtov O, Berns L, Werbin B, Tamir L (1980) Serum lipids and lipoprotein concentrations during the acute phase of myocardial infarction. Atherosclerosis 35: 433
35. Gillet MP, Besterman EM (1975) Plasma concentration of lysolecithin and other phospholipids in the healthy population and in men suffering from atherosclerotic disease. Atherosclerosis 22: 111
36. Berlin R, Oldfelt CO, Vikrot O (1969) Acute myocardial infarction and plasma phospholipid levels. Acta Med Scand 185: 439
37. Avogaro P, Bittolobon G, Corrolato G, Quinci GP, Samson A (1978) Variation in apolipoproteins B and A during the course of myocardial infarction. Eur J Clin Invest 8: 121
38. Ryder RE, Hayes TM, Mulligan IP, Kingswood JC, Williams S, Owens DR (1984) How soon after myocardial infarction should plasma lipid values be assessed? Br Med J 289: 1651
39. Björntorp P, Malmerona R (1960) Serum cholesterol in patients with myocardial infarction in younger ages. Acta Med Scand 168: 151
40. Tibbin G, Cramer K (1963) Serum lipids during the course of an acute myocardial infarction and one year afterwards. Acta Med Scand 174: 451
41. Kirkeby K (1972) Disturbance in serum lipids and in their fatty acid composition following acute myocardial infarction. Acta Med Scand 192: 523

DNA Polymorphism for the Genetic Analysis of Atherosclerosis

D. J. Galton

Introduction

Coronary atherosclerosis - one of the major health problems of our time - arises from a complex interaction between environmental and genetic factors. Evidence for genetic factors comes from many studies reporting a strong familial aggregation of the disease. A heritability (that is the proportion of phenotypic variance that can be attributed to additive genetic factors) of 0.63 for coronary artery disease of early onset in family studies has been reported [1]. Twin studies have revealed a higher concordance rate of the disease in monozygotic than in dizygotic pairs. In one representative study of coronary artery disease occurring before the age of 60, concordance rates were 0.83 and 0.22 for mono- and dizygotic twin pairs, respectively, the disease end point being angina pectoris and/or myocardial infarction [2].

There is now a mass of clinical, epidemiological and experimental data to implicate altered metabolism of lipoproteins in the aetiology of atherosclerosis. In rare instances, a simple monogenic disorder such as a defect in the cell surface receptor for endocytosis of low-density lipoproteins (LDL) can strongly predispose to the development of premature atherosclerosis [3]. However, in the majority of cases it is not possible to identify single genetic determinants and it is likely that several major genes may contribute to the manifestation of the disease. It will be of great interest to map which of the major genes segregate with the trait. This may allow identification from birth of individuals who are predisposed to develop premature atherosclerosis.

The most likely candidates for genetic variants predisposing to atherosclerosis are those coding for the lipid transport proteins; and the next section summarises recent information on the apolipoprotein gene family.

The Apolipoprotein Genes

Use of recombinant DNA techniques has identified the chromosomal locations of all the major apolipoprotein genes and permitted a detailed study of their genomic structure. The apolipoprotein (apo) genes are dispersed amongst four chromosomes (Fig. 1). There is a cluster of three on the long arm of chromosome 11 (apo A-I, C-III and A-IV). Another cluster occurs on chromosome 19 (apo C-I, C-II and E; together with the LDL receptor). Two others are located on chromosome 1 (apo A-II) and on the short arm of chromosome 2 (apo B).

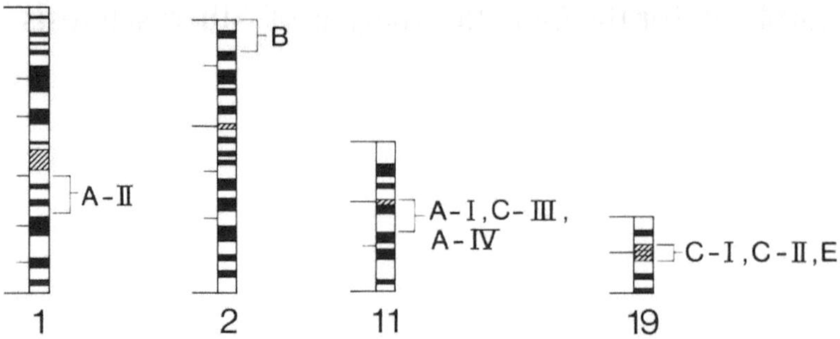

Fig. 1. Chromosomal localisation of the apolipoprotein multigene family. A map of human chromosomes 1, 2, 11 and 19 showing approximate assignments of the apolipoprotein genes (see [5, 7]). Apolipoproteins AI, AII, C-I, etc. are corresponding gene loci

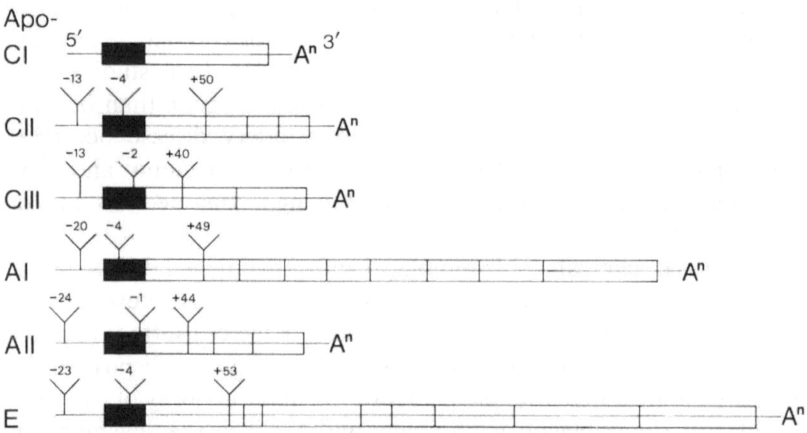

Fig. 2. Genomic structures of the apolipoprotein multigene family. The intron-exon organisation of members of the apolipoprotein gene family. *Solid boxes,* leader sequence; *open boxes,* exons; *Y,* site of introns that are spliced out; *A*^{n}, polyadenine tail. *Numbers* above intron sites are base-pairs from start codon. (Data from [5, 7])

There are considerable nucleotide sequence homologies amongst the apolipoprotein genes, and it is possible they arose from a common ancestral gene by duplications or conversion events. Thus their genomic structures reveal the presence of three introns in strikingly similar positions. One is within the 5′ untranslated region of the gene; the second within the leader sequence; and the third intron within the coding part of the gene. These divide the gene into four exons; and the fourth exon is variably expanded by internal repeat units of approximately 66 base pairs (Fig. 2). These may code for aminoacid sequences that form the amphipathic helix and be responsible for the lipid-binding properties of these apolipoproteins. A possible scheme for the evolution of this multigene family is presented in Fig. 3. The common ancestral gene may have been very similar to the present-day apolipoprotein C-I in structure and length. Then, by a series of gene duplications, the other genes

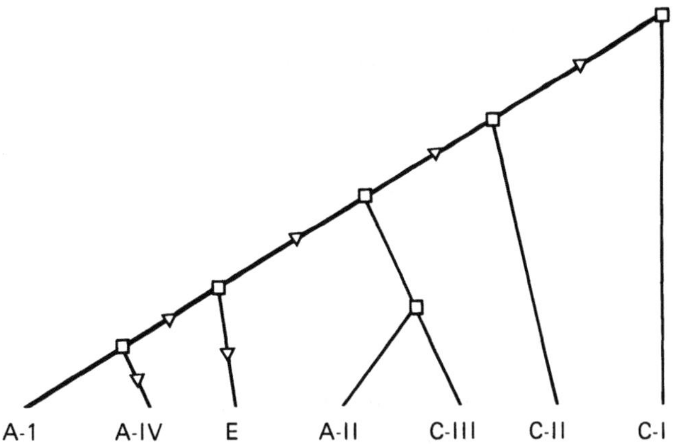

Fig. 3. Evolution of the apolipoprotein gene family. A hypothetical scheme for the evolution of the apolipoprotein genes. The ancestral gene was probably similar to apo C-I. Gene duplication (□) led to apo C-II. Duplication of 22 codons in exon 3/4 (△) diversified the length. (Modified from [5])

were formed and diversified by variable duplication of stretches of codons within their fourth exons.

Genetic Polymorphisms

Mutations are a fundamental way of altering the genome and in some instances can produce a deleterious change in gene function. Such mutations may gradually become eliminated from the gene pool of the population under the influence of natural selection on the resulting phenotype. However, occasionally a mutation will arise that may have some selective advantage over the common allele and may gradually increase in frequency to the point of permanent fixation in the population [4]. When the frequency of the uncommon variant occurs to an appreciable extent that cannot be accounted for by new mutations (arbitrarily taken as more than 1%) it is called a polymorphic variant. A genetic polymorphism is therefore the occurrence in the same population of two or more alleles at one locus, each occurring at an appreciable frequency and not accounted for by new mutations. The DNA polymorphism may not occur within structural genes. It has been calculated [6] that one in every 100 nucleotides may be variable in flanking regions of the gene or in spacer regions (i.e. intergenic DNA). This makes the extent of DNA polymorphisms much greater than observed for protein polymorphisms.

Genetic polymorphisms constitute a basic component of hereditary variation in natural populations on which evolutionary forces operate. A polymorphic variant that is of minor selective disadvantage, and may be declining in frequency, may become a selective advantage if the prevailing environmental conditions alter slightly. This therefore provides a means whereby populations can evolve in different directions. In general, the greater the genetic variation inherent in a natural population, the greater the opportunities for evolutionary change.

From a preliminary analysis (human genomic probes have only been available since the mid-1970s) there is clearly a large amount of genetic polymorphism in human populations. Some of this polymorphism may be impermanent, representing a transient phase of molecular evolution. The rarer of the variant alleles could be in the process of increasing or decreasing in frequency, under the influence of natural selection and/or by random genetic drift. Alternatively, the polymorphism may be permanent, i.e. in equilibrium with the common form.

Detection of Polymorphisms

DNA polymorphisms can be detected if the mutation directly affects the recognition site of a restriction endonuclease, either creating a new site or abolishing an old one. In either case a different-sized DNA fragment will be produced (Fig. 4). More than 100 restriction enzymes are available, each with different nucleotide sequence specifities, and each enzyme is of potential use for detecting new polymorphisms. This is currently providing a wealth of new genetic markers for clinical studies. Alternatively, a DNA polymorphism can be produced by variable insertions of repetitive sequences within a short stretch of the genome. This leads to DNA fragments produced by digestion with restriction enzymes of highly variable length (Fig. 4).

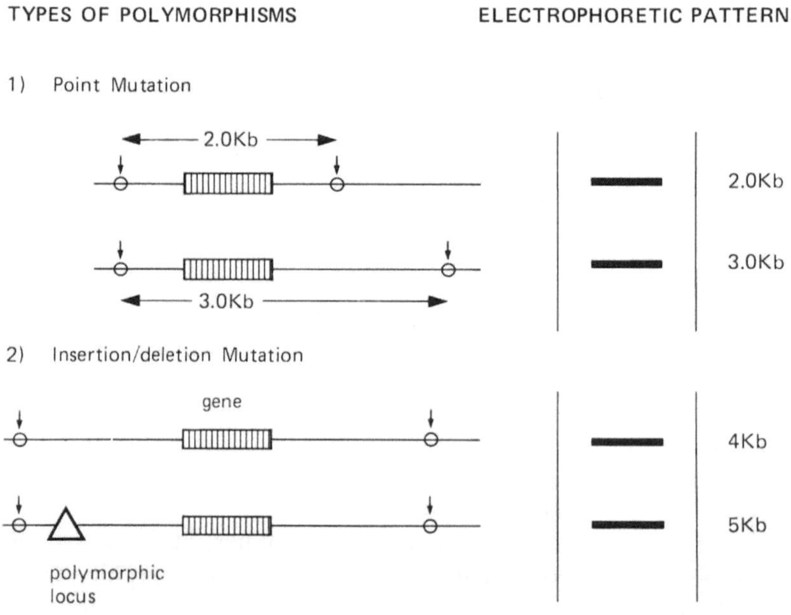

Fig. 4. Types of DNA polymorphisms revealed by Southern blotting. This scheme illustrates a hypothetical gene *(hatched bar)* digested with the restriction enzyme *(O)* together with the blotting patterns after gel electrophoresis of the DNA fragments. One type of polymorphisms is due to nucleotide substitutions *(panel 1)*. The other is due to variable DNA insertions at the polymorphic locus (Δ) as in *panel 2*

The most useful method to detect DNA polymorphisms is by "Southern blotting" [17]. Usually leucocyte DNA is digested with various restriction enzymes and fractionated according to size on agarose or polyacrylamide gel. The DNA on the gel is denatured with alkali, neutralised with Tris buffer and transferred by capillary flow to a nitrocellulose or other filter - the blotting process. The filter now carries a "print" of the DNA from the gel that can be hybridised to a labelled gene probe and then visualised by autoradiography. This probe can be a cloned DNA sequence or a synthetic oligonucleotide. Using different restriction enzymes, this method can generate far more allelic variants than is possible by a study of protein polymorphisms. It is now possible to take a gene which has no protein variants associated with it and in a relatively short time discover several DNA variants at that locus. Such DNA variants may be due to mutations in introns, exons, flanking sequences or spacer DNA. The latter can be in linkage disequilibrium with nucleotide variation within the coding region of structural genes and can be of diagnostic value.

Genetic Polymorphisms Related to Atherosclerosis

An early locus to be studied for population associations with coronary artery disease was the apo A-I-C-III-A-IV gene cluster on the long arm of chromosome 11. This region appears to be relatively prone to new mutations and DNA rearrangements. The apo A-I and A-IV genes (that are closely related) have been separated by the interposition of the apo C-III gene in the opposite orientation to both; and intra-strand recombination has been described between the A-I and C-III genes. There are also multiple restriction site polymorphisms along the genome over a distance of approximately 14 kb [7]. These occur in exons, introns and flanking sequences as described in Fig. 5. These sites reveal a complex pattern of linkage associations. Linkage analysis has been done using haplotypes of pairs of allelic sites. The degree of linkage disequilibrium is not a simple function of the relative physical distance between sites over a region of 14 kb. For example the Sst 1 and Pvu II restriction site polymorphisms are close together yet appear in linkage equilibrium; the Sst 1 and Msp 1 sites are further apart yet show linkage disequilibrium. The simplest explanation is that the processes of mutation and genetic drift are primarily responsible for the observed associations. The relative role of differential selection on haplotypes is difficult to assess. The effects of recombination over such

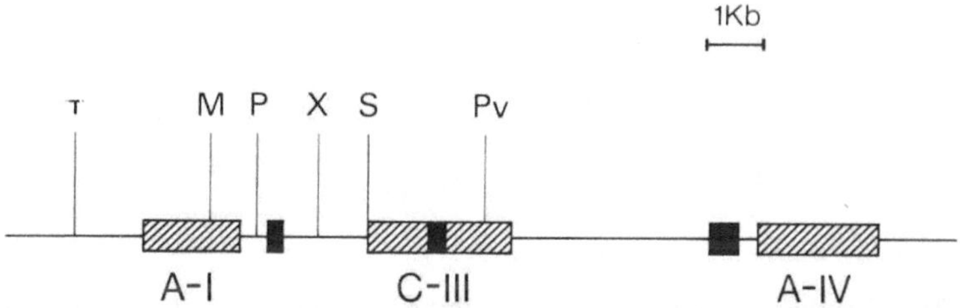

Fig. 5. Restriction map of the A-I/C-III/A-IV genes showing multiple polymorphic sites indicated. *Hatched bars* are exons/introns and spacer DNA are *lines*. *Solid boxes* are repetitive elements. *Pv*, Pvu II; *S*, Sst 1; *X*, Xmn 1; *P*, Pst 1; *M*, Msp 1; *T*, Taq 1

short distances are potentially less significant than mutation and drift/selection in the formation of new haplotypes [9].

Apo C-III Polymorphisms

Exon 4. A DNA polymorphism for the restriction enzyme Sst 1 occurs in the fourth exon 39 base pairs from the C terminal codon [10]. It is due to a C to G transversion and can be used to identify two alleles, S1 and S2, by Southern blotting. The frequency distribution of this polymorphism has been extensively studied in different ethnic populations as well as in disease groups [11]. In a study of coronary artery disease defined by coronary angiography [12] the frequency of the rare allele (S2) rose from 6% ($n=68$) in the controls to 22% ($n=61$) in severely affected subjects (Fig. 6). A similar study has been performed with young survivors of myocardial infarction [13]. The variant (S2) allele was found in 4% ($n=47$) of healthy controls compared to 21% ($n=48$) of infarction subjects (Fig. 6).

Intron 1. There is a Pvu II site polymorphism in the first intron of the apo C-III gene giving rise to two alleles of respective frequencies 0.79 and 0.21 in a population in the Federal Republic of Germany [8]. The frequency of the rare allele is increased in subjects ($n=155$) with coronary artery disease as defined by angiography compared to healthy controls with a relative incidence of 3.5 (calculated by the method of Woolf).

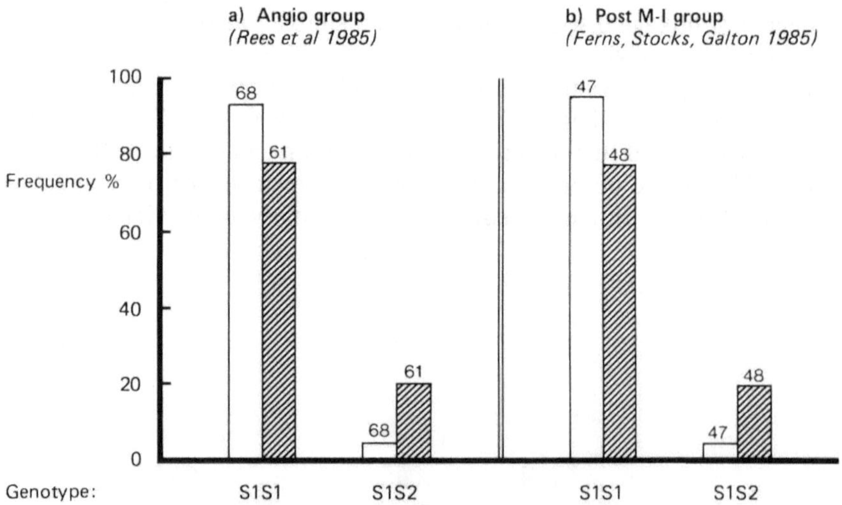

Fig. 6. Distribution of an Sst 1 polymorphism in the apolipoprotein C-III gene in early-onset coronary artery disease. Genotype frequencies are presented in patient groups with either severe or minimal coronary artery disease defined by angiography (see [12]); or in survivors of myocardial infarction (see [13])

The Apo A-I Gene

This gene is situated 2.6 kb upstream from the apo C-III gene and is transcribed in the opposite orientation. There is a Pst 1 site polymorphism 314 base-pairs from the 3′ end of the apo A-I gene. The frequency of the rare (P2) allele in randomly selected controls was 4% (n=123) and was 3.3% in 30 subjects with no evidence of coronary disease by angiography. By contrast, in 88 patients with coronary disease prior to the age of 60 years (defined by angiography) the P2 allele occurred in 31.8% (p<0.0001) of subjects [14]. This at present is the strongest genetic marker reported for coronary artery disease.

The next stage in these studies is to examine haplotype combinations of polymorphic restriction sites to see if they constitute stronger genetic markers for atherosclerosis [15]. The A-I-C-III-A-IV cluster with multiple restriction site polymorphisms can provide valuable genetic markers since polymorphic sites that are physically close together can show a number of haplotype combinations [18]. These can act as multi-allelic markers and may provide better identification of any putative atherogenic loci in their vicinity.

A possible interpretation of the above studies is that these DNA polymorphisms at the A-1-C-III locus are harmless mutations but are acting as linkage markers for a deleterious atherogenic allele in this region. The reasons why the linkage markers vary amongst three populations (Federal Republic of Germany, Britain and North America) could be that: (a) the atherogenic allele has mutated several times during evolution and hence associates with different background polymorphisms in different populations as a result; or (b) there have been recombinational events between the atherogenic allele and the different polymorphic restriction sites. The mutation therefore can spread to a different background of chromosomal polymorphisms. The latter is somewhat unlikely in view of the short physical distances between the various linkage markers.

There are also other examples in the apolipoprotein gene family where multiple mutations have probably occurred. For example the apolipoprotein C-II gene mutation producing familial apo C-II deficiency is linked to one allele of a Taq 1 polymorphism in a North Italian pedigree, but to the other allele in a Dutch pedigree [16]. The apo C-II gene has probably mutated twice to account for these different allelic associations. A similar situation may have arisen with the putative atherogenic allele on the long arm of chromosome 11.

Conclusion

These studies represent first attempts to identify major alleles that segregate with the inheritance of premature coronary artery disease. Identification of these atherogenes may allow prediction from an early age of individuals who are predisposed to develop premature atherosclerosis. Thereafter treatment could be instituted to modify environmental factors that interact with such high-risk genes to produce disease. One of the most important applications of this area of genetic research is a more precise appreciation of the environmental factors that interact with the genome to predispose to atherosclerosis. Finally, information on the major atherogenic loci may lead to newer forms of therapy directed against possible deleterious gene products.

Acknowledgements. Financial support for these studies has come from the Medical Research Council, Wellcome Trust and British Diabetic Association and is gratefully acknowledged. Financial support from the Fritz-Thysson-Foundation is also gratefully acknowledged.

References

1. Nora JJ, Lortscher RH, Spangler RD, Nora AH, Kimberley WJ (1980) Genetic-epidemiologic study of early-onset ischaemic heart disease. Circulation 61: 503-508
2. Berg K (1983) Genetics of coronary heart disease. In: Steinberg, Bearn, Motulsky, Childs (eds) Progress in medical genetics vol V. Saunders, Philadelphia
3. Brown MS, Goldstein JL (1976) Receptor mediated control of cholesterol metabolism. Science 191: 150-154
4. Galton DJ (1985) Molecular genetics of common metabolic disease. Arnold, London
5. Luo CC, Li WH, Moore MN, Chan L (1986) Structure and evolution of the apolipoprotein multigene family. J Mol Biol 187: 325-340
6. Jeffreys AJ (1979) DNA sequence variants in the G, A, S and B globin genes of man. Cell 18: 1-10
7. Breslow JL (1985) Human apolipoproteins: molecular biology and genetic variants. Annu Rev Biochem 54: 699-727
8. Frossard PM, Coleman R, Funke H, Assmann G (1986) Molecular genetics of the human apo A1-CIII-AIV gene complex: application to detection of susceptibility to atherosclerosis (to be published)
9. Barker D, Holm T, White R (1984) A locus on chromosome 11p with multiple restriction site polymorphisms. Am J Hum Genet 36: 1159-1171
10. Rees A, Shoulders CC, Stocks J, Galton DJ, Baralle FE (1983) DNA polymorphism adjacent to the human apoprotein A-I gene. Lancet II: 444-447
11. Rees A, Sharpe C, Stocks J, Shoulders CC, Baralle FE, Galton DJ (1985) DNA polymorphism in the apo AI/CIII gene cluster. J Clin Invest 76: 1090-1095
12. Rees A, Stocks J, Williams LG, Caplin JL, Jowett NI, Camm AJ, Galton DJ (1985) DNA polymorphisms in the apolipoprotein CIII and insulin genes and atherosclerosis. Atherosclerosis 58: 269-275
13. Ferns GAA, Stocks J, Ritchie C, Galton DJ (1985) Genetic polymorphisms of apolipoprotein CIII and insulin in survivors of myocardial infarction. Lancet I: 300-303
14. Ordovas JM, Schaefer EJ, Salem D et al. (1986) Apolipoprotein AI gene polymorphism associated with premature coronary artery disease and familial hypoalphalipoproteinaemia. N Engl J Med 314: 671-677
15. Rees A, Stocks J, Paul H, Ohuchi Y, Galton DJ (1986) Haplotypes identified by DNA polymorphisms at the apolipoprotein AI/CIII gene locus and hypertriglyceridaemia. Hum Genet 72: 168-171
16. Humphries SE, Williams LG, Stalenhoef AF, Baggio G, Crepaldi G, Galton DJ, Williamson R (1984) Familial apolipoprotein CII deficiency: a preliminary analysis of the gene defect in three independent individuals. Hum Genet 67: 151-156
17. Southern EM (1975) Detection of specific sequences among DNA fragments separated by gel electrophoresis. J Mol Biol 98: 503-514
18. Ferns GAA, Galton DJ (1986) Haplotypes of the human apoprotein AI-CIII-AIV gene cluster in coronary atherosclerosis. Hum Genet 73: 245-249

Lipoproteins

Chylomicron Catabolism and Uptake by the Liver

E. Windler and H. Greten

Chylomicrons carry lipids of intestinal origin to peripheral tissues and the liver. The lipids are of two sources. First, there are the endogenous lipids of desquamated intestinal epithelial cells and the bile. Secondly, exogenous lipids of dietary origin are absorbed. This latter source is the most important for triglycerides, while much of the cholesterol and phospholipids follow the conservative cycle of endogenous lipids being reabsorbed. As the quantity of triglycerides determines the size of chylomicron particles, postprandially their diameter rises up to 2000 Å or more. That is why chylomicrons are postprandially easily recognized in the blood stream, although they are continuously secreted. The particles produced in the fasting state are much smaller with a diameter in the range of 500 Å, which is similar to that of very low density lipoproteins (VLDL) of hepatic origin. For this reason these "small chylomicrons" are also referred to as "intestinal VLDL", which gives rise to confusion as the catabolic pathways of chylomicrons and VLDL differ considerably [1].

Small chylomicrons provide more surface area per volume as compared to large chylomicrons, so that surface material such as cholesterol and phospholipids of endogenous origin can be transported in the lymph even in the nonabsorptive state. For the triglycerides added postprandially to these chylomicrons there is a need for only small amounts of additional surface material. This is also true for the apolipoproteins, which reside on the surface of the particles as well. Since there is only one molecule of apolipoprotein B per chylomicron, it is not surprising that the synthesis of apolipoprotein B remains constant during fat absorption. Quantitatively the most important apolipoprotein of chylomicrons is apolipoprotein A-I, the synthesis of which also does not depend on the functional state of the intestine. It is abundant with manifold more molecules on each chylomicron than apolipoprotein B. Its function in chylomicron metabolism, however, is not known with certainty. Findings in the disease apolipoprotein A-I deficiency suggest a critical role in the absorption of vitamin E and essential fatty acids. After transfer from chylomicrons to high density lipoproteins (HDL) in the blood stream, apolipoprotein A-I activates lecithin: cholesterol acyltransferase (LCAT), although it does not seem to be essential for this. It may rather be crucial for the structure of HDL. Chylomicrons, therefore, may play an important role as vehicles for the transport of apolipoprotein A-I from the place of synthesis to HDL [2]. From this it appears that apolipoprotein B is the only known protein synthesized by the intestine in appreciable amounts that is of significance for the metabolism of chylomicrons. It is a smaller species that contains only 48% of the amino acids as compared with the apolipoprotein B of low density lipoproteins (LDL), termed B-48. Its synthesis is essential for the formation and secretion of chylomicrons. In contrast to VLDL, particles with apolipoprotein

B-48 cannot be converted to LDL but are exclusively taken up by the liver for their final catabolism [3].

Four more apolipoproteins that regulate the intravascular catabolism of chylomicrons are absorbed by the chylomicrons upon their entrance into the blood stream. Small amounts of these apolipoproteins are already bound by chylomicrons during their passage in the mesenteric lymph. These proteins are small enough to be filtered from the blood into the lymph. Thus, even lymph chylomicrons do not reflect the original state as they are secreted by enterocytes. Closer to the original particles are chylomicrons harvested from mesenteric lymph of hypolipemic animals. The vastly lowered levels of apolipoproteins allow only minimal filtration of apolipoproteins into the lymph [4].

The chylomicrons from such animals mainly contain the apolipoproteins B, A-I, and A-IV. These chylomicrons can be taken up by the liver at appreciable rates. Thus, a mechanism is needed to allow time for the intravascular catabolism of chylomicrons. Upon entry into the blood stream the A apolipoproteins are transferred from chylomicrons to HDL and C apolipoproteins are taken up in return. This occurs even without catabolism, merely by contact of these two lipoproteins. Thus, this exchange appears to be a matter of distribution due to affinity of these apolipoproteins to both lipoproteins. However, there seem to be physicochemical differences between these two particles. While all of the A apolipoproteins are transferred to HDL, there is a balance of distribution between chylomicrons and HDL for the C apolipoproteins. From this it appears that the affinity of HDL to the A apolipoproteins is much higher than to the C apolipoproteins. Apolipoprotein E is also distributed among HDL and chylomicrons in plasma. The interesting point is that the ratio of apolipoprotein E and the C apolipoproteins changes during the intravascular catabolism of chylomicrons, indicating that there is a differential alteration of the affinity to these proteins. This has been shown to be of extraordinary functional importance [5] (Fig. 1).

In order to allow sufficient time for triglyceride hydrolysis by lipoprotein lipase in the capillary bed, a factor that inhibits the premature uptake of chylomicrons from the blood stream had to be postulated. The observation that the C apolipoproteins are absorbed by the chylomicrons upon their entry in the blood stream, but are removed from the particles before their hepatic uptake, made them appear possible

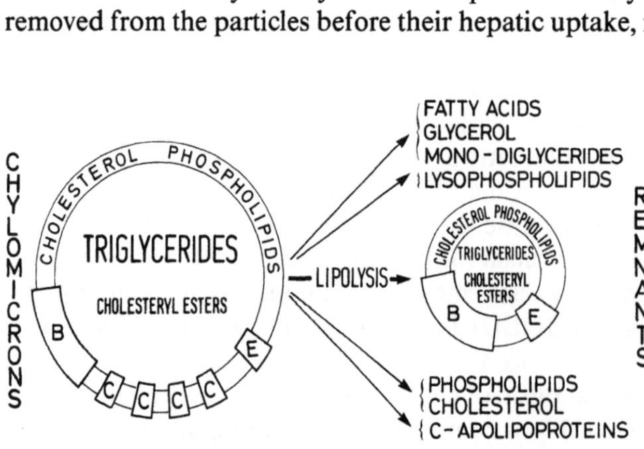

Fig. 1. Changes of lipid and apolipoprotein constituents during remnant formation by lipolysis of chylomicrons. (From [10] with permission of the publishers)

candidates. Direct evidence for such a capability of the C apolipoproteins to act as inhibitors for the hepatic uptake of chylomicrons was gained in studies with chylomicrons and their remnants, in which they were enriched in C apolipoproteins in vitro. The unfractionated C apolipoproteins from humans and rats as well as the individual C apolipoproteins C-II, C-III-0, and C-III-3 from rats and C-I, C-II, C-III-1, and C-III-2 from humans were able to inhibit the uptake of the chylomicrons or their remnants by isolated perfused rat livers. This effect is independent of the presence of apolipoprotein E. This was derived from the following observations: C apolipoproteins showed independently an inhibitory effect whether apolipoprotein E was, totally or to varying degrees, displaced from the particles by C apolipoproteins or whether apolipoprotein E was retained on the particle or even increased in parallel with the C apolipoproteins. In agreement with these experiments, addition of apolipoprotein E to chylomicrons in the presence of C apolipoproteins did not lead to enhanced uptake by the liver in contrast to the effect of addition of apolipoprotein E to chylomicrons which were deficient in C apolipoproteins. From this observation it was concluded that the C apolipoproteins act not only irrespectively of the amount of apolipoprotein E, but even dominate over the ability of apolipoprotein E to induce hepatic uptake [6].

While all of the C apolipoproteins inhibit the hepatic removal of chylomicrons from the blood stream, it is only apolipoprotein C-II that plays an additional role as an activator of lipoprotein lipase. This enzyme resides on the endothelial surface of the capillaries. Structural analysis of apolipoprotein C-II revealed that it comprises three functional regions. One is responsible for the binding of the apolipoprotein to the outer surface of lipoproteins. Two others mediate the interaction with lipoprotein lipase: one of them acts as a binding site for the enzyme, while the other catalyzes the enzymatic reaction of triglyceride hydrolysis. The fatty acids produced are taken up by peripheral tissues for the most part, yet one-third or more may be removed by the liver. A structurally different triglyceride hydrolase is found attached to the endothelial cells of the hepatic sinusoids. This enzyme is termed hepatic triglyceride lipase (HTGL). Experiments taking advantage of antibodies raised against the purified enzyme showed a substantial increase in plasma triglycerides after injection of antiserum. Experiments conducted in vivo and in vitro allowed the conclusion that this enzyme is responsible for the lipoprotein triglyceride hydrolysis, yet it may act at a later stage of the cascade from triglyceride-rich lipoproteins to their triglyceride-poor, cholesterol-rich remnants. In contrast to lipoprotein lipase, HTGL does not rely on an activator, i.e., it is independent of apolipoprotein C-II. Thus HTGL may still be active in the late stage of remnant formation, when the C apolipoproteins are already transferred to HDL [6, 7].

It was shown that alterations of the lipid composition are no prerequisites for the hepatic uptake of chylomicrons, and the intravascular catabolism is exclusively regulated by changes of the apolipoprotein composition. Yet it appeared possible that changes of the lipid composition are responsible for changes in the apolipoproteins, as the apolipoproteins bind to the surface lipids. The amount of apolipoprotein E per particle increases several-fold during remnant formation. At the end of the triglyceride hydrolysis apolipoprotein E may comprise almost half of the protein constituents. In contrast, the structural changes during remnant formation lead to transfer of the C apolipoproteins to HDL. This may be in part due to dimunition of the surface area because of reduction in particle size. However, this may account for no more than 40%–50%. Thus, additional mechanisms had to be investigated. Four lines of evidence suggest a connection between C apolipoproteins and lysophosphatidylcholine. First, triglyceride-rich lipoproteins of density $(d) < 1.006$ g/ml in human plasma contain less lysophosphatidylcholine but much more C apolipoprotein than the fraction of $d = 1.006$–1.0019 g/ml, which represents remnant particles. This was true in the fasted as well as in the postprandial state. Intravenous injection of heparin leads to enhanced triglyceride hydrolysis due to activation of lipoprotein lipase. This is accompanied by a loss of C apolipoproteins from the triglyceride-rich lipoproteins, while lysophosphatidylcholine increases. Secondly, the same inverse relationship between lysophosphatidylcholine and C apolipoproteins was observed when human chylomicrons isolated from chylothorax were hydrolyzed by incubation in postheparin plasma in vitro. Thirdly, comparable results were obtained when rat chylomicrons were compared with remnants produced in functionally hepatectomized rats. Fourthly, even experiments with artificial triglyceride-phospholipid emulsions yielded the same correlation. The emulsion is able to absorb C apolipoproteins, but this affinity is greatly reduced after hydrolysis in postheparin plasma, which leads to a rise in the content of lysophosphatidylcholine. Additionally these experiments documented that the connection between C apolipoproteins and lysophosphatidylcholine is independent of the structure of the lipoprotein and its content of cholesterol. Rather, in all of the cases mentioned an increase in lysophosphatidylcholine and a decrease in C apolipoproteins were the only consistent changes during triglyceride hydrolysis [8] (Fig. 2).

Beyond this observed correlation a causal relationship had to be established. Therefore, chylomicrons were enriched in lysophosphatidylcholine by incubation with this phospholipid in vitro. This results in an exchange of lysophosphatidylcholine for phosphatidylcholine with no other change in the lipid composition, whereas the amount of C apolipoproteins decreases. This could be shown with rat as well as human chylomicrons. Concentrations of lysophosphatidylcholine equal to those in remnant particles are sufficient to induce a loss of some 50% of the C apolipoproteins. Reincubation of these chylomicrons enriched in lysophosphatidylcholine with even high concentration of C apolipoproteins does not result in restoration of the original content in C apolipoproteins. From this follows that lysophosphatidylcholine appears to decrease the affinity of chylomicrons or their remnants to the C apolipoproteins. Thus, a deminution of particle size and the relative increase in lysophosphatidylcholine during remnant formation are sufficient to account for a

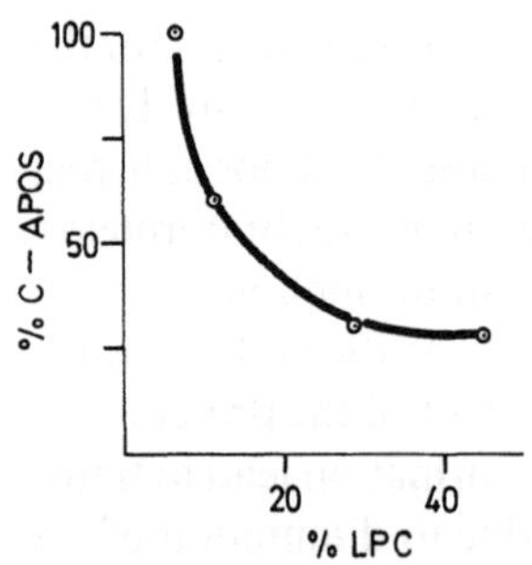

Fig. 2. Effect of lysophosphatidylcholine *(LPC)*, added by incubation to rat small chylomicrons in vitro, on the contents in C apolipoproteins *(C-APOS)*

total loss in C apolipoproteins although in vivo other changes such as the concentration of cholesterol may also contribute [8].

The rise of lysophosphatidylcholine in chylomicrons during triglyceride hydrolysis may be due to two mechanisms. More than three-quarters of the phospholipids may leave the chylomicrons during remnant formation. According to their affinity, the individual phospholipids will leave the particles to variable extents. Relatively more lysophosphatidylcholine may be retained on the particles. A second source of lysophosphatidylcholine is the hydrolysis of phosphatidylcholine. Phospholipase A activity has been attributed to both lipoprotein lipase and HTGL. The mechanism of the interaction of lysophosphatidylcholine with the binding of apolipoproteins to the lipoprotein surface is not certain. Competition between the surface components, as well as destabilization of the surface structure due to the unique physicochemical characteristics of lysophosphatidylcholine that differ from other phospholipids, may lead to interference with the binding of the apolipoproteins. Thus both may be important factors. The effect of lysophosphatidylcholine differs among the various C apolipoproteins. More obvious in rats than in man, apolipoprotein C-II is more sensitive to the interaction with lysophosphatidylcholine than apolipoprotein C-III. Thus, it can be expected that apolipoprotein C-II is the first apolipoprotein that is lost from the newly formed remnant particles. Since it functions as the activator of lipoprotein lipase, triglyceride hydrolysis would cease at this point. When all of the C apolipoproteins are transferred from the remnant particle to HDL, their inhibitory effect on the hepatic uptake is abolished and immediate removal from the circulation by the liver results [6, 8].

In previous work it could be shown that it is the apolipoprotein E which directs chylomicrons to the liver after hydrolysis of the component triglycerides. Isolated perfused livers take up the apolipoprotein E-rich remnant particles at a manifold higher rate than the parent chylomicrons. This is independent of the size of the remnant particle, as remnants of large and small chylomicrons may differ considerably in diameter, but are removed by the liver at comparably high rates. As the composition of chylomicrons changes in many ways during the formation of remnants, it was essential to show that it is apolipoprotein E that plays a crucial role in the hepatic uptake. This was possible by using small chylomicrons from the mesenteric lymph of hypolipidemic rats. As outlined above chylomicrons from such rats are only slightly contaminated by plasma apolipoproteins. These chylomicrons contain no more than one molecule of apolipoprotein E per every three particles on an average and very few C apolipoproteins. Uptake of these particles by perfused livers is slow and limited. After enrichment with apolipoprotein E, size and chemical composition is unaltered. These modified chylomicrons, however, are rapidly removed from the perfusate, comparably to what is observed with chylomicron remnants. Thus, these experiments demonstrate that neither triglyceride hydrolysis with the accompanying changes of lipid composition nor decrease in size are prerequisites for efficient hepatic uptake. Rather, direct evidence is provided that apolipoprotein E by itself is able to induce a rapid uptake by the liver [4].

Indirect evidence supports the view that this concept is also true in man. In most cases of dysbetalipoproteinemia, a structural abnormality of apolipoprotein E can be detected. Most often homozygosity of a mutant apolipoprotein E is found, which is termed apolipoprotein E-2 because of its unique position in isoelectric focusing electrophoresis. In the circulation of such patients, particles that resemble remnants, accumulate suggesting impeded hepatic uptake. By means of isolated perfused rat livers it was demonstrated that lipoproteins containing this abnormal apolipoprotein E are less efficiently removed from the circulation by the liver than particles containing normal apolipoprotein E [9].

In binding studies it could be shown that lipoproteins containing apolipoprotein E are able to interact with the LDL receptor of hepatocytes. As can be expected for binding to specific receptors, binding curves were curvilinear and saturable. Apolipoprotein E-containing particles had a much higher affinity than LDL. The various apolipoprotein E-containing lipoproteins and LDL competed for the binding. The reaction was calcium dependent and pronase sensitive due to the protein structure of the receptor. In these studies it could also be demonstrated that the inhibitory effect of the C apolipoproteins on the hepatic uptake is due to interference with the interaction of apolipoprotein E and the receptor. Thus, the transient uptake of C apolipoproteins by chylomicrons entering the blood stream yields a specific mechanism which determines the time of circulation. The removal of the C apolipoproteins, induced by an increase in lysophosphatidylcholine, acts as a signal for the final hepatic uptake. In addition to the LDL receptor, chylomicrons bind to a receptor that only recognizes apolipoprotein E. This apolipoprotein E receptor is not regulated like the LDL receptor [10, 11].

The catabolism of chylomicrons takes place in the hepatocytes. Autoradiographic studies clearly excluded endothelial cells or Kupffer's cells as a major site of catabolism. In electronmicroscopic studies the event of uptake by clathrin-coated pits could be visualized. After this internalization the resultant endocytic vesicles combine to make larger multivesicular bodies which are transported to the region of Golgi. At this point, primary lysosomes fuse with the multivesicular bodies and shed their enzymes among the lipoproteins leading to hydrolysis. Thus, exogenous cholesterol is transported by chylomicrons to the liver and may influence the hepatic cholesterol synthesis as well as the LDL receptor activity [12, 13].

Acknowledgement. This research was supported by the Deutsche Forschungsgesellschaft.

References

1. Windler E, Beil U, Greten H (1986) Der Dünndarm als Lipidstoffwechselorgan. In: Caspary WF (ed) Struktur und Funktion des Dünndarms in Diabetes Form I. Excerpta Medica, Amsterdam (to be published)
2. Green PHR, Glickman RM (1981) Intestinal lipoprotein metabolism. J Lipid Res 22: 1153-1173
3. Kane JP, Hardman DA, Paulus HE (1980) Heterogeneity of apolipoprotein B: isolation of a new species from human chylomicrons. Proc Natl Acad Sci USA 77: 2465-2469
4. Windler E, Chao Y, Havel RJ (1980) Regulation of the hepatic uptake of triglyceride-rich lipoproteins in the rat. J Biol Chem 255: 8303-8307
5. Windler E, Chao Y, Havel RJ (1980) Determinants of hepatic-uptake of triglyceride-rich lipoproteins and their remnants in the rat. J Biol Chem 255: 5475-5480
6. Windler E, Havel RJ (1985) Inhibitory effects of C apolipoproteins from rats and humans on the uptake of triglyceride-rich lipoproteins and their remnants by the perfused rat liver. J Lipid Res 26: 556-565

7. Schrecker O, Greten H (1979) Activation and inhibition of lipoprotein lipase - studies with artificial lipoproteins. Biochim Biophys Acta 572: 244-256
8. Windler EET, Preyer S, Greten H (1986) Influence of lysophosphatidylcholine and the C-apolipoprotein content of rat and human triglyceride-rich lipoproteins during triglyceride hydrolysis. J Clin Invest 78: 658-666
9. Havel RJ, Chao Y, Windler EE, Kotite L, Guo LSS (1980) Isoprotein specificity in the hepatic uptake of apolipoprotein E and the pathogenesis of familial dysbetalipoproteinemia. Proc Natl Acad Sci USA 77: 4349-4353
10. Windler EET, Därr WH, Greten H (1986) Removal of chylomicron remnants by the hepatic LDL receptor - possible contribution of the low density lipoprotein receptor. In: Greten H, Windler E, Beisiegel U (eds) Receptor-mediated uptake in the liver. Springer, Berlin Heidelberg New York Tokyo, pp 91-96
11. Hui DY, Brecht WJ, Hall EA, Friedman G, Innerarity TL, Mahley RW (1986) Isolation and characterization of the apolipoprotein E receptor from canine and human liver. J Biol Chem 261: 4256-4267
12. Jones AL, Hradek GT, Hornick C, Renaud G, Windler EET, Havel RJ (1984) Uptake and processing of remnants of chylomicrons and very low density lipoproteins by rat liver. J Lipid Res 25: 1151-1158
13. Greten H, Windler E (1985) Physiologie und Pathophysiologie des Lipoproteinstoffwechsels - Beziehung zu Hyperlipämien und Arteriosklerose. Internist 26: 399-404

Lipoprotein Lipase, Synthesis and Regulation

O. Stein, Y. Stein, G. Friedmann, and T. Chajek-Shaul

Synthesis and Secretion of Lipoprotein Lipase

Lipoprotein lipase (LPL), the key enzyme in the catabolism of chylomicron and very low-density lipoprotein (VLDL) triacylglycerol is present in the heart in two compartments, one intracellular, the other situated on the cell surface [1]. The surface compartment has been localized to the plasma membrane of endothelial cells, and it is also the site of action of the enzyme. LPL in the rat heart is delivered to its site of action by a vesicular transport, which can be inhibited by colchicine [2]. The cellular origin of the enzyme, whether it is synthesized in the myocardial muscle cells, or in the mesenchymal cells of the interstitium, which comprises the capillary endothelium, pericytes and fibroblasts, has been disputed. It has been shown that cultured cells derived from newly born rat heart [3] are capable of synthesizing LPL [4]. With the help of microscopy and cytochemistry it has been established that such cultures contain two types of cells, one which represents the cardiac myocytes (M), the other which comprises the mesenchymal cells (F). It has become possible to differentiate between the two cell types with the help of "preplating" [5] and to obtain cultures with a preponderance of one cell type.

LPL activity was determined in heart cells which had been cultured for 3-11 days. The enzyme activity was inhibited 92.7% by addition of 1 *M* NaCl and 77.7% by addition of protamine sulfate. In the absence of serum the loss of activity was 85.7% [6]. As shown in Table 1, enzyme activity increased with time in culture in the three cell preparations studied (F_1, F_2, and M), but was highest in the F_1 preparation at all time intervals. The presence of LPL on the cell surface was also demonstrated with the help of its native substrate, i.e., triacylglycerol present in VLDL [7]. The hydrolysis of the labeled VLDL triacylglycerol was compared in the F_1 and M cultures, and was up to 10 times faster in the F_1 cultures than in M cultures.

Table 1. Lipoprotein lipase activity in cultured mesenchymal (F) and myogenic (M) cells of rat hearts. (Adapted from [6])

Days in culture	Lipoprotein lipase activity (nmol fatty acid released-mg cell protein-h^{-1})		
	F_1	F_2	M
3	136.3 ± 16.4	55.9 ± 16.5	34.3 ± 2.4
5	441.0 ± 18.9	171.5 ± 25.8	29.0 ± 3.7
8	650.0 ± 84.3	262.5 ± 35.0	107.0 ± 8.2
11	799.5 ± 87.9		98.9 ± 16.4

In analogy to the findings in the perfused heart, LPL could be released from cultured heart cells into the medium by a brief exposure to heparin. While a very small release of LPL was observed in heparin-free medium, addition of heparin resulted in a sharp increase in enzyme release within the first 3 min. The heparin-releasable activity amounted to 20%-30% of total cellular LPL and was inhibited 90% by 1 *M* NaCl. Exposure of the heart cells to heparin resulted in a continuous release of enzyme, so that 30 min after addition of heparin more than 80% of the enzyme activity was found in the medium; at 3 h total enzyme activity doubled, and about 95% was found in the medium [6].

The transport of LPL in the cultured heart cells is affected by colchicine in analogy to the findings in the intact rat hearts [2]. Pretreatment of the cells with colchicine for 4 h resulted in a pronounced decrease in heparin-releasable activity, while the residual activity remained high in the colchicine-treated cells. Thus, enzyme synthesis was not impaired but its transport to the cell surface was inhibited by the treatment with the drug [6].

Role of Glycosylation of Lipoprotein Lipase

Because LPL is a glycoprotein, the role of the sugar moiety in enzyme activity was studied. Reduction in LPL activity was observed when 2-deoxyglucose was added to the culture medium [8]. The inhibition of enzyme activity was apparent after 2 h of incubation and progressed more rapidly at later time intervals. While no interference with the incorporation of [^{3}H]leucine into total cellular protein was observed, a marked and progressive fall occurred in the incorporation of labeled glucosamine, mannose and galactose into glycoproteins [8].

Asparagine-linked glycoproteins can be divided into two main types, high mannose and complex oligosaccharide containing glycoproteins. Tunicamycin interferes with N-glycosylation, by inhibiting the formation of dolichol-linked oligosaccharide [9]. The conversion of high mannose to a complex oligosaccharide form requires the trimming of 4-6 mannose residues and addition of the terminal oligosaccharide, a process that occurs in the distal portion of the Golgi complex [9]. Monensin, an Na^+ ionophore, was shown to block this process and inhibit incorporation of galactose into various secretory glycoproteins [10]. When tunicamycin was added to the heart cell cultures, a 3-h pretreatment was required to demonstrate the fall in LPL activity [8]. This was probably due to a slow intracellular penetration of the antibiotic. However, after this lag period a 60%-70% fall in enzyme activity and a 50% reduction in the incorporation of labeled glucosamine and mannose into glycoproteins occurred, while protein synthesis decreased by only 9%.

In order to learn about the role of terminal glycosylation in the expression of LPL activity and in the translocation of the enzyme to the cell surface use was made of monensin [11]. In cultured rat preadipocytes, in which LPL is secreted spontaneously into the culture medium(without addition of heparin), monensin treatment permitted the investigation of the role of the terminal oligosaccharide in the secretion of the enzyme. The availability of an antiserum to rat adipose tissue LPL enabled us to investigate whether synthesis of inactive LPL occured when glycosylation was inhibited either by monensin or tunicamycin [11]. A 70% reduction of

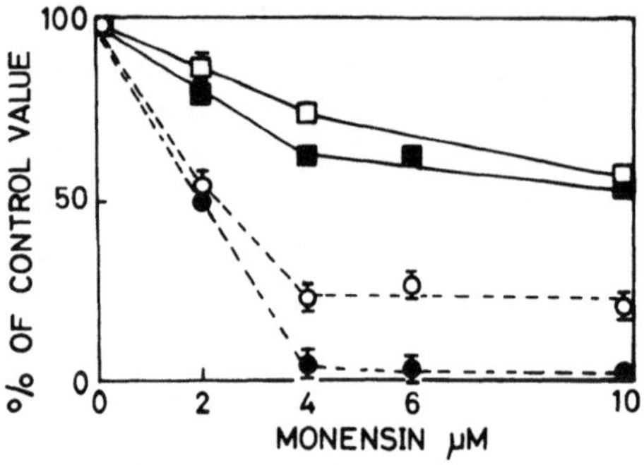

Fig. 1. Effect of monensin on lipoprotein lipase secretion by rat preadipocytes. The cells were cultured in medium containing 20% serum, with last medium change on day 7. On day 8, increasing concentrations of monensin were added and incubation was carried out for 3 or 24 h. During the last 20 min, 5 μCi ^{3}H-leucine was present in the culture medium of some dishes. Values are means ± SE of triplicate dishes (○-----●, lipoprotein lipase activity; □——■, protein synthesis; *open symbols,* 3 h, and *closed symbols,* 24 h. (Adapted from [11])

LPL activity in the culture medium occurred after 3 h of treatment of preadipocytes with 6 μ*M* monensin (Fig. 1), at a time when only 20% inhibition of cellular protein synthesis was seen. This fall in LPL activity in the culture medium was apparently not due to rapid degradation of secreted LPL, as very little proteolytic degradation of ^{125}I-milk LPL was seen in media of cultured preadipocytes and it was not increased by monensin. Thus it seems that monensin inhibited secretion of LPL into the culture medium, as well as the formation of the heparin-releasable fraction, which may be considered an immediate precursor pool of the secreted enzyme. The intracellular enzyme activity was identified as LPL by inhibition with 1 *M* NaCl and by antiserum to rat adipose tissue LPL. After 4 h, monensin caused a 77% reduction in the incorporation of leucine into LPL, which was commensurate with the 75% fall in LPL activity in the medium (Table 2). At the same time, cellular activity did not change or increase. Tunicamycin on the other hand, caused only a 50% decrease in enzyme synthesis, with a 98% fall in LPL activity. Since tunicamycin almost completely abolished mannose incorporation into glycoproteins, it appears that nonglycosylated LPL cannot express enzyme activity. The finding of incorporation of mannose into newly synthesized LPL in monensin-treated cells and a high mannose to galactose ratio (Table 3), indicates that enzyme activity can be expressed even when the processing of the glycoprotein is arrested in the high-mannose form [11].

What is then the role of terminal glycosylation in the LPL system? In the present study, it was not possible to ascertain whether any of the non-glycosylated LPL, which is synthesized in the presence of tunicamycin, is secreted into the medium. The lack of LPL activity in the culture medium of monensin-treated cells indicated that in contradistinction to cathepsin D [12], LPL is apparently not secreted in the high-mannose form. These results could indicate that terminal glycosylation may be the obligatory step for the secretion of the enzyme from the cell.

Although several studies on the purification of heart LPL have been performed, no agreement has been reached regarding the molecular weight of the enzyme and the values ranged between 34, 60, or 73 kilodaltons [13–15]. When rat hearts were

Table 2. Effect of monensin and tunicamycin on incorporation of ^{3}H-leucine into lipoprotein lipase. (Adapted from [11])

Treatment	Lipoprotein lipase activity (nmol fatty acid released/h)			^{3}H-Leucine incorporation into:	
	Medium	3 min heparin-releasable	Cellular	Total protein	Immunoadsorbable LPL
				DPM[a]	DPM
Control	1497 ± 87	269 ± 16	597 ± 60	1.29×10^6	1150
Monensin	499 ± 46	20 ± 2	732 ± 52	0.93×10^6	469
Tunicamycin	115 ± 18	16 ± 6	87 ± 24	1.08×10^6	672

[a] DPM: disintegrations per minute.

Rat preadipocytes were cultured for 8-9 days in medium containing 20% serum. On the day of the experiment MEM medium devoid of leucine was used. The cells were exposed to tunicamycin 5 μg/ml for 24 h and to monensin 6 μ*M* for 4 h. During the last 20 min, 5 μCi ^{3}H-leucine was added, then the medium was taken off, the cell layer washed 3 times with phosphate-buffered solution (PBS) and the cells were incubated for 3 min in PBS containing 5 units/ml heparin. Thereafter, the cells were scraped into PBS, homogenized and aliquots were taken for trichloroacetic acid (TCA) precipitation and protein determination. For the determination of ^{3}H-leucine incorporation into LPL, eight dishes of control and eight dishes of monensin-treated cells were pooled and subjected to immunoadsorption. Data are from duplicate gels which agreed within 10%. Values for LPL activity are mean ± SE of triplicates.

Table 3. Effect of monensin on incorporation of ^{14}C-mannose and ^{3}H-galactose into LPL. (Adapted from [11])

Experiment	Treatment	Incorporation of labeled sugars into glycoproteins, DPM					
		Total			Immunoadsorbable LPL		
		^{3}H--galactose	^{14}C--mannose	^{14}C/^{3}H	^{3}H--galactose	^{14}C--mannose	^{14}C/^{3}H
1	Control	1.09×10^6	1.2×10^6	1.1	11375	1719	0.15
	Monensin	0.97×10^6	2.1×10^6	2.1	6294	5663	0.90
2	Control	0.81×10^6	0.9×10^6	1.1	14213 ± 296	1998 ± 78	0.14
	Monensin	0.86×10^6	1.8×10^6	2.1	4975 ± 778	4792 ± 350	0.96

		Lipoprotein lipase activity (nmol fatty acid released h^{-1} $dish^{-1}$)		
		Medium	3 min heparin--releasable	Cellular
1	Control	4481 ± 294	951 ± 30	566 ± 33
	Monensin	96 ± 15	0	1042 ± 85
2	Control	2920 ± 210	820 ± 34	438 ± 30
	Monensin	37 ± 16	0	896 ± 72

Rat preadipocytes cultured from 9 days were incubated for 24 h with ^{3}H-galactose (5 μCi/ml) and ^{14}C-mannose (2 μCi/ml), and 6 μ*M* monensin (where appropriate). Thereafter, the medium was removed, the cells washed with PBS and incubated with heparin, 5 units/ml PBS for 3 min at room temperature. LPL activity and incorporation of labeled sugars into total proteins and into LPL were determined as described in Methods. Values are means of duplicates in experiment and means ± SE of triplicates in experiment. 2. All values of LPL are means ± SE of triplicates.

perfused with heparin for 2 min at 4 °C, the LPL activity in the perfusate was inhibited by antiserum to rat adipose tissue LPL. By immunoblotting, the LPL derived from the functional pool of the heart was found to be a protein with an apparent molecular weight of 69 kilodaltons [16]. Using radiation inactivation, Garfinkel et al. [17] found a functional molecular weight for rat heart LPL of 127 kilodaltons, which seems to constitute a dimer. We were able to show that the lower molecular weight protein of 28 kilodaltons can be derived from the 69 kilodalton protein by incubation of the perfusate at 37 °C for 24 h, and therefore is not a physiological derivative of the enzyme but a degradation product [16]. Recently, Socorro and Jackson reported a similar observation with bovine milk LPL; a protein of 18–22 kilodaltons was derived from the 55-kilodalton enzyme after 24 h incubation at 37 °C [18].

Hormonal Regulation of Lipoprotein Lipase

Hormonal regulation of LPL was studied extensively in the intact animal and was shown to vary with the tissue studied [19]. The culture system seemed to provide a convenient tool to study hormonal regulation of LPL synthesis. Addition of hydrocortisone to the culture medium resulted in an increase in LPL activity at all stages of culture [20]. LPL activity did not increase after addition of insulin to the complete culture medium. When the cells were cultured in the presence of medium containing 5% serum (serum poor), the increase in LPL activity between day 3 and 6 was much lower. A significant rise in LPL activity was encountered by the addition of hydrocortisone and insulin to the serum-poor medium. When serum-poor medium replaced 20% serum containing medium, between day 6 and 7 of culture a fall in enzyme activity occurred which could be prevented by hydrocortisone with or without the addition of insulin [20].

The mechanism underlying the reciprocal control of LPL of adipose tissue and heart by fasting and feeding has been attributed in part to the effects of insulin and catecholamines but is still unclear [21]. Cultured neonatal rat heart cells [6] as well as rat preadipocytes [22] which synthesize LPL were used as models to examine the possible role of cyclic adenosine monophosphate (cAMP) in the regulation of enzyme activity. The response of the heart cell cultures to cholera toxin, IBMX, and dibutyryl (db) cAMP during the first 3–6 h of incubation was variable. No decrease in LPL activity was encountered after incubation with cholera toxin while with IBMX or dbcAMP the reduction in enzyme activity was 25%–30% [23]. After 24-h incubation with these three effectors, an increase in LPL activity was seen in the heart cell cultures, which ranged between 100% and 250% (Table 4). In cholera toxin-treated cultures, the rise in LPL was preceded by a four-fold increase in the cellular concentration of cAMP, but cAMP returned to basal levels at the time of maximal increase of LPL [23]. Incubation of heart cell cultures with dbcAMP for 24 h resulted in a six-fold increase of heparin-releasable LPL activity while residual activity was doubled. The dbcAMP-induced heparin-releasable and residual LPL activity had the same half-life as the basal activity, indicating that the rise in LPL was due to an increase in enzyme synthesis [23].

Table 4. Effect of cAMP effectors on LPL activity in the mesenchymal rat F_1 heart cell cultures. (Adapted from [23])

Additions to cultures	Lipoprotein lipase activity nmol fatty acid released/mg cell protein/h		
	Control	+1 *M* NaCl	− Serum
None	851 ± 12[a]	2 ± 0.9	68 ± 3
435 μ*M* dibutyryl cyclic AMP	2271	0	175
100 μ*M* 3-isobutyl-1-methyl-xanthine	1271 ± 101[b]	26 ± 15	112 ± 20
1 μg/ml each of cholera toxin + ganglioside GM_1	1413 ± 54[c]	7 ± 3.9	109 ± 4

All incubations were carried out for 24 h. Values are mean ± SD of triplicate dishes. Control determination of enzyme activity under standard conditions. +1 *M* NaCl, assay in the presence of 1 *M* NaCl; − Serum, assay without rat serum.
Superscripts: a vs. b and a vs. c $P < 0.001$.

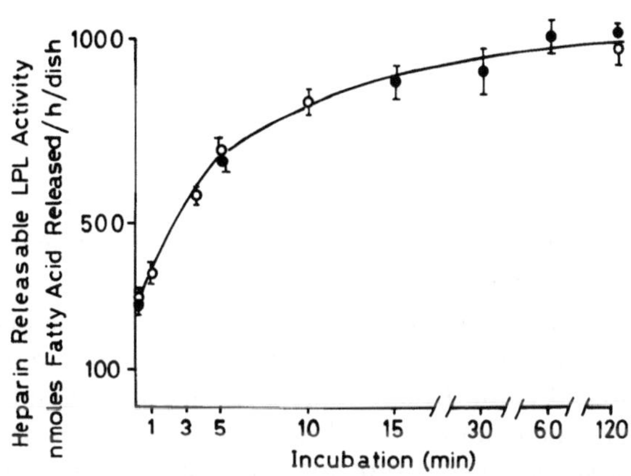

Fig. 2. Time course of isoproterenol effect on the heparin-releasable lipoprotein lipase activity. *Conditions* were as in Table 5. Incubation was carried out with 10^{-7} *M* isoproterenol. Values are means ± SE of triplicate dishes in two different experiments (0)

Using the perfused rat heart, it was shown that stimulation of the β-adrenergic receptor for 2 or 4 h with norepinephrine resulted in an increase in heparin-releasable LPL activity [24]. Recently, a short term β-adrenergic stimulation of rat parotid acinar cells was shown to increase N-linked protein glycosylation [25]. Thus it was important to investigate whether glycosylation of LPL in heart cell cultures can be modulated by isoproterenol. Using immunoadsorption, it also became possible to determine whether β-adrenergic stimulation affects only enzyme activity or the synthesis and processing of the glycoprotein molecule as well. Within 3–5 min there was a relatively rapid effect of isoproterenol on heparin-releasable LPL activity (Fig. 2). This effect was due mainly to the redistribution of enzyme activity between

Table 5. Prevention of the isoproterenol-induced increase in heparin-releasable LPL activity in heart cell cultures by propranolol. (Adapted from [26])

Additions to cultures	Lipoprotein lipase activity (nmol fatty acid released h^{-1} $dish^{-1}$)	
	Heparin releasable	Cellular
None	185 ± 14	1435 ± 205
10^{-7} *M* isoproterenol	488 ± 22	1251 ± 113
10^{-5} *M* propranolol	187 ± 14	1491 ± 22
10^{-5} *M* propranolol + 10^{-7} *M* isoproterenol	205 ± 16	1538 ± 28

Heart cells were cultured for 11 days and on day 12, 10^{-5} *M* propranolol was added to some dishes for 1 h. Thereafter, 10^{-7} *M* isoproterenol was added and incubation was carried out for an additional 2 h. For determination of heparin-releasable LPL activity, at the end of incubation the medium was collected and the cultures were incubated for 3 min at room temperature with 0.5 ml F_{10} medium containing 20% serum and 5 units/ml heparin. An assay for LPL activity was performed on 0.1 ml medium. For the determination of cellular LPL activity, the heparin-containing medium was removed and the cell layer was washed with PBS, scraped with 1 ml 0.025 *M* NH_3/NH_4Cl buffer (pH 8.1) containing 1 unit/ml heparin, and homogenized at 0 °C. An assay for LPL activity was performed on 0.1 ml cell homogenate. Values are means ± SE of triplicate dishes.

the intracellular and surface-related, functional compartment, with no change in total enzyme activity (Table 5).

The isoproterenol effect could be abolished completely by pretreatment of the cultures with propranolol, indicating that it represented a β-adrenergic receptor-linked event. At later time intervals, activation of the adenylate cyclase system by isoproterenol or dbcAMP influenced the incorporation of labeled mannose and galactose in glycoproteins of the cultured heart cells in analogy to the findings with parotid cells [25]. However, even after 2 h of pretreatment no increase in immunoadsorbable LPL synthesis was seen. Pretreatment of the cells with isoproterenol for 2 h resulted in a rise in the ratio of $^3H/^{14}C$ in LPL after labeling with ^3H-galactose and ^{14}C-mannose. Thus it seems that in addition to the enhancement of N-linked protein glycosylation, which occurs in the endoplasmic reticulum, activation of the adenylate cyclase system could also affect later events in glycoprotein processing, i.e., trimming of mannose and terminal glycosylation.

As was discussed above, inhibition of N-linked glycosylation by tunicamycin prevents the expression of LPL activity, even though the protein part of the enzyme continued to be synthesized. On the other hand, monensin treatment, which interferes mainly with terminal processing of glycoproteins, resulted in an almost complete disappearance of secretable LPL, while the intracellular enzyme retained full activity [11]. On the basis of these findings, it seems that mannose processing and terminal glycosylation affect mainly the transformation of the enzyme from a "storage" form into a functional form situated at the cell surface. Exposure of the cultures to isoproterenol for 24 h resulted in an increase in total LPL activity and a concomitant increase in the synthesis of enzyme protein.

Thus it appears that one may distinguish three effects of isoproterenol and cAMP on LPL. The first effect results in an increase in the heparin-releasable fraction, which becomes measurable 3 min after exposure to the effector. The second effect, discernible after 2 h, involves protein glycosylation and results in the appearance of LPL with a ratio of ^{3}H-galactose to ^{14}C-mannose which is up to three times higher than in the enzyme produced in the control cultures. The third effect becomes apparent after a longer lag period and results in enhancement of synthesis of new enzyme.

References

1. Chajek T, Stein O, Stein Y (1976) Interaction of concanavalin A with membrane-bound and solubilized lipoprotein lipase of rat heart. Biochim Biophys Acta 431: 507
2. Chajek T, Stein O, Stein Y (1975) Interference with the transport of heparin-releasable lipoprotein lipase in the perfused rat heart by colchicine and vinblastine. Biochim Biophys Acta 388: 260
3. Harary I, Farley B (1963) In vitro studies on single beating rat heart cells. Part 1 (Growth and organization). Exp Cell Res 29: 451
4. Pinson A, Frelfin C, Padieu P (1973) The lipoprotein lipase activity in cultured beating heart cells of the postnatal rat. Biochimie 55: 1261
5. Pollinger IS (1970) Separation of cell types in embryonic heart cell cultures. Exp Cell Res 63: 78
6. Chajek T, Stein O, Stein Y (1978) Lipoprotein lipase of cultured mesenchymal rat heart cells. I. Synthesis, secretion and releasability by heparin. Biochim Biophys Acta 528: 456
7. Chajek T, Stein O, Stein Y (1978) Lipoprotein lipase of cultured mesenchymal rat heart cells. II. Hydrolysis of labeled very low density lipoprotein triacylglycerol by membrane-supported enzyme. Biochim Biophys Acta 528: 466
8. Friedman G, Stein O, Stein Y (1980) Lipoprotein lipase activity in cultured mesenchymal rat heart cells. Part 5. Effect on enzyme activity of the glycosylation inhibitors, 2-deoxyglucose and tunicamycin. Atherosclerosis 36: 289
9. Elbein AD (1983) Inhibitors of lipoprotein synthesis: Methods Enzymol 98: 135–154
10. Tartakoff AM (1983) Perturbation of vesicular traffic with the carboxylic ionophore monensin. Cell 32: 1026
11. Chajek-Shaul T, Friedman G, Knobler H, Stein O, Etienne J, Stein Y (1985) Importance of the different steps of glycosylation for the activity and secretion of lipoprotein lipase in rat preadipocytes studied with monensin and tunicamycin. Biochim Biophys Acta 837: 123
12. Pohlmann R, Kruger S, Hasilik A, von Figura K (1984) Effect of monensin on intracellular transport and receptor mediated endocytosis of lysosomal enzymes. Biochem J 217: 649
13. Chung J, Scanu AM (1977) Isolation, molecular properties, and kinetic characterization of lipoprotein lipase from rat heart. J Biol Chem 252: 4202
14. Twu JS, Garfinkel AS, Schotz MC (1975) Rat heart lipoprotein lipase. Atherosclerosis 22: 463
15. Ehnholm C, Kinnunen PJ, Huttunen JK, Nikkila EA, Ohta M (1975) Purification and characterization of lipoprotein lipase from pig myocardium. Biochem J 149: 649
16. Friedman G, Chajek,Shaul T, Etienne J, Stein O, Stein Y (1986) Characterization of the lipoprotein lipase in the functional pool of rat heart by immunoblotting. Biochim Biophys Acta 875: 397
17. Garfinkel AS, Kempner ES, Ben-Zeev O, Nikazy J, James SJ, Schotz MD (1983) Lipoprotein lipase: size of the functional unit determined by radiation inactivation. J Lipid Res 24: 775
18. Socorro L, Jackson RL (1985) Monoclonal antibodies to bovine milk lipoprotein lipase. Evidence for proteolytic degradation of the native enzyme. J Biol Chem 260: 6324
19. Robinson DS (1970) The function of the plasma triglycerides in fatty acid transport. Compr Biochem 18: 51

20. Friedman G, Stein O, Stein Y (1978) Lipoprotein lipase of cultured mesenchymal rat heart cells. III. Effect of glucocorticoids and insulin on enzyme formation. Biochim Biophys Acta 531: 222
21. Cryer A (1981) Tissue lipoprotein lipase activity and its action in lipoprotein metabolism. Int J Biochem 13: 525
22. Bjorntorp P, Karsson M, Pertoft H, Pettersson P, Sjostrom L, Smith LL (1978) Isolation and characterization of cells from rat adipose tissue developing into adipocytes. J Lipid Res 19: 316
23. Friedman G, Chajek-Shaul T, Stein O, Stein Y (1983) Modulation of lipoprotein lipase activity in cultured rat mesenchymal heart cells and preadipocytes by dibutyryl cyclic AMP, cholera toxin and 3-isobutyl-1-methylxanthine. Biochim Biophys Acta 752: 106
24. Stam H, Hulsmann WC (1984) Effects of hormones, amino acids and specific inhibitors on rat heart heparin-releasable lipoprotein lipase and tissue neutral lipase activities during long-term perfusion. Biochim Biophys Acta 794: 72
25. Kousvelari E, Grant SR, Baum BJ (1983) β-Adrenergic receptor regulation of N-linked protein glycosylation in rat parotid acinar cells. Proc Natl Acad Sci USA 80: 7146
26. Friedman G, Chajek-Shaul T, Stein O, Noe L, Etienne J, Stein Y (1986) β-Adrenergic stimulation enhances translocation, processing and synthesis of lipoprotein lipase in rat heart cells. Biochim Biophys Acta 877: 112–120

Structural and Clinical Aspects of the Plasma Phospholipid Subclasses

V. Blaton and D. Hollez

Introduction

The presence of phospholipid (PL) in plasma lipoproteins, in the arterial wall, and in atherosclerotic lesions has been well demonstrated by both biochemical and histochemical investigations. Metabolic studies have shown that most PL within the arterial wall is synthesized endogenously, and the mechanism of such synthesis has been explored. However, changes of the PLs and their precise role within the lipoproteins remain uncertain.

While total cholesterol, triglycerides, and apoproteins have been extensively used as biochemical parameters for the study of spontaneous and experimental atherosclerosis, the literature dealing with the fourth class of lipoprotein components is rather scarce. However, there are indications that the plasma levels of some PLs and the distribution of PLs between the lipoprotein classes might be relevant to the diagnosis of atherosclerosis and other diseases. The lack of information about PLs is mainly due to the difficulties which have to be overcome to determine total PL, and even more to analyse single PLs, as solvent extraction, one- or two-dimensional thin-layer chromatography (TLC), and scanning or elution of individual fractions may have to be done.

Predictive Value of Plasma and High-Density Lipoprotein PL

In order to clarify the clinical significance of plasma PL in hyperlipoproteinemia and to analyse the phospholipid fatty acids we used a conventional TLC procedure. Lipids were extracted and re-extracted with chloroform - methanol (2:1, v/v) in the presence of 2 g/$CaCl_2$/l. For separation of polar lipids by TLC we used a mixture of $CHCl_3$, CH_3OH, HAc, H_2O, in proportions of 50:25:8:2. For quantitative analysis of the phospholipid subclasses we sprayed with perchloric acid and heated the plate for 10 min at 180 °C to char. The different PLs were scraped off and the PL content determined based on the colour reaction with ammonium heptamolybdate in the presence of ascorbic acid [1]. We analyzed the percentage PL distribution in different types of hyperlipoproteinemia. Phosphatidylcholine (PC) and sphingomyelin (Sphm) are the major PL subclasses and we observed an increase of PC in type IV hyperlipoproteinemia and a decrease in type II. Sphm increased in type II and decreased in type IV hyperlipoproteinemia. A further differentiation of the PL subclasses were obtained with the low-density lipoproteins (LDL, $1.019 < \text{density} < 1.063$), and high-density lipoproteins (HDL, $1.063 < \text{density} < 1.210$).

Each lipoprotein fraction has a different phospholipid profile and the highest Sphm content was found in the LDL_2 fraction. In type II hyperlipoproteinemia the Sphm concentration was only significantly increased in HDL [2].

In experimental studies we investigated and compared the normal plasma PL levels in human and non-human primates [3]. For all species PC and Sphm are the major phospholipid subclasses. However, in the baboon and the rhesus the Sphm concentration is only half that in humans and chimpanzees. Phosphatidylinositol (PI), phosphatidylserine (PS) and phosphatidylethanolamine (PET) are minor components and are at very similar concentrations except for PET which is much higher in the non-human primates. The differences observed in the PL subclasses may be related to structural and compositional differences between the individual apolipoproteins, although this remains to be clarified and include the higher percentage of PC and the lower Sphm content of the old world representatives.

The fast resolution of structurally similar components by TLC was a first step in the development of valuable screening techniques for lipids in biological materials. However, the quantitation of TLCs has not yet been solved and is still limited by the dependency of staining and charring procedures on the type of lipid, the size, the homogeneity and thickness of the layer itself, and the lack of linearity over a wide range of concentrations. Nevertheless, the ease and sensitivity of photodensitometric methods have proved their popularity by multiple application in the study of lipids. TLC with flame ionization detection (TLC - FID) was an important advance in the analysis of lipids, with great potential for application in clinical chemistry enabling quantitative screening of hyperlipidemia. The drawbacks of this method are its insensitivity and the size of sample needed. These limitations can partially be avoided by the use of a suitable internal standard [4]. However, chromatographic methods are not widely used in clinical laboratories because of their complexity, and the need to measure the phosphorus content of each PL.

Enzymatic assays are now available to assay plasma and lipoprotein PL. We have described a method for direct enzymatic determination of PC and Sphm in serum, and presented data comparing our results with those obtained by the choline oxidase and metavanadate methods of analysis for the choline and phosphorus liberated enzymatically from serum PC and Sphm. Phospholipase C and sphingomyelinase from *B. cereus* are used to liberate phosphorylcholine, from which inorganic phosphorus is hydrolyzed by the action of alkaline phosphatase [5]. A procedure suitable for screening purposes has also been developed for determination of the above two PLs in HDL. It entails precipitation of apolipoprotein - B - containing lipoproteins from native serum with $MgCl_2$ - phosphotungstic acid and, subsequently, specific enzymatic determination of the individual phospholipids in the supernatant.

The diagnostic value of HDL phosphatidylcholine (HDL-PC) was examined in company employees in Westfalia within the framework of an epidemiological study [6]. HDL-PC values were found to be age independent, higher in women than in men, and with a log-normal distribution. HDL PC correlated positively with HDL cholesterol (HDL-C; $r=0.61$) within both sexes. The ratio of HDL-C : HDL-PC is increased with increasing HDL-C values or decreasing serum triglyceride values. The reason for this may lie in the different lipid composition of HDL subfractions HDL_2 and HDL_3 and the negative correlation between HDL_2 and very low-density lipoproteins. Work is in progress to assay PC and Sphm ratios in HDL and HDL components by enzymatic methods in order to use them as indicators of changes in the composition and concentration of HDL subfractions.

Relationships of Plasma PL Subclasses

Serum HDL lipoproteins remove free cholesterol from peripheral tissues. This is followed by cholesterol esterification by lecithin-cholesterol acyltransferase (LCAT) and transport of cholesterol to the liver, the organ primarily responsible for its metabolism and excretion. There is a close interaction between apoprotein, PL, and free cholesterol in HDL and it can be expected that the PL components play an active part in the transport and incorporation into HDL of cholesterol.

In vitro studies have shown that the PL present at the surface of serum lipoproteins is accessible to the action of phospholipases, indicating that all PLs except for Sphm are cleaved into their lyso derivatives and the fatty acids accepted by serum albumin. Treatment with unsaturated PLs affects mostly the composition of the HDL_3 fraction, which is therefore characterized by a more fluid outersurface and a denser core. The new HDL_3 particles act as a better carrier of cholesterol from cells, playing a protective role in the development of atherosclerosis [7]. LCAT is activated by unsaturated phospholipids [8]. The actual mechanism for the fatty-acid transferase reaction to cholesterol is not known but it probably requires apo A-I as a cofactor and a substrate concentration ratio of lecithin to cholesterol of 3:1 or 4:1. The inhibition by apo A-II of the LCAT reaction is related to the capacity of this apoprotein to displace apo A-I from the surface of HDL.

PLs play an important role in the action of lipid-modifying enzymes, and lipoprotein PLs are also involved in interactions with cell membranes, although these have not been clearly defined. Exchange and transfer processes ensure equilibration of PLs between lipoprotein and cell membranes and facilitate the movement of cholesterol from cellular membranes to plasma. In vitro studies have suggested that PLs have an additional specific role in lipoprotein-cell interactions through their transformation into lyso-forms. The generation of these lyso-phosphatides may imitate biochemical events related to the lipoprotein-dependent regulation of cell metabolism [9]. PLs are at the center of the interactions between lipoproteins and lipid-modifying enzymes, and probably also between lipoproteins and cells. More information is needed to know how they may modulate the interaction between lipoproteins and metabolic events within the cell.

References

1. Blaton V, De Buyzere M, Declercq B, Pracetyo A, Vanderkelen G, Delanghe J, Spincemaille J (1984) Effect of polyunsaturated isocaloric fat diets on plasma lipids, apolipoproteins and fatty acids. Atherosclerosis 53: 9-20
2. Blaton V, Peeters H (1976) The non-human primates as models for studying atherosclerosis. Studies on the chimpanzee, the baboon and the Rhesus maccacus. In: Day C (ed) Atherosclerosis drug discovery. Plenum, New York, pp 33-63
3. Noel C, Marcel Y, Davignon J (1972) Plasma phospholipids in the different types of primary hyperlipoproteinemia. J Lab Clin Med 79: 611-621

4. Van Tornout P, Vercaemst R, Caster H, Lievens MJ, De Keersgieter W, Soetaway F, Rosseneu M (1979) Use of 1-octadecanol as an internal standard for plasma lipid quantitation on chromazods. J Chromatogr 164: 222-227
5. Blaton V, De Buyzere M, Spincemaille J, Declercq B (1983) Enzymic assay for phosphatidylcholine and sphingomyelin in serum. Clin Chem 29: 806-809
6. Assmann G (1982) Lipid metabolism and atherosclerosis. Schattauer, Stuttgart, pp 166-167
7. Rosseneu M, Declercq B, Vandamme D, Vercaemst R, Soeteway F, Peeters H, Blaton V (1979) Influence of oral polyunsaturated and saturated phospholipid treatment on the lipid composition and fatty acid profile of chimpanzee lipoproteins. Atherosclerosis 32: 141-153
8. Blaton V, Vandamme D, Peeters H (1974) Activation of lipoprotein lipase in vitro by unsaturated phospholipids. FEBS Lett 44: 185-188
9. Scanu AM (1983) Phospholipids in serum lipoproteins. In: Avogaro P, Mancini M, Ricci G, Paoletti R (eds) Phospholipids and atherosclerosis. Raven, New York, pp 91-97

Irregular Working Hours and Lipid Levels in Men

G. de Backer, M. Kornitzer, M. Dramaix, H. Peeters, and F. Kittel

Introduction

The literature on the overall health effects of irregular working hours is extensive. However, the relationship between work rhythm and cardiovascular diseases (CVD) has rarely been studied.

Results from some studies [1, 2] indicate that irregular working hours are related to an increased risk of CVD. This relationship seems to be specific since shift work was not related to any of the other major diagnoses. In other studies no relationship between work rhythm and CVD has been observed [3, 4]. In a recent review of the problem it was concluded that the evidence of a relationship between shift work and elevated CVD risk cannot yet be considered conclusive [5].

If irregular working hours increase the coronary risk it is not clear if this relationship is direct or indirect. Data from experimental studies suggest that the cholesterol metabolism has a circadian rhythm [6]. Disturbances of these rhythms could theoretically result in dyslipoproteinemias and therefore increase the coronary risk [7, 8]. Irregular working hours could also have an indirect influence on the lipids through different eating patterns or differences in physical activity.

Work rhythm by itself could have an influence on the cardiovascular system since it interacts with many negative work environment variables which could by themselves increase the coronary risk [1].

Considering the paucity of data on this important issue, it was decided to start an epidemiological study on the subject.

Working Hypothesis

It was postulated that irregular working hours are apt to influence blood lipids directly or indirectly. Therefore it was postulated that subjects who worked under different work rhythms also had different blood lipid levels independently of other variables that are known to affect blood lipids.

Design

A cross-sectional epidemiological survey was carried out although it was recognized from the beginning that a longitudinal prospective survey would have been preferable and necessary if the prevalence study favoured the working hypothesis.

Groups that differ in the regulation of working hours were compared. A male population group aged 25–40 years was selected. Older age groups were excluded to avoid a selection of men who already had CVD, resulting in a job selection bias due to existing disease. Younger age groups were excluded to avoid subjects who had only worked for 1 or 2 years in a particular work rhythm.

As we were well-aware of the fact that blood lipid levels are influenced by other environmental factors, it was decided to measure dietary habits, smoking habits, the pattern of leisure time physical activity, body mass index (BMI), and psychosocial variables as possible confounders.

Methodology

Employers with different working hour regulations were asked to participate. If they agreed, the personnel department was asked to provide a list of all the men aged 25–40 years. All eligible men were invited by letter to participate in the study.

The screening visit included:

- Questionnaires on medical history, smoking habits, drug intake, professional class, and subjective symptoms.
- The Minnesota leisure time physical activity questionnaire [9] was administered by a trained technician. This questionnaire results in an activity metabolic index (AMI) which equals kilocalories if one assumes that the basal metabolic rate equals 60 kcal/h.
- Psychological tests: the behavior pattern type A described by Rosenman and Friedman was assessed by the Bortner test [10]. The higher the Bortner scale, the more one is inclined towards type A behaviour. A job stress questionnaire was applied in order to measure specifically psychological constraints on the job; this questionnaire had already been used in other Belgian epidemiological surveys. The more positive the job stress score, the higher the stress level.
- Dietary interview: a 24-h food intake record method was used to assess nutritional habits.
- Anthropometric data: height and weight were measured by trained technicians using standardized methods.
- Blood lipid measurements: a blood sample was drawn from an antecubital vein in supine position. All blood samples were taken in fasting condition during morning hours at the end of the screening visit and before the start of work. For subjects working shift or irregular hours the screening visit was scheduled when they were working in a shift starting in the morning hours. Blood lipid measurements were made using standardized methods. Low-density lipoprotein (LDL) cholesterol was calculated by the Friedewald formula.

Statistics

Differences between groups were studied by analyses of variance and covariance and by stepwise discriminant analysis using the SPSS package.

Results

Subjects were recruited from seven Belgian industries. A total of 1324 men aged 25–40 years were eligible; 909 (69%) agreed to participate. Among these 401 were employed in a normal day work system (group A). 243 in a three-shift work system (group B), and 238 in a heterogeneous system consisting of 24 h at work, 24 h off, 24 h at work, and 48 h off (group C); the latter were all professional firemen. Only 27 men were employed in a two-shift work system. Because of the small number they were not considered as a separate group and not included in the present analysis.

In Table 1 the lipid levels of the three groups are compared. Significant differences were observed: group C had an adverse lipid profile with higher total cholesterol and LDL cholesterol levels, a lower high-density lipoprotein (HDL) cholesterol level and a lower HDL cholesterol/non-HDL cholesterol ratio.

The groups were compared for age, BMI, smoking, and dietary habits, leisure time, physical activity, job stress, and type A behavior pattern as possible confounders. These results are presented in Tables 2 and 3.

The three groups were strictly comparable in age and height. There was a slight difference in weight and BMI: it increased from being the lowest in group A being the highest in group C. Group C also scored higher in the job stress questionnaire. The type A behavior pattern expressed by the Bortner scale was also more pronounced in group C.

Regarding dietary habits, subjects from group C took more of their calories from saturated fat and less from polyunsaturated fats; so, the dietary polyunsaturated/saturated (P/S) ratio was different between the groups. There was also a trend towards a higher consumption of dietary cholesterol and of alcohol in group C. Smoking was significantly different between the groups with extreme differences

Table 1. Comparison of lipid levels in three different work rhythm groups

Lipids		Groups according to work rhythm			p^a
		A $n=401$	B $n=243$	C $n=238$	
Total cholesterol (mg%)	mean	204	201	220	<.001
	SD	38	40	40	
HDL cholesterol (mg%)	mean	47.2	45.6	43.4	<.001
	SD	12.2	11.1	11.6	
ln triglycerides (mg%)	mean	4.6	4.7	4.7	NS
	SD	.5	.6	.6	
LDL cholesterol (mg%)	mean	134	132	151	<.001
	SD	35	37	35	
$\frac{\text{HDL cholesterol}}{\text{Non-HDL cholesterol}} \times 100\%$	mean	32	32	26	<.001
	SD	13	13	11	

[a] Based on ANOVA. NS, not significant.

Table 2. Comparison of possible confounders in the three different work rhythm groups

Possible confounders		Groups according to work rhythm			p^a
		A	B	C	
Age (years)	mean	32.4	32.3	32.7	NS
	SD	4.1	4.0	4.2	
Weight (kg)	mean	75.0	75.4	77.2	<.05
	SD	9.5	10.8	9.7	
Height (cm)	mean	174	174	174	NS
	SD	6	7	7	
Body mass index (kg/m^2)	mean	24.7	24.9	25.4	<.05
	SD	2.9	3.1	2.8	
Job stress score	mean	− .14	− .36	+ .78	<.001
	SD	2.0	1.9	2.6	
Bortner scale	mean	172	174	184	<.001
	SD	34	33	39	

[a] Based on ANOVA. NS, not significant.

Table 3. Comparison of possible confounders in the three work rhythm groups

		Groups according to work rhythm			p
		A	B	C	
Dietary habits					
Saturated fat (% kcal)	mean	17.4	17.4	19.4	<.001
	SD	5.3	5.9	7.3	
Polyunsaturated fat (% kcal)	mean	6.1	6.7	5.5	=.01
	SD	3.1	4.1	3.6	
Dietary P/S ratio	mean	.41	.43	.33	<.05
	SD	.37	.32	.28	
Cholesterol (mg)	mean	461	442	505	.06
	SD	294	262	343	
Alcohol (g)	mean	20.7	20.8	25.7	.09
	SD	26.7	28.4	36.2	
Smoking habits					
Cigarette smokers	(%)	40	48	57	<.001
Leisure time physical activity					
Total score, AMI	mean	372	403	516	<.001
	SD	300	376	414	

from 40% to 57% between day workers and group C. Group C was more active during leisure time, reflected in a higher leisure time activity score.

In order to study the relationship between irregular working hours and serum lipids independently of other factors, multivariate analyses were done. In Table 4 the three groups are compared for serum lipids by analysis of covariance after adjust-

Table 4. Differences in serum lipids between the three work rhythm groups by analysis of covariance after adjustment for smoking habits, leisure time activity score, body mass index, job stress score, Bortner scale, dietary alcohol, and dietary cholesterol

Serum lipids		Groups according to work rhythm			p
		A	B	C	
Total cholesterol (mg%)	mean	205	202	220	<.001
HDL cholesterol (mg%)	mean	46.7	45.1	43.8	.025
ln triglycerides (mg%)	mean	4.6	4.7	4.7	NS
LDL cholesterol (mg%)	mean	134	132	151	<.001
$\frac{\text{HDL cholesterol}}{\text{Non-HDL cholesterol}} \times 100\%$	mean	32	31	27	<.001

NS, not significant.

ment for smoking, leisure time activity, BMI, job stress, Bortner scale, dietary cholesterol, and alcohol.

Total cholesterol and LDL cholesterol were significantly higher in group C independently of all other variables. Among the covariates the leisure time activity score and the BMI were also significantly related to total cholesterol and LDL cholesterol: leisure time activity in a negative sense, BMI in a positive sense.

Part of the variance of total (13%) and LDL cholesterol (11%) were explained by the differences in the work rhythm, leisure time activity, and BMI.

HDL cholesterol and the HDL cholesterol/non-HDL cholesterol ratio were significantly different between the groups independently of all other variables. Among the covariates, BMI and smoking were negatively and alcohol positively related with HDL cholesterol and with the HDL cholesterol/non-HDL cholesterol ratio. Part of the variance of HDL cholesterol (6.4%) and of the HDL cholesterol/non-HDL cholesterol ratio (15%) were explained by the differences in work rhythm. BMI, smoking, and alcohol consumption. Triglyceride levels were not significantly different between the three groups.

Besides these analyses of variance, stepwise discriminant analyses were performed to study in a multivariate way the characteristics which distinguished the subjects working in the three groups. For this purpose, the following variables were always fed into the analysis: job stress score, leisure time physical activity score, dietary P/S ratio, smoking habits, Bortner scale, BMI, dietary cholesterol, dietary alcohol; in addition, one lipid variable was introduced into each discriminant analysis.

Total cholesterol, HDL cholesterol, LDL cholesterol, and the HDL cholesterol/non-HDL cholesterol ratio were found to be significant discriminators between the three groups in each analysis. As an example, the LDL cholesterol results are presented in Table 5. Among all the variables that were fed into the analysis, the LDL cholesterol was selected as the most powerful discriminator. Besides LDL cholesterol five other variables were selected as significant discriminators between the three groups: job stress score, leisure time physical activity score, dietary P/S ratio, smoking habits, and the Bortner scale. Using these classification factors to perform an a posteriori group classification gave a 52% correct classification into the three groups.

Table 5. Stepwise discriminant function analysis comparing the three work rhythm groups. Classification function coefficients and signification of F to remove the variable from the equation

	Classification function coefficients			*p*
	A	B	C	
Constant	-57.536	-58.684	-62.987	
LDL cholesterol	.0631	.0602	.0767	<.001
Job stress score	-.608	-.632	-.447	<.001
Leisure time activity score	.00673	.00663	.00768	<.001
Dietary P/S	2.80	3.07	1.84	<0.01
Smoking	2.48	2.89	3.17	<.001
Bortner scale	.157	.158	.164	<.05

Discussion

In most epidemiological studies within homogeneous population groups interindividual differences in blood lipid levels are poorly explained. The low order or no correlation found between nutrition and cholesterol levels in such studies has been attributed to a large intraindividual variability in nutritional habits and to homogeneous eating habits in single population groups.

Only 9% of the variance of serum cholesterol in a Belgian middle-aged population group was explained by factors such as relative weight (3.5%), regional differences (reflecting nutritional differences?), job activity, systolic blood pressure, age, and socioeducational class [11]. Although genetics play an important role in explaining interindividual differences in lipids, results from other studies suggest that stress, work rhythm and environmental factors may be related to blood lipid levels [12, 13].

If indeed, lipoprotein metabolism in men is regulated by a circadian system it could well be that a disregulation of normal work rhythm affects that system resulting in differences in blood lipid levels. In the literature only a few observations support this view. In an experimental study of day workers who were suddenly rescheduled to temporary night work the cholesterol level increased and fell back on return to day work [8]. In two other cross-sectional studies higher lipid levels were found among shift workers [14, 15]. In a study among Californian accountants elevated cholesterol levels were found when these subjects were exposed to extra job stress during certain periods of the year [16].

In the present study blood lipids were compared in three groups of men, comparable in age structure but different in work rhythm. One group (C) consisted of firemen with a specific work schedule: 24 h at work, 24 h off, 24 h at work, and 48 h off. This group of men showed differences from the other groups in all the determined blood lipids except triglycerides. However, they also differed in other factors that are known to affect blood lipid levels, such as BMI, nutrition, smoking habits, and leisure time phyisical activity. Some of these differences could partly explain some part of the observed difference in lipids: subjects in group C were more obese, smoked more, consumed more cholesterol and saturated fat and less polyunsaturated fat. These differences could explain to some extent a higher total and LDL cholesterol level and the lower HDL cholesterol level. On the other hand, group C was more active during leisure time and consumed more alcohol. From these differences one would expect a higher HDL cholesterol and a lower total cholesterol level in group C.

When the Keys formula is used as a guide for estimating the possible effect of the nutritional differences on total cholesterol between group C and the others a difference of 5.8 mg% is expected while 17.9 mg% is observed.

The confounding effects of obesity, smoking, nutrition, and physical activity were studied in multivariate analyses. These results indicate that the differences in serum lipids between the work rhythm groups are hardly affected when all possible confounders are considered. The differences in serum lipids are substantial and indicate a greater coronary risk in the men working in the most heterogeneous work rhythm. The fact that subjects in group B showed no differences in serum lipids from subjects in group A suggests that night work by itself or classical shift work does not influence plasma lipids. It is therefore difficult to speculate on the mechanisms whereby group C has an adverse lipid profile. It is not explained by the classical environmental factors that are known to be related with lipids. It could still be related to the work rhythm being particularly disturbed in group C. Differences in work rhythm induce differences in the pattern of food intake and this could adversely affect the circadian rhythm of lipid metabolism.

It has been shown that irregular working hours influence the diurnal pattern of catecholamine excretion [8]. Catecholamines are known to give rise to hemoconcentration. However, the hematocrit was strictly comparable between the three groups in our study; so, hemoconcentration cannot explain the differences in serum lipids. It could have something to do with other environmental factors, typical for group C. From the study it can be concluded that a relationship exists between work-related factors and serum lipids in group C. The working hypothesis should be further tested in prospective epidemiological surveys where subjects should be examined at recruitment into industries with various work rhythms and where their lipid profiles should be followed over time to study the effect of work rhythm independently of other changes that occur after starting work.

Acknowledgement. This work was supported by EEC grant No. 723, art. 1-1b.

References

1. Akerstedt T, Alfredsson L, Theorell T (1986) An aggregate study of irregular work hours and cardiovascular disease. In: Haider M, Koller M, Cervinka R (eds) Night and shiftwork: long-term effects and their prevention. Lang, Frankfurt, pp 419-424
2. Koller M (1983) Health risks related to shift work. Int Arch Occup Environ Health 53: 59-75
3. Taylor PJ, Pocock PJ (1972) Mortality of shift and dayworkers 1956-1968. Br J Ind Med 29: 201-207
4. Angersback D, Knauth P, Loskant H, Karvonen MJ, Undeutsch K, Rutenfranz J (1980) A retrospective cohort study comparing complaints and disease in day and shift workers. Int Arch Occup Environ Health 45: 127-140
5. Akerstedt T, Knutsson A, Alfredsson L, Theorell T (1984) Shiftwork and cardiovascular disease. Scand J Work Environ Health 10: 409-414

6. Mlekusch W (1982) Circadian rhythms of plasma lipid metabolites in rats adapted to a day or night feeding schedule. Nut Rep Int 25: 789-797
7. Parker TS, Brown C, Kolb M, McNamara DJ, Ahrens EH (1984) Mevalonic acid in human plasma: relation to cholesterol synthesis and circadian rhythm. Circulation 64 [Suppl IV]: 1032
8. Theorell T, Akerstedt T (1976) Day and night work: changes in cholesterol, uric acid, glucose and potassium in serum and in circadian patterns of urinary catecholamine excretion. Acta Med Scand 200: 47-53
9. Taylor HL, Jacobs DR Jr, Schucker B, Knudsen J, Leon AS, De Backer G (1978) A questionnaire for the assessment of leisure time physical activities. J Chronic Dis 31: 741-755
10. Bortner RW, Rosenman RH (1967) The measurement of pattern A behavior. J Chronic Dis 20: 533-535
11. Kornitzer M, Dramaix M, De Backer G, Thilly C (1977) The Belgian multifactor preventive trial in CVD: cholesterolemia and psychosociobiological variables. Hart Bull 8: 147-154
12. Kurppa K, Hietanen E, Klockars M, Partinen M, Rantanen J, Rönnemaa T, Viikari J (1984) Chemical exposures to work and cardiovascular morbidity. Scand J Work Environ Health 10: 381-388
13. Theorell T, Alfredsson L, Knox S, Perski A, Svensson J, Wahler D (1984) On the interplay between socioeconomic factors, personality and work environment in the pathogenesis of cardiovascular disease. Scand J Work Environ Health 10: 373-380
14. Thelle DS, Forde OH, Try K, Lehmann EH (1976) The Tromso heart study. Acta Med Scand 200: 107-118
15. Knuttson A, Zamore K (1982) Nagra medicinska och sociala aspekter pa skiftarbete vid Ortvikers Pappersbruk. Stressforskningsrapporter no 148. Karolinska, Institutet, Stockholm
16. Friedman M, Rosenman R, Carroll V (1958) Changes in the serum cholesterol and blood dotting time in men subjected to cyclic variation of occupational stress. Circulation 17: 852-861

Identification and Computer Modeling of Functional Domains in Plasma Apolipoproteins

M. Rosseneu, H. de Loof, R. Brasseur, and J. M. Ruysschaert

Introduction

The protein moiety of the lipoproteins consists of several proteins named "apolipoproteins," which have several physiological functions, including lipid binding, receptor binding, and enzyme activation. The sequences of most of the apolipoproteins have been reported and increasing efforts have been devoted to the interpretation of these sequences. The localization and characterization of functional domains, responsible for the properties listed above, has become especially relevant for the understanding of their physiological functions. Sequencing of the smaller apolipoproteins, apo AI, AII, CI, CII, CIII, was initially carried out by conventional protein sequencing [1], while the elucidation of the sequence of the larger apolipoproteins has required the use of molecular biological techniques [2]. The interpretation of these sequences is expected to reveal both, features common to all apolipoproteins such as lipid-binding domains, and specific characteristics for some of the apolipoproteins, such as receptor-binding and enzyme-activating regions.

Theoretical calculations based on prediction of the protein secondary structure and on calculation of the hydrophobicity index and hydrophobic moment have been applied to the prediction of functional domains in proteins [3]. We have applied these methods to the apolipoprotein sequences, and further carried out a modeling of the functional domains interacting with phospholipids, through an energy minimalization technique [4].

The results of this theoretical approach, applied to apo AI, AII, AIV, CII, E, and B, will be described and analysed in this paper.

Lipid-Binding Segments in Apolipoproteins

The lipid-binding properties of the soluble apolipoproteins, with the exception of apo B, have been attributed by Segrest et al. [5] to amphipathic helices present in these proteins. These helical domains, with a clear separation of hydrophobic and hydrophilic residues on the two faces of the helices, are able to interact with both the hydrophobic and hydrophilic parts of the phospholipids.

The hydrophobic moment of a protein segment was calculated according to the procedure of Eisenberg et al. [3]. As the hydrophobic moment is a function of the periodicity in the protein structure, this parameter was calculated assuming different values for the angle at which the side chains emerge from the backbone, when the segment is viewed down its axis. This angle can assume any value from 0° for a helix with an infinite repeat, to 180° for a straight segment of β-structure. We also used a modification of the method of Finer-Moore and Stroud [6] in which the hydrophobic moment calculated under all angles is plotted for all consecutive segments of the sequence.

The method described above was applied to detect amphiphilic helices within the apolipoprotein sequences. As these amphiphilic helices are involved in lipid binding, we compared the results of the modified Finer-Moore plots to the experimental data reported in the literature [7].

An example of such a plot is shown in Fig. 1 A for apo AII. The existence of two lipid-binding domains in apo AII was documented from experiments with synthetic peptides [7]. One domain is located in the NH_2-terminal region, around residues 12–31, while the second domain encompassing residues 50–58 lies in the COOH-terminal region of the protein. The modified Finer-Moore plot for apo AII shows two pronounced maxima at an angle of 100°, which match exactly the two lipid-binding domains detected experimentally. In the classical Eisenberg [3] plot, a cluster of several helices with a high hydrophobic moment and a relatively high mean hydrophobicity value appears, corresponding to the helices responsible for phospholipid binding. According to their relative position on this plot and the

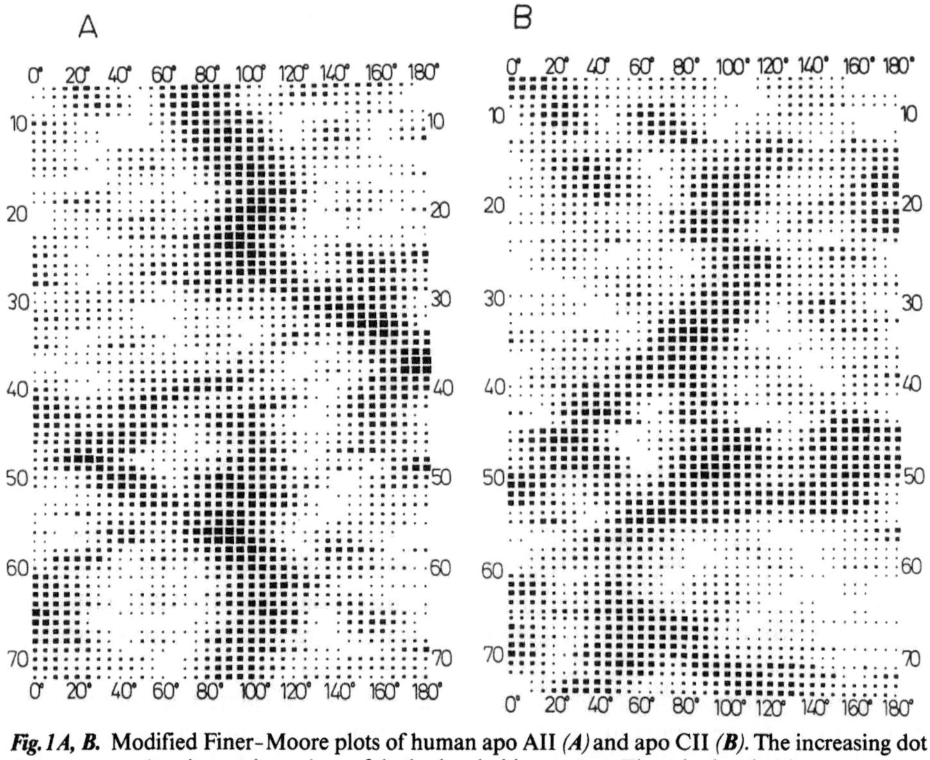

Fig. 1A, B. Modified Finer-Moore plots of human apo AII *(A)* and apo CII *(B)*. The increasing dot size corresponds to increasing values of the hydrophobic moment. These hydrophobic moments are plotted for different angles (*x* axis) as a function of the midpoint of the segments used (*y* axis)

nomenclature used by Eisenberg [3] these helices should be classified as "surface seeking" helices.

Some of these features were also shared by the hydrophobicity profiles of other small apolipoproteins in which phospholipid-binding domains have been identified experimentally. There is evidence that residues 45-55 of apo CII are involved in phospholipid binding and activation of lipoprotein lipase at high phospholipid packing [1, 7]. On the modified Finer-Moore plot (Fig. 1 B) this region shows a maximum around 100°.

This theoretical approach therefore seems in good agreement with the experimental data available on the lipid-binding properties of these natural and synthetic peptides.

Activation Properties of Apolipoproteins for the Lecithin: Cholesterol Acyltransferase

Lecithin: cholesterol acyltransferase (LCAT; EC. 2.3.1.43) is the enzyme responsible for cholesterol esterification in serum. Several high-density lipoprotein (HDL) apolipoproteins have activator properties towards this enzyme, being apo AI the most efficient activator, followed by apo AIV, apo CI and apo E [8]. The structural requirements for LCAT activation have not been clearly defined yet. A correlation between the available experimental data and the hydrophobicity profiles of these sequences was searched for.

A plot of the average of all hydrophobic moments for 11-residue segments of the polypeptide is shown on Fig. 2 A for human apo AI, apo AII and apo AIV. All three proteins bind phospholipids to form complexes [1] and have a pronounced maximum at an angle of about 100°, corresponding to an amphiphilic helical structure as described above for apo AII. However, in the plots of human apo AI and apo AIV, a second maximum of similar magnitude appears at an angle of 160°-170°. In apo AII, which has no activator properties, this extra peak is very weak, while the peak at 100° is relatively more important.

An additional test of our theoretical approach lies in an analysis of synthetic "model" peptides designed for their lipid-binding properties, and which have also the ability to activate the LCAT enzyme. The hydrophobicity profiles of the LAP-20 peptide [7] and of that described by Fukushima et al. [9], are shown in Fig. 2 B, together with the profile of a 20-residue segment of apo AII (residues 51-70) located in a lipid-binding domain. Although the hydrophobicity profiles of the two model peptides have peaks of different magnitude, their overall shape is the same and both show a peak at 160°. In contrast, the lipid-binding segment of apo AII lacks the peak at around 160°.

This theoretical approach seems sensitive enough to differentiate between the various amphipathic helices and provides a better insight in the functional domains of the apolipoproteins.

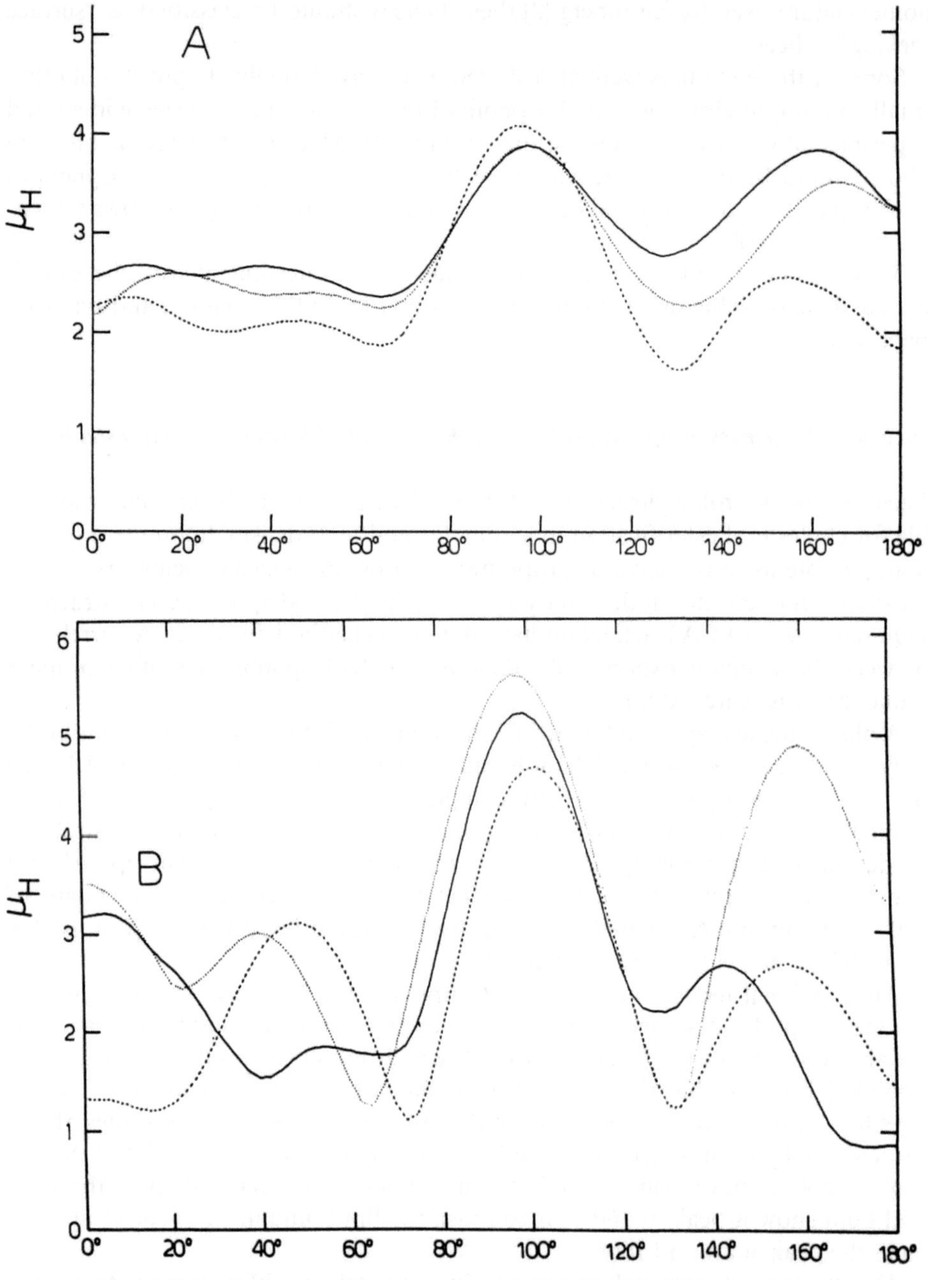

Fig. 2A, B. Average of the modified Finer-Moore hydrophobicity plots for: *A* human apo AI (——), apo AII (-----), and apo AIV (·····), and *B* two synthetic lipid-binding peptides, LAP-20 (-----) [7] and the docosapeptide described by Fukushima et al. [9] (·····), and a lipid-binding domain of apo AII (——) (residues 51-70)

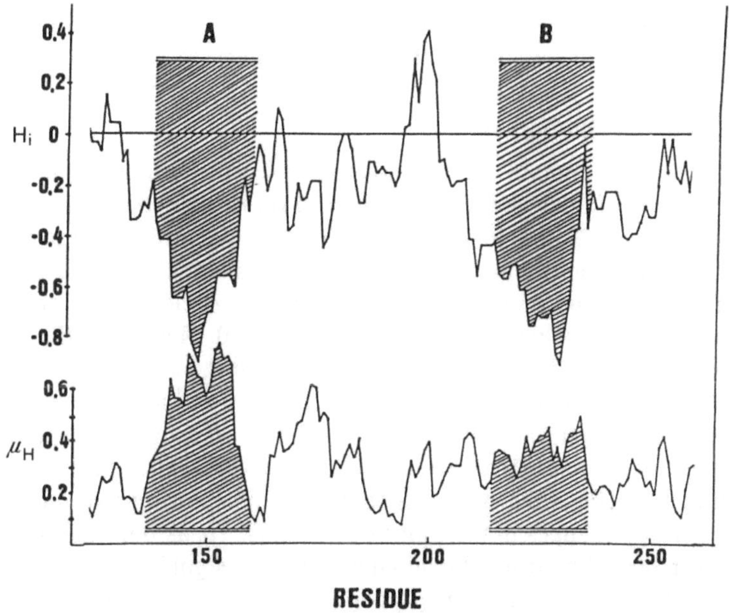

Fig. 3. Hydrophobicity profile of residues 100-250 of human apo E. Plot of μ_H and H_i as functions of the midpoint of the 11-residue segments used for the calculations. The *shaded areas* (residues 136-160 and 214-236) correspond to the two clusters (*A* and *B*) described in the text

Prediction of Receptor-Binding Domains in Apolipoproteins

We applied the mean hydrophobicity and hydrophobic moment calculations to predict the receptor-binding domains in apo E, and to evaluate the effect of mutations in the apo E sequence on the receptor-binding properties of the mutants [10]. The mean α-helical hydrophobic moment (μ_H) and mean hydrophobicity (H_i) were calculated according to the procedure of Eisenberg et al. [3]. A segment of 11 residues was moved through the protein sequence and the mean hydrophobicity and mean hydrophobic moment per segment were calculated. These two parameters were plotted as a function of the mid-point of the segment along the sequence (Fig. 3). μ_H was also plotted versus H_i for all possible segments, except for those containing a proline residue, as this has a strong helix-breaking capacity (Fig. 4A).

Several helices with a relatively high hydrophobicity ($-0.2 < H_i < 0.4$) and hydrophobic moment ($0.3 < \mu_H < 0.65$) can be detected in the μ_H versus H_i plot of apo E (Fig. 4A). Such helices can also be found in other apolipoproteins and were suggested to be involved in lipid binding [5]. The most striking feature of these plots (Figs. 3, 4) is, however, the appearance of two clusters of residues with a very low hydrophobicity ($H_i < -0.55$), together with a very high ($\mu_H > 0.52$, cluster A) to intermediate ($0.29 < \mu_H < 0.46$, cluster B) hydrophobic moment. Using Fig. 3 these residues can easily be located as belonging to the regions 136-160 and 214-236 with the following sequences:

Arg-Leu-Ala-Ser-His-Leu-Arg-Lys-Leu-Arg-Lys-Arg-Leu-Leu-Arg-Asp-Ala-Asp-Asp-Leu-Gln-Lys-Arg-Leu-Ala

for the first cluster and for the second cluster:

Leu-Arg-Ala-Arg-Met-Glu-Glu-Met-Gly-Ser-Arg-Thr-Arg-Asp-Arg-Leu-Asp-Glu-Val-Lys-Glu-Gln-Val

This first domain corresponds to the receptor-binding domain of apo E as proposed by Mahley et al. [11]. In order to get further confirmation of the involvement of residues 136-160 in the receptor binding we carried out the same calculations for all known apo E mutants. The substitutions affecting the receptor-binding activity all affected the plot of apo E in domain A. A close-up of this region for normal apo E and three mutations is shown in Fig. 4B. The plot of the Arg-158→Cys mutation (Fig. 4C), decreasing the receptor-binding activity to less than 2% [11], shows that the mean hydrophobicities of the 11-residue segments with mid-points at 153-155 increase from about −0.57 to −0.32 while their mean hydrophobic moments decrease from about 0.72 down to 0.63. The Cys-112→Arg, Arg-142→Cys mutation (Fig. 4D), with less than 20% receptor-binding activity, also results in extensive changes in the plot of μ_H against H_i, as both the hydrophilicity and the mean helical hydrophobic moment decrease significantly. The modifications in the plot for a third mutation (Lys-146→Gln) are less extensive (Fig. 4E). The mean hydrophobicities of this site do not exceed −0.5 and experimental data showed that this mutation retains 40% receptor-binding activity.

We could detect a similar cluster of hydrophilic residues at positions 128-152 in the rat apo E sequence (Fig. 4F). This domain is exactly aligned with residues 136-160 of human apo E.

The second domain has not yet been directly implicated in receptor binding, although the existence of a second binding region interacting with the β-VLDL receptor has already been proposed [11]. An additional possibility might be that the A and B domains together form the receptor-binding site of apo E. This would explain why protein cleavage at position 199 has a profound effect on receptor binding. Heparin binding [12] has recently been demonstrated to occur in these regions.

The first receptor-binding domain of apo E has a strong homology with that proposed by Knott et al. [13] and further confirmed by Yang et al. [14] for apo B.

Modeling of Functional Domains in Apolipoproteins

The elucidation of the complete apo B sequence through DNA recombinant technologies has led to a further search of specific functional domains for this huge apolipoprotein (molecular weight 512.723 daltons).

We applied a semi-empirical conformational analysis to two distinct domains of apo B, selected as follows. The COOH-terminal peptide (residues 4507-4536) was selected in view of its hydrophobicity and since the COOH-terminal residue of apo B is masked in LDL. The second peptide (residues 4154-4189) was identified as an amphipathic helix with a significant homology with the amphipatic helices identified in the smaller apolipoproteins.

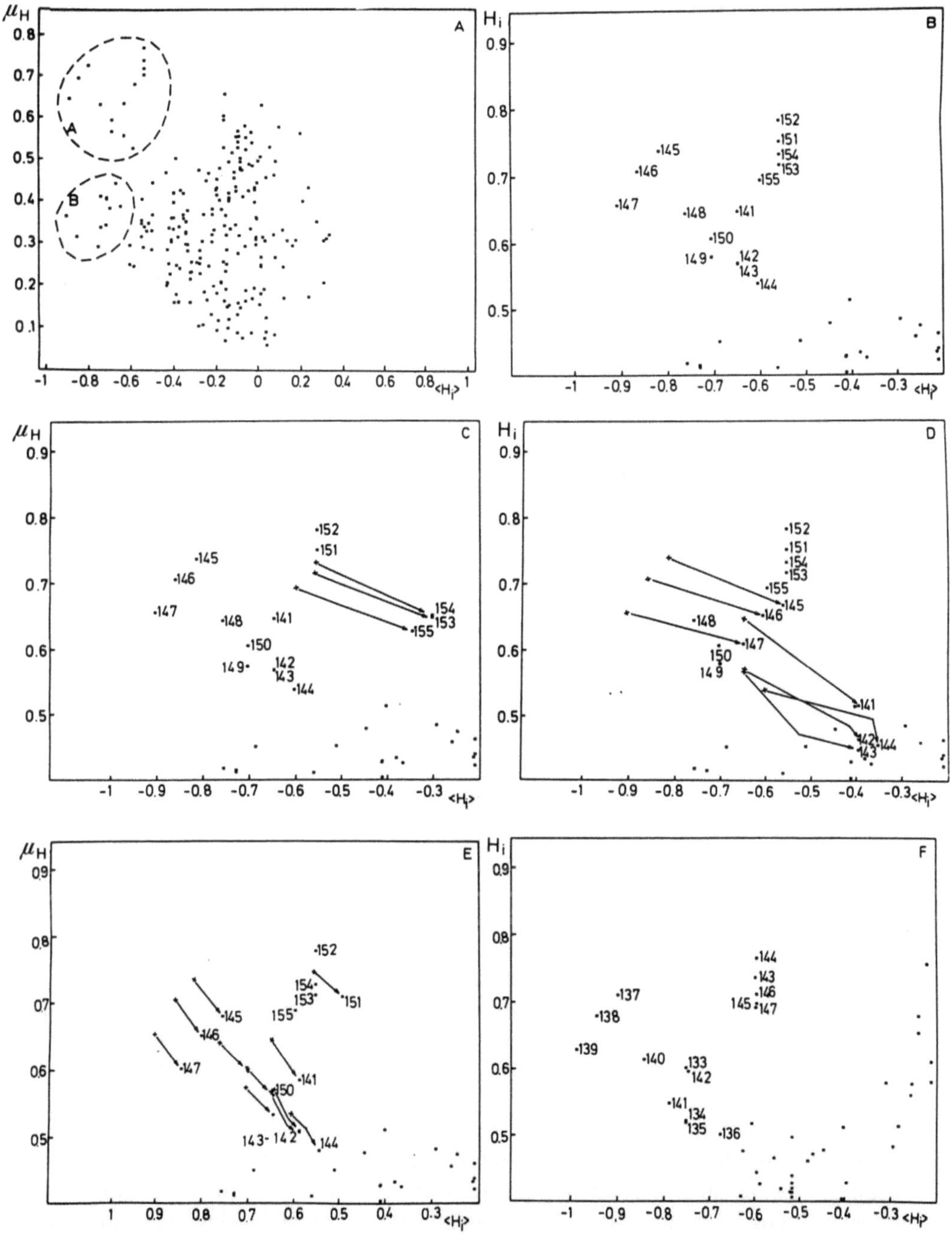

Fig. 4. ***A*** Plot of H_i (x-axis) against μ_H (y axis) for all 11-residue segments of apo E, except for those containing a proline residue. The two clusters of residues involved in receptor binding (*A* and *B*) are circled. ***B–F*** Representations of the receptor-binding domain of apo E, around cluster A, on an expanded scale (x axis (H_i) -1 to -0.2, and y axis (μ_H) 0.3 to 1.0). ***B*** Normal apo E; ***C*** Arg-158→Cys; ***D*** Cys-112→Arg, Arg-142→Cys; ***E*** Lys-146→Gln mutant. The *arrows* indicate the displacement of some residues compared with their position in the plot of normal apo E. ***F*** Rat apo E

The procedure for conformational analysis has been described previously [4]. Space-filling structures of polypeptides were based on the Chou and Fasman prediction of the secondary structure [4] and on assigning to the torsional angles the values classically associated with the α-helix, β-sheet and β-turn structures. From the energy of transfer of single atoms, or groups of atoms, from a hydrophobic into a hydrophilic medium, we defined the hydrophilic center (C_W) and hydrophobic center (C_{HC}). The polypeptide was oriented with the line joining the hydrophilic and hydrophobic centers perpendicular to the interface.

The total conformational energy of the polypeptide-phospholipid complex was calculated as the sum of the London-Van der Waals energy of interaction between nonmutually bonded atoms, the electrostatic interaction between atomic point charges, and the transfer energy.

The 4173-4189 peptide has an amphipathic helical structure with a segregation of the hydrophobic and hydrophilic residues on each side of the helix. In contrast to the COOH-terminal peptide, this peptide lies parallel to the interface, with its hydrophilic residues towards the aqueous phase. The hydrophobic and hydrophilic energies of transfer are 190 and 201 kcal/mol respectively. The distance between hydrophobic and hydrophilic centers is 0.116 nm. The amphipathic helix (residues 4173-4189) was assembled with seven dipalmitoylphosphatidylcholine (DPPC) molecules (Fig. 5). A minimal energy of interaction between the peptide and DPPC, of −14 kcal/mol lipid, was calculated when the peptide is orientated parallel to the interface.

Similar calculations carried out with synthetic model peptides such as LAP-20 [7] and the peptide synthesized by Fukushima et al. [9], yielded comparable conformations and interaction energies (−19 kcal/mol). However, the apo B amphipathic helix is more hydrophobic (Fig. 5) and the 1-2 and 1-4 alternation of charged residues is less pronounced. The interaction between hydrophobic residues and acyl chains extends up to 6th methyl group of the fatty acid. The hydrophilic residues are located above the P-N dipole of the phosphocholine head group.

The COOH-terminal peptide of apo B (residues 4517-4536) in its most probable conformation, a β-sheet structure, is orientated perpendicular to the interface. This is due to the large distance (0.354 nm) between the hydrophobic and hydrophilic centers. The hydrophobic (E_{trj}) and hydrophilic (E_{tri}) transfer energies associated with the peptide amount to 181 and 215 kcal/mol respectively.

In the presence of phospholipids, this peptide lies parallel to the acyl chains of the six DPPC molecules. The last three residues, Ile-4534, Ile-4535, Leu-4536, can penetrate into the lipid phase, past the DPPC acyl chains, and might interact with the cholesteryl esters of the LDL core. Residues 4527-4533 interact with the DPPC acyl chains. The lipid-water interface lies close to the Leu-4527 residue. Residues Tyr-4524, Met-4525, and Lys-4526 are located at the level of the phospholipid head groups. In such a structure, Tyr-4524 and Lys-4526 can interact with three phosphate groups located on the same side of the β-sheet while Met-4525 can interact with the carboxyl group of glycerol on the other side (Fig. 5). The more hydrophilic residues (4517-4523) are no longer in contact with the lipids and are located in the aqueous phase.

The energy of interaction between this peptide and DPPC amounts to −22 kcal/mol lipid in the crystalline state and to −21 kcal/mol in the fluid state, compared to

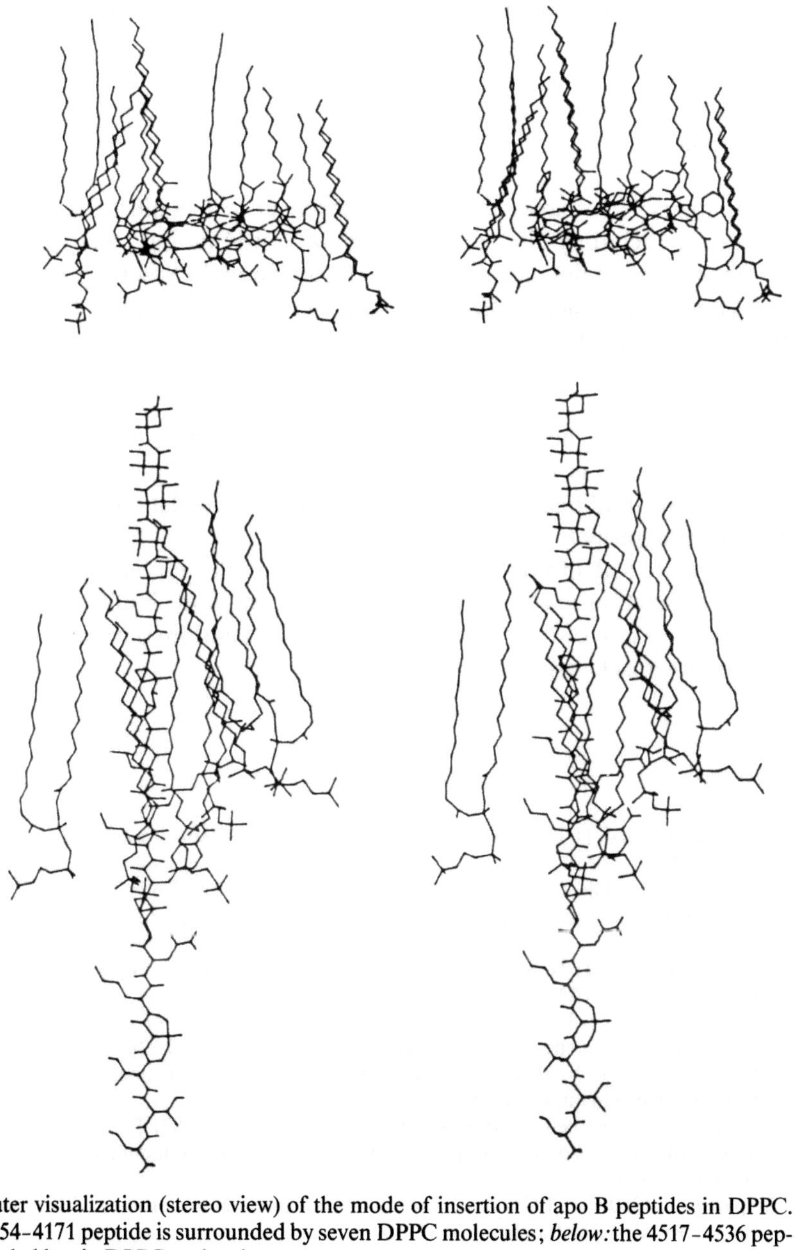

Fig. 5. Computer visualization (stereo view) of the mode of insertion of apo B peptides in DPPC. *Above:* The 4154–4171 peptide is surrounded by seven DPPC molecules; *below:* the 4517–4536 peptide is surrounded by six DPPC molecules

−13 kcal/mol for pure DPPC [4]. This configuration, characterized by a large energy of interaction with the lipids, is very stabile and this might account for the masking of the COOH-terminal residue in LDL.

The validity of these calculations and modeling was confirmed by turbidity and fluorescence measurements showing that the COOH-terminal peptide is able to perturb the phospholipid bilayer more, and possibly to induce a fusion of DMPC small vesicles, suggestive of a different orientation compared with a classical amphipathic helix.

Conclusion

In summary, we have presented theoretical calculations on apolipoprotein sequences, including the identification of lipid-binding, receptor-binding, and enzyme-activating domains, and we have compared the results of these calculations with experimental data, whenever available. The predictions of the lipid-binding and enzyme-activating domains of these apolipoproteins were in agreement with the data reported in the literature about the corresponding properties of natural and synthetic peptides. The receptor-binding activity of several apo E mutants was also in agreement with the "in vitro" measurements and with the defects observed "in vivo" in the patients. Finally, the modeling of the apo B peptides and their conformation in the lipid phase is supported by the available data on apo B solubility and lipid-binding properties.

This theoretical approach can therefore be usefully applied to the analysis of the structure-function relationship in apolipoproteins, and should contribute to a better understanding of their physiological function and involvement in the development of atherosclerosis.

References

1. Gotto A, Pownall H, Havel R (1986) Introduction to the plasma lipoproteins. Methods Enzymol 128: 3-41
2. Chen SH, Yang CH, Chen PF, Setzer D, Tanimura M, Li WH, Gotto A, Chan L (1986) The complete cDNA and amino acid sequence of human apolipoprotein B-100. J Biol Chem 261: 12918-12921
3. Eisenberg D (1984) Three-dimensional structure of membrane and surface proteins. Ann Rev Biochem 53: 595-623
4. Brasseur R, Ruysschaert JM (1986) Conformation and mode of organisation of amphiphilic membrane components: A conformational analysis. Biochem J 238: 1-11
5. Segrest J, Jackson R, Morrisett J, Gotto A (1974) A molecular theory of lipid-protein interactions in the plasma lipoproteins. FEBS Lett 38: 247-253
6. De Loof H, Rosseneu M, Brasseur R, Ruysschaert JM (1987) Functional differentiation of amphiphilic helices of the apolipoproteins by hydrophobic moment analysis. Biochim Biophys Acta 911: 45-52
7. Sparrow J, Gotto A (1981) Apolipoprotein lipid interactions: studies with synthetic polypeptides. CRC Crit Rev Biochem 13: 87-107
8. Jonas A (1986) Synthetic substrates of lecithin:cholesterol acyltransferase. J Lipid Res 27: 689-698
9. Fukushima D, Yokoyama S, Kroon D, Kezdy F, Kaiser E (1980) Chain length-function correlation of amphiphilic peptides. J Biol Chem 255: 10651-10657
10. De Loof H, Rosseneu M, Brasseur R, Ruysschaert JM (1986) Use of hydrophobicity profiles to predict receptor binding domains on apolipoprotein E and the low density lipoprotein apolipoprotein (B-E) receptor. Proc Natl Acad Sci USA 83: 2295-2299
11. Mahley A, Innerarity T, Rall C, Weisgraber K (1984) Plasma lipoproteins: apolipoprotein structure and function. J Lipid Res 25: 1277-1294

12. Cardin A, Hirose N, Blankenship D, Jackson R, Harmony J, Sparrow D, Sparrow J (1986) Binding of a high reactive heparin to human apolipoprotein E: identification of two heparin-binding domains. Biochem Biophys Res Commun 134: 783-789
13. Knott T, Rall S, Innerarity T, Jacobson S, Urdea M, Levy-Wilson B, Powell L, Pease R, Eddy R, Nakai H, Byers M, Priestley L, Robertson E, Rall L, Betsholtz, Shows T, Mahley B, Scott J (1985) Human apolipoprotein B: structure of carboxyl-terminal domains, sites of gene expression and chromosomal localization. Science 230: 37-43
14. Yang CY, Chen SH, Gianturco S, Bradley W, Sparrow J, Tanimura M, Li WH, Sparrow D, De Loof H, Rosseneu M, Lee FS, Gu ZW, Gotto A, Chan L (1986) Sequence, structure, receptor-binding domains and internal repeats of human apolipoprotein B-100. Nature 323: 738-742

New Perspectives in Human Apolipoprotein B Metabolism

J. Shepherd and C. J. Packard

Recent developments in our understanding of human apolipoprotein B (apo B) metabolism have led to the emergence of new concepts linking this polypeptide to the pathogenesis of atherosclerosis. For, although it has long been known that raised plasma concentrations of the protein circulating in association with low-density lipoproteins (LDL) are linked to increased risk of ischaemic heart disease, less emphasis has been placed on the potential involvement of apo B in particles of lower density like very low- and intermediate-density lipoproteins (VLDL and IDL). Now, their impact on the atherogenic process is becoming more and more evident. For example, whereas LDL in itself is unable to induce foam cell formation in cultured macrophages, subfractions of VLDL do have this propensity [1]. Clearly then, we ought not only to attempt to delineate the factors which govern the concentration of LDL in the plasma, but should also focus attention on its metabolic precursors, VLDL and IDL. Fortunately, B protein constitutes an integral component of these precursors and remains associated with them throughout their lifetime. It is therefore a useful marker of their metabolic fate. We have taken advantage of such knowledge to follow the metabolism of subpopulations of particles within human VLDL, IDL and LDL. Our studies [2, 3] have shown that the spectrum, within the Sf 0-400 flotation interval, is substantially heterogeneous and is subject to regulation at multiple points. Our evidence suggests that receptors may be implicated in these regulatory processes [4].

Apo B - Associated Cholesterol Transport

Seventy per cent of plasma cholesterol in normal individuals circulates with LDL in the Sf 0-12 flotation range. Only small amounts appear in the less dense VLDL and IDL species. But, since the turnover rates of these particles are several times that of LDL, the flux of cholesterol through them is greater than their steady-state concentrations suggest. In fact, it seems that as much cholesterol is delivered to the liver by remnants of VLDL and chylomicron particle metabolism as is via LDL [5]. It is tempting to speculate that active, receptor-mediated hepatic removal of these species represents part of a protective mechanism since, as noted above, they have the potential of generating foam cells if they are allowed to come in contact with peripheral tissue macrophages. Two experiments of Nature support this contention. First, individuals suffering from the homozygous form of familial hypercholesterolaemia (FH) and lacking functional receptors for LDL accumulate significant amounts of VLDL remnants in their plasma and, interestingly, deposit substantial quantities of cholesteryl ester in their tissue macrophages [6]. This undoubtedly predisposes to their particularly florid pattern of atherosclerosis. Of course, the gross increase in their plasma LDL plays a major contributory role in this regard, but it should be noted that other individuals with type III hyperlipoproteinaemia, who show similar defects in VLDL remnant metabolism leading to accumulation of these particles in their circulation in the absence of an increase in LDL, also develop premature, accelerated atherosclerosis [7]. The discussion which follows examines in some detail the processes by which the levels of VLDL and their metabolic products are controlled in normal and hyperlipidaemic individuals and attempts to define how they vary in response to therapeutic intervention.

Control Points in Apo B Metabolism

Figure 1 delineates those points on the delipidation cascade which have been identified as contributing to the metabolic regulation of apo B-containing particles in man.

Regulation Point 1: Synthesis of VLDL

The liver is responsible for the secretion of triglyceride-rich apo B-containing particles into the bloodstream. From early studies [8] it was envisaged that the protein first appeared in the largest particles which were precursor to smaller VLDL and ultimately LDL. In this process, the particle is remodelled, the triglyceride in its

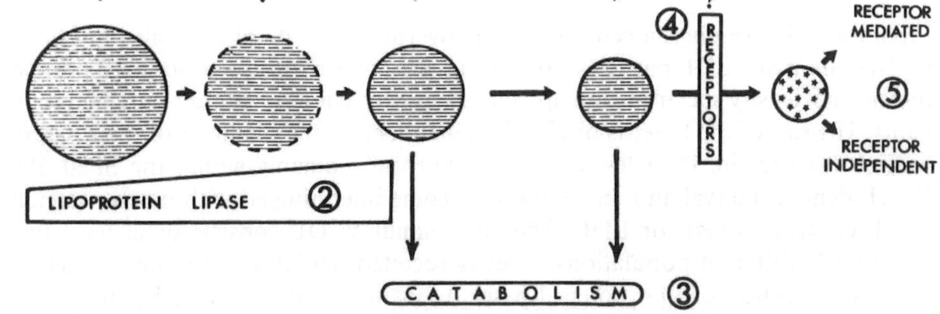

Fig. 1. Sites of regulation of apolipoprotein B metabolism. Five points of regulation on the VLDL delipidation cascade are considered: ① synthesis of very low-density lipoproteins; ② lipoprotein lipase and VLDL catabolism; ③ catabolism of VLDL remnants; ④ involvement of receptors in IDL-LDL conversion; ⑤ receptor-mediated and receptor-independent LDL catabolism

core being effectively replaced by cholesteryl esters. However, subsequent and more sophisticated studies using [^{14}C]leucine to locate the sites of introduction of B protein into the VLDL cascade led to a reassessment of this model [9]. It now appears that VLDL is synthesised in a spectrum of sizes over the entire flotation range from Sf 20 to Sf 400. This being so, it is reasonable to speculate that not all VLDL particles are in metabolic equilibrium with one another [10]. They may therefore be destined for a variety of fates. In experiments conducted in our laboratory we were able to confirm this premise by demonstrating that particles of Sf 100–400 exhibited different metabolic properties from smaller lipoproteins of Sf 20–100 [3]. The larger particles both in normal and hyperlipidaemic patients were subject to direct removal from the circulation without being converted to LDL. Smaller VLDL particles of Sf 20–100 were the main source of the latter. It follows then that small variations in the spectral distribution of VLDL particles which are secreted can alter dramatically the apparent metabolic properties of the entire lipoprotein class. For example, it is known that type IV hyperlipoproteinaemic individuals synthesise more of the large triglyceride-rich particles. Proportionally less of their VLDL is therefore converted to LDL, so that the metabolic link between VLDL and LDL is to all appearances deranged [11]. In other words, apparent differences in VLDL handling between normal and hyperlipoproteinaemic individuals may in actuality reflect disproportionate production of particles within the Sf 20–400 spectrum rather than derive from a fundamental qualitative alteration in B protein metabolism. This being so, it becomes important to unravel how the various therapeutic modalities used to lower blood lipids might influence not only the net production rate of B protein in VLDL but also the distribution of particles within the spectrum. In a recent study of the effects of bezafibrate on lipoprotein turnover in type III hyperlipoproteinaemic subjects [12] we noted that plasma lipids fell to normal in association with an overall reduction in VLDL apo B synthesis. However, the decrement in large VLDL (five-fold) was proportionally greater than that in smaller particles (two-fold), largely due to a greater limitation on the rate of synthesis of the former.

Regulation Point 2: Lipoprotein Lipase and VLDL Catabolism

Lipoprotein lipase plays a central role in governing the rate of catabolism of large triglyceride-rich VLDL particles. As the triglyceride is hydrolysed, so the B protein transits the density spectrum and appears in smaller, cholesteryl ester-enriched remnants. The size of the latter is obviously dependent on the diameter of their parent nascent lipoprotein. Particles of Sf 200–400 form remnants within the Sf 20–100 VLDL density interval and, in so doing, become intermingled with newly secreted small VLDL destined for LDL. Therefore small VLDL consists of at least two intrinsically different populations – newly secreted particles and remnants generated by the action of lipoprotein lipase. Activation of the enzyme by drugs like bezafibrate reduces plasma triglyceride levels by increasing the rate of catabolism of large VLDL [2, 12]. The clearance rate of small VLDL is not materially changed by therapy.

Regulation Point 3: Catabolism of VLDL Remnants

We have seen how the processing of large triglyceride-rich particles is primarily under the control of lipoprotein lipase while small VLDL are less affected by the enzyme. Several lines of evidence suggest that membrane receptors may be more involved in the metabolism of the latter. In order to examine this possibility we followed the fate of VLDL after it had been treated with 1,2-cyclohexanedione to block its putative receptor interaction [4]. Briefly, large VLDL of Sf 100-400 was isolated from the plasma of normal and hypertriglyceridaemic subjects and divided into two aliquots which were labelled separately with ^{125}I and ^{131}I. The latter was then exposed to 1,2-cyclohexanedione to block the arginyl residues on its protein moiety as described previously for LDL. The flow of B protein in both tracers, followed from VLDL through IDL to LDL, is illustrated in Fig. 2. Modification of the VLDL had little effect on the rate of transit of the protein from large VLDL into remnants of Sf 12-100, consistent with the premise that lipoprotein lipase governs this process. At this point, however, the clearance rates of the two tracers became divergent, chemical modification retarding catabolism. As we had found previously, B protein-containing particles derived from large VLDL were virtually eliminated from the plasma at this stage. Whatever was converted to LDL appeared in and decayed from that fraction more slowly following cyclohexanedione treatment.

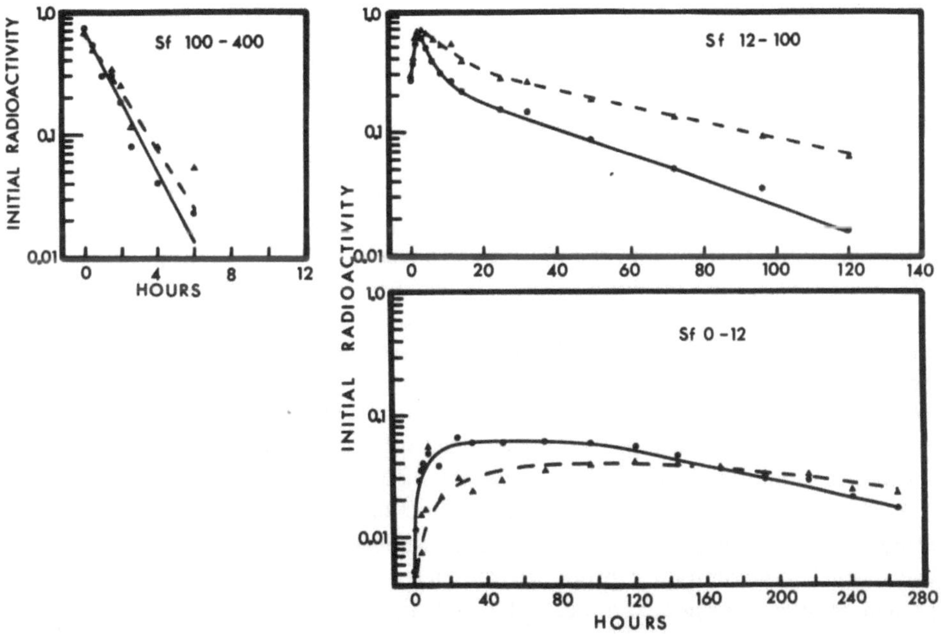

Fig. 2. Role of receptors in apo B metabolism. Autologous ^{125}I-native and ^{131}I-cyclohexanedione-treated Sf 100-400 VLDL were injected into a normal subject and the flow of apolipoprotein B radioactivity was followed from this fraction through Sf 12-100 lipoproteins to LDL of Sf 0-12. Native lipoprotein: ●, observed; — calculated. CHD-treated lipoprotein: ▲, observed; --- calculated

These data are consistent with the view that the metabolism of VLDL takes place in at least two distinct stages - lipolysis of newly secreted VLDL particles to form remnants followed, possibly, by receptor-mediated processing of the latter. The kinetic properties of VLDL as a whole therefore depend on the interplay between these two activities.

Regulation Point 4: The Involvement of Receptors in IDL-LDL Conversion

The sequence of events responsible for the conversion of IDL to LDL is not clearly defined. Obviously, lipase may be involved, since lipid hydrolysis is integral to the phenomenon. But, as noted above, lipoprotein receptors also apparently play a part. Support for this idea has come from a study of VLDL-IDL-LDL conversion in homozygous FH subjects [13] (Packard et al., unpublished observations). Some of these individuals take as long as 9 days to generate LDL from IDL instead of the usual 12-24 h seen in normal subjects. By inference we must therefore implicate the LDL receptor in the processing of apo B from IDL to LDL. This would be a novel role for the receptor since classically it has been envisaged purely as a unidirectional pathway responsible for the degradative assimilation of lipoprotein particles by cells. If it does facilitate the remodelling of IDL to LDL one would have to postulate a mechanism whereby it operates reversibly to bind and release lipoproteins without initiating their destruction. It is conceivable that it is responsible for binding the lipoprotein at a site immediately adjacent to the lipolytic enzyme found on hepatocyte membranes.

Regulation Point 5: Receptor-Mediated and Receptor-Independent LDL Catabolism

In man approximately one-half of LDL catabolism occurs by a receptor-mediated process. The activity of the receptor varies in response to genetic factors, diet, hormones and drug therapy and the mechanisms whereby these stimuli produce their effects are now quite well-understood. Less clear however, are the events responsible for the remaining 50% of LDL catabolism. They form the focus of ongoing research since they appear to be intimately involved in atherogenesis. Their activity can be gauged by following the rate of plasma clearance of cyclohexanedione-treated, receptor-blocked LDL. Metabolic studies from the laboratory of Ginsberg et al. [14] would implicate the monocyte-macrophage system in this process. They showed that patients with myeloproliferative disorders exhibit hypercatabolism of LDL due to activation of pathways which function independently of the receptor. Drug-induced remission from the diseases resulted in suppression of these pathways which concomitantly produced an increment in plasma LDL. It is well-known, to quote another example, that grossly hypertriglyceridaemic subjects overcatabolise LDL. We have shown that this again derives from hyperactivity of the receptor-independent mechanism [15]. Reduction of plasma triglyceride levels in such patients redirects LDL into the receptor pathway, thereby arguably reducing the atherogenic potential of the hypertriglyceridaemic state in these patients. The change in plasma LDL which follows triglyceride-lowering drug therapy is known to be dependent on the recipient's initial LDL level which, as we have seen above, is partly governed by the patient's triglyceride status. Thus, it is not particularly surprising that compounds which lower plasma LDL in normotriglyceridaemic hypercholesterolaemic patients commonly raise this fraction in their hypertriglyceridaemic normocholesterolaemic counterparts.

References

1. Mahley RW, Innerarity TL, Brown M, Ho YK, Goldstein JL (1980) Cholesteryl ester synthesis in macrophages: stimulation by βVLDL from cholesterol fed animals of several species. J Lipid Res 21: 970-980
2. Shepherd J, Packard CJ, Stewart JM, Atmeh RF, Clark RS, Boag DE, Carr K, et al. (1984) Apolipoprotein A and B (Sf 100-400) metabolism during bezafibrate therapy in hypertriglyceridaemic subjects. J Clin Invest 74: 2164-2177
3. Packard CJ, Munro A, Lorimer AR, Gotto AM, Shepherd J (1984) Metabolism of apolipoprotein B in large triglyceride-rich VLDL of normal and hypertriglyceridaemic subjects. J Clin Invest 74: 2178-2192
4. Packard CJ, Boag DE, Clegg RJ, Bedford DK, Shepherd J (1985) The effects of 1,2 cyclohexanedione modification on the metabolism of very low density lipoprotein apoprotein B: potential role of receptors in intermediate density lipoprotein catabolism. J Lipid Res 26: 1058-1065
5. Packard CJ, Shepherd J (1986) Cholesterol 7α-hydroxylase: involvement in hepatobiliary axis and regulation of plasma lipoprotein levels. In: Fears R, Sabine JR (eds) Cholesterol 7α-hydroxylase. CRC Press, Boca Raton, pp 147-165
6. Goldstein JL, Brown MS (1978) Familial hypercholesterolemia: pathogenesis of a receptor disease. Johns Hopkins Med J 143: 8-16
7. Brown MS, Goldstein JL, Fredrickson DS (1983) Familial type 3 hyperlipoproteinemia. In: Stanbury JB, Wyngaarden JB, Fredrickson DS, Goldstein JL, Brown MS (eds) The metabolic basis of inherited disease. McGraw-Hill, New York, pp 655-671
8. Berman M, Hall M, Levy RI, Eisenberg S, Bilheimer DW, Phair RD, Goebel RH (1978) Metabolism of apo B and apo C lipoproteins in man: kinetic studies in normal and hyperlipoproteinemic subjects. J Lipid Res 19: 38-56
9. Fisher WR, Zech LA, Bardalaye P, Warmke G, Berman M (1980) The metabolism of apolipoprotein B in subjects with hypertriglyceridemia and polydisperse LDL. J Lipid Res 21: 760-774
10. Fisher WR (1982) Apolipoprotein B kinetics in man: concepts and questions. In: Berman M, Grundy SM, Howard BV (eds) Lipoprotein kinetics and modeling. Academic, New York, pp 43-68
11. Reardon MF, Fidge NH, Nestel PJ (1978) Catabolism of very low density lipoprotein in man. J Clin Invest 61: 850-860
12. Packard CJ, Clegg RJ, Dominiczak MH, Lorimer AR, Shepherd J (1986) Effects of bezafibrate on apolipoprotein B metabolism in type III hyperlipoproteinemic subjects. J Lipid Res (in press)
13. Soutar AK, Myant NB, Thompson GR (1982) Metabolism of very low density and intermediate density lipoproteins in patients with familial hypercholesterolaemia. Atherosclerosis 43: 217-231
14. Ginsberg H, Goldberg IJ, Wang-Iverson P, Gitler E, Lee NA, Gilbert HS, Brown WV (1983) Increased catabolism of native and cyclohexanedione modified LDL in subjects with myeloproliferative diseases. Arteriosclerosis 3: 233-241
15. Shepherd J, Caslake MJ, Lorimer AR, Vallance BD, Packard CJ (1984) Fenofibrate reduces LDL catabolism in hypertriglyceridemic subjects. Arteriosclerosis 5: 162-168

Fish Eye Disease: Implications for the Understanding of Cardiovascular Disease and Plasma Lipoprotein Metabolism

L. A. Carlson and L. Holmquist

A New Familial Disease - Fish Eye Disease

In 1975 a 61-year-old women was referred to one of us (L. A. C.) because of hypertriglyceridemia. The note of referral came from the Dermatology department and indicated that she had suffered from mild acrodermatitis atroficans Herxheimer, which condition had healed with penicillin treatment.

At the very moment when the patient entered through the door in the outpatient department one was, at a distance of 5 meters, struck by the extremely unusual appearance of her eyes. Interest in the patient grew rapidly when she said that her father as well as two of her sisters had the same eye condition. Apparently this was a unique familial eye disease! The patient told that in the small village in northern Sweden where the family lived, the villagers, with an unbeatable combination of good observation and popular humor, called them *"the family with fish eyes."* And indeed, the eyes of all three patients that we have seen have had a very close resemblance to those of boiled fish. Hence the syndrome with the characteristic corneal opacities and the unique dyslipoproteinemia (vide infra) was called "fish eye disease" [1, 2]. The initial patient will be referred to as FED 1.

One of the sisters of FED 1 was investigated in 1976, at the age of 77 years. She had identical corneal opacities and dyslipoproteinemia to FED 1, which proved the familial nature of fish eye disease.

In 1978 there was then a most unusual and fortunate *lex duplex*. A patient visited the outpatient department at the eye clinic of the Karolinska hospital because of visual impairment. Dr. Bo Philipsson, to whom we had referred FED 1, made a tentative diagnosis of fish eye disease and so referred a third patient with that condition, FED 2, to us [3]. The families of FED 1 and FED 2 have been traced back to the 17th century and there is no evidence for consanguinity between them.

Dyslipoproteinemia

The dyslipoproteinemia of fish eye disease affects all three major plasma lipoproteins and its features are summarized in Table 1. The concentrations of cholesterol and triglycerides in the very low-density lipoprotein (VLDL) fraction are moderately elevated. In the low-density lipoprotein (LDL) class there is a high but normal concentration of cholesterol. However, these LDLs are abnormally enriched with triglycerides. The most marked divergences from the normal lipoprotein pattern are present in the high-density lipoprotein (HDL) class. The plasma concentration of

Table 1. Basic characteristics of the dyslipoproteinemia of fish eye disease: concentration of serum lipids and of serum lipoprotein constituents

Serum cholesterol	Serum triglyceride	VLDL	LDL	HDL
Normal	Moderately elevated	Moderate elevation of cholesterol and triglycerides	Normal cholesterol, elevated triglycerides	Cholesterol and apolipoproteins reduced by 90%
		Normal molar ratio of cholesterol to triglycerides	Normal electrophoretic mobility	Normal electrophoretic mobility
		Normal electrophoretic mobility		Abnormally small particle size

this density class is reduced by 90%. In addition, the HDL particles are abnormally small [2].

Clinical Features

The only characteristic clinical symptoms of fish eye disease are the pronounced corneal opacities. These bilaterally symmetric opacities seem to be visible to others in the teens but do not cause visual impairment until middle age, whereafter the vision gradually deteriorates to a state which makes corneal transplantation necessary. In our two patients, FED 1 and FED 2, corneal transplantation was performed at the ages of 64 and 73 years respectively. Now, 8 and 5 years later respectively, the transplants are clear and the vision of both patients is substantially improved.

Lipid Risk Factors and Premature Atherosclerosis

In the first family where the father and three of his daughters had the eye disease there is no history of *premature* atherosclerotic vascular disease. The father, whose serum lipid levels were never investigated, died suddenly at age 76 from a "heart attack." One of the sisters who was healthy died at age 37 from an accident. The oldest afflicted sister that had the same dyslipoproteinemia as FED 1 [2] suffered from a myocardial infarction when 77 years old. She died suddenly 1 year later. No autopsy was performed. When first seen in 1975–1976, FED 1, then 63 years old, had no symptoms of atherosclerotic vascular disease. However, her ECG during and after an exercise load, which was normal in 1976, showed ST-segment depressions in 1977 that were compatible with coronary insufficiency. At that time her blood pressure, earlier around 150/85 mmHg, varied between 190/120 and 180/100 mmHg, and treatment with saluretics was started. Since 1980 she has had a permanent left bundle branch block. A mild effort-angina, responding well to long-acting nitrates, started at age 70. FED 1, who is a widow without children, lives on her own and takes good care of herself.

FED 2 when first seen in 1978 appeared clinically hypothyroid and had an elevated serum concentration of thyroid-stimulating hormone (TSH). Substitution with thyroxin slightly lowered the cholesterol concentration of the serum as well as of LDL, but had no effect on the low levels of HDL [2]. In 1983 a third-degree atrioventricular block necessitated implantation of a pacemaker. In 1984 a type II diabetes was diagnosed and treatment with glibenclamid was started.

It is evident that fish eye disease is not associated with premature atherosclerosis in spite of the dramatically reduced levels of plasma HDL cholesterol. Decreasing levels of HDL cholesterol in plasma have been shown to be strongly associated with increased risk of myocardial infarction. In the Framingham study the risk of women to suffer from a myocardial infarction increased 10-fold when the concentration of HDL cholesterol decreased from 1.8 to 0.8 mmol/l [4]. However, the extremely low HDL cholesterol levels in fish eye disease (0.1-0.2 mmol/l) have evidently not been associated with an increased risk of myocardial infarction in our few patients. Furthermore, the patients are hypertriglyceridemic, which according to the Stockholm Prospective Study is a risk factor in females for myocardial infarction [5]. Also, various "atherogenic indices" calculated on different lipoprotein constituents are very high in fish eye disease. As an example, the ratio of the concentration of LDL cholesterol to that of HDL is around 20 in our patients, compared with a normal value of around 2.

The lack of increased risk of atherosclerosis in fish eye disease, in spite of the very low plasma levels of HDL, is intriguing. This issue becomes even more intriguing when we consider the pattern of HDL subfractions. There is considerable evidence that the risk of myocardial infarction relates principally to changes in HDL_2 rather than total HDL (for review, see [6]). By ultracentrifugation at a density of 1.125 kg/l we have demonstrated that the majority of HDL in fish eye disease belongs to the HDL_3 fraction. The amount of HDL_2 cholesterol in plasma from FED 1 and FED 2 corresponded to 1% and 4%, respectively, of that in plasma from normal females [2]. After polyacrylamide gradient gel electrophoresis of the lipoproteins from plasma of the patients with fish eye disease, no particles were visible in the region to which HDL_2 usually migrates. The virtually complete absence of HDL_2 in fish eye disease and the lack of premature atherosclerosis are difficult to reconcile with the hypothesis that HDL_2 plays an important role in protection against atherosclerosis. However, it is possible that the abnormally small HDL particles associated with fish eye disease may be protective against atherosclerosis. In this connection it should be stressed that the net sterol balance and the biliary lipid composition seem normal in FED 1 [7]. This indicates that the liver is provided with adequate amounts of cholesterol as substrate for bile acid production.

Tangier disease is another familial disease with very low levels of HDL [8], and in this condition also there appears to be no strikingly increased risk of atherosclerosis [9]. However, Tangier disease differs inter alia from fish eye disease in that plasma levels of LDL are low and those of VLDL are normal.

Lecithin-Cholesterol Acyl Transferase

At the first visit of FED 1 the immediate supposition was that we might be dealing with a case of deficiency of lecithin-cholesterol acyl transferase (LCAT), the disease described by Norum and Gjone in 1967 [10], but neither the detailed clinical picture

Table 2. Main findings indicating normal LCAT activity in fish eye disease (approximate values)

	Fish eye disease	LCAT deficiency	Normal
Percentage of esterified plasma cholesterol	60	10	65
Plasma cholesterol esterification rate (% of normal)	100	0–10	100
Percentage of linoleic acid in plasma cholesteryl esters	60	10	60

nor the biochemical analyses could confirm that. Our main findings that ruled out LCAT deficiency in fish eye disease are listed in Table 2. The search for the basic metabolic defect in this condition then went along other, "non-LCAT"-related lines.

Plasma Lipid Metabolising Activities

Early studies of fish eye disease indicated that the post-heparin activities in plasma of lipoprotein lipase and hepatic lipase were normal. These findings are well in accordance with the characteristic differences between the dyslipoproteinemias that are due to lack of these lipases and the one present in fish eye disease. The hallmark of the lipidemia caused by lack of lipoprotein lipase is the accumulation of huge amounts of chylomicrons in plasma, and this is not a feature of fish eye disease.

One very significant difference between fish eye disease and lack of hepatic lipase concerns HDL. A 90% reduction of plasma HDL cholesterol in fish eye disease sharply contrasts with the normal HDL cholesterol level in hepatic lipase deficiency [11, 12]. Furthermore, as demonstrated by gradient gel electrophoresis the particle size of the HDL is abnormally small in fish eye disease, but is extremely large in deficiency of hepatic lipase [12].

Lipid transfer protein activities assayed in lipoprotein-depleted plasma from the patients with fish eye disease [13], as well as net lipid transfer between lipoproteins in the same plasmas supplemented with normal HDL (L. Holmquist and L. A. Carlson, unpublished manuscript), were normal. Apparently there is no deficiency of known cholesteryl ester transfer or lipid transfer activities in fish eye disease.

Apolipoproteins

No qualitative abnormalities of the HDL apolipoproteins from patients with fish eye disease were revealed upon polyacrylamide disc gel electrophoresis or isoelectric focusing [14]. Furthermore, high-resolution two-dimensional electrophoresis also showed an apparently qualitatively normal apolipoprotein A-I (apo A-I) isoform pattern in this condition [15]. The apo A-I pattern in fish eye disease is quite different from that in other dyslipoproteinemias with low HDL levels, such as apo A-I_{Milano} [16, 17], apo A-$I_{Giessen}$ [16], apo A-$I_{Marburg}$ [16, 17], and Tangier disease [18].

Composition of HDL

A detailed compositional analysis of isolated HDL from plasma of the patients with fish eye disease revealed one striking abnormality [14]. The relative amount of cholesterol that was esterified was very low, only 20% against the normal 80%. Apparently, the relative amounts of cholesteryl esters are normal in VLDL and LDL, but abnormally low in HDL. This unexpected finding forced us to reconsider the possibility of some kind of hitherto unknown abnormality of LCAT activity in fish eye disease, in spite of the earlier findings (Table 1) which indicated normal LCAT activity.

α- and β-LCAT Activities

The current concept of the action of LCAT holds that the enzyme primarily acts on the free cholesterol of a subfraction of HDL (for reviews see [19, 20]). It was impossible to reconcile this view with the biochemical findings in fish eye disease. To explain the lack of esterification of HDL cholesterol but normal esterification of VLDL and LDL cholesterol in fish eye disease we hypothesized that *there exist in normal plasma two LCAT activities, one - α-LCAT activity - esterifying the free cholesterol of HDL and the other - β-LCAT activity - esterifying that of combined VLDL and LDL.* The normal relative cholesteryl ester content of VLDL and LDL but abnormally low such content of HDL might then be due to the presence of a functioning β-LCAT and the existence of a specific lack of α-LCAT in fish eye disease.

The incubation experiments performed to test the above hypothesis unambiguously showed that plasma from the patients with fish eye disease indeed lacks the ability, present in normal plasma, to esterify the free cholesterol of normal as well as fish eye disease HDL [21]. Furthermore, the free cholesterol of HDL from fish eye disease was rapidly esterified by normal plasma [21]. At the same time the small particle size of the HDL was normalized. Fish eye disease is accordingly the first condition with a demonstrated deficiency of α-LCAT activity. Pig plasma, which lacks lipid transfer protein activities, also readily esterifies the cholesterol of fish eye disease HDL and simultaneously enlarges these HDL particles into a normal range [22], further indicating that modification of lipid transfer proteins is not an explanation of the abnormal HDL in fish eye disease.

After the demonstration of the specific lack in plasma from patients with fish eye disease of the ability to esterify the free cholesterol of both autologous and homologous HDL (α-LCAT deficiency), it was felt important to verify the presence of β-LCAT activity in human plasma. When plasmas depleted of HDL, both from normal subjects and from patients with fish eye disease, were incubated in vitro there was a rapid esterification of the free cholesterol of combined VLDL and LDL [23]. Hence, there is β-LCAT activity in normal human plasma as well as in the plasma of patients with fish eye disease.

Lessons from Fish Eye Disease

What may we learn from these studies of the very rare fish eye disease? Clinically these patients have shown us that it is not universally true that a very low level of HDL cholesterol, in particular of HDL_2 cholesterol, is a factor increasing the risk of atherosclerotic vascular disease. Furthermore, a new deficiency of a plasma cholesterol esterifying activity has been discovered in the plasma of these patients; this seems to give new clues to a more complete understanding of the complex "metabolic plasma cholesterol-cholesteryl ester axis." Both the clinical and biochemical lessons will hopefully stimulate new tests of the current clinical and biochemical hypotheses, thereby expanding the horizons of atherosclerosis research.

Acknowledgement. Supported by grants from the Swedish Medical Research Council 19X-204 and Nordisk Insulinfond.

References

1. Carlson LA, Philipson B (1979) Fish-eye disease, a new familial condition with massive corneal opacities and dyslipoproteinaemia. Lancet II: 921-3
2. Carlson LA (1982) Fish eye disease: a new familial condition with massive corneal opacities and dyslipoproteinaemia. Eur J Clin Invest 12: 41-53
3. Carlson LA (1979) A further case of fish-eye disease. Letter to the Editor. Lancet II: 1376-7
4. Gordon T, Castelli WP, Hjortland MC, Kannel WB, Dawber TR (1977) High density lipoprotein as a protective factor against coronary heart disease. The Framingham study. Am J Med 62: 707-14
5. Carlson LA, Böttiger LE (1985) Risk factors for ischaemic heart disease in men and women. Results of the 19-year follow-up of the Stockholm prospective study. Acta Med Scand 218: 207-11
6. Gidez LI, Eder HA (1984) The clinical significance of plasma high-density lipoproteins. In: Miller NE, Miller GJ (eds) Clinical and metabolic aspects of high-density lipoproteins. Elsevier, Amsterdam, pp 415-450
7. Angelin B, Carlson LA (1986) Bile acids and plasma high density lipoproteins: biliary lipid metabolism in fish eye disease. Eur J Clin Invest 16: 157-62
8. Herbert PN, Gotto AM, Fredrickson DS (1978) Familial lipoprotein deficiency. In: Stanbury JB, Wyngarden JB, Fredrickson DS (eds) The metabolic basis of inherited disease, 4th edn. McGraw-Hill, New York, p 544
9. Schaefer EJ, Zech LA, Schwartz DE, Brewer HB (1980) Coronary heart disease prevalence and other clinical features in familial high-density lipoprotein deficiency (Tangier disease). Ann Intern Med 93: 261-6
10. Norum KR, Gjone E (1967) Familial plasma lecithin: cholesterol acyltransferase deficiency. Biochemical study of a new inborn error of metabolism. Scand J Clin Lab Invest 20: 231-7
11. Breckenridge WC, Little JA, Alaupovic P et al. (1982) Lipoprotein abnormalities associated with a familial deficiency of hepatic lipase. Atherosclerosis 45: 161-79
12. Carlson LA, Holmquist L, Nilsson-Ehle P (1986) Deficiency of hepatic lipase activity in post-heparin plasma in familial hyper-α-triglyceridemia. Acta Med Scand 219: 435-47
13. Calvert GD, Carlson LA (1983) Plasma lipid transfer in fish-eye disease. Acta Med Scand 213: 253-4
14. Carlson LA, Holmquist L (1983) Studies on high density lipoproteins in fish eye disease. Acta Med Scand 213: 177-82
15. Marshall T, Williams KM, Holmquist L, Carlson LA, Vesterberg O (1985) Plasma apolipoprotein pattern in fish-eye disease examined by high-resolution two-dimensional electrophoresis. Clin Chem 31: 2032-5

16. Uterman G, Feussner G, Franceschini G et al. (1982) Genetic variants of Group A apolipoproteins. Rapid methods for screening and characterisation without ultracentrifugation. J Biol Chem 257: 501-7
17. Menzel HJ, Kladetzky RG, Assmann G (1982) One-step screening method for the polymorphism of apolipoproteins A-I, A-II, and A-IV. J Lipid Res 23: 915-22
18. Sprecher DL, Taam L, Brewer HB (1984) Two-dimensional electrophoresis of human plasma apolipoproteins. Clin Chem 30: 2084-92
19. Norum KR, Berg T, Helgerud P, Drevon CA (1983) Transport of cholesterol. Physiol Rev 63: 1343-419
20. Marcel YL (1982) Lecithin: cholesterol acyltransferase and intravascular cholesterol transport. Adv Lipid Res 19: 85-136
21. Carlson LA, Holmquist L (1985) Evidence for deficiency of high density lipoprotein lecithin: cholesterol acyltransferase activity (α-LCAT) in fish eye disease. Acta Med Scand 218: 189-96
22. Holmquist L, Carlson LA (1986) In vitro normalization of cholesteryl ester content and particle size of fish eye disease high density lipoproteins. Acta Med Scand (in press)
23. Carlson LA, Holmquist L (1985) Evidence for the presence in human plasma of lecithin: cholesterol acyltransferase activity (β-LCAT) specifically esterifying free cholesterol of combined pre-β- and β-lipoproteins. Acta Med Scand 218: 197-205

Diabetes

Vascular Growth Factors and Atherogenesis in Diabetes Mellitus

T. Koschinsky and F. A. Gries

Severe and premature atherosclerosis often occurs in type 1 as well as in type 2 diabetic patients. The diabetes-specific reasons for this are still poorly understood [1]. Within the various pathomechanisms that are involved in the development of macrovascular disease, alterations in the growth of arterial wall cells have received increased attention, and abnormally increased growth of vacular cells is well-established as an intrinsic part of atherogenesis [2]. This paper will focus on the potential relevance of vascular growth stimulating factors that could initiate or accelerate growth of human arterial wall cells, in relation to atherogenesis in diabetes mellitus.

In this regard, it has to be kept in mind that in vivo cell growth is usually regulated by the combined effects of various growth-stimulating and -inhibiting factors. Therefore, increased vascular cell growth in diabetes could be due to an increase of the stimulator(s) and/or to a decrease of the inhibitor(s). But until now, factors inhibiting growth of vascular cells have not been studied in relation to diabetes mellitus. In addition, vascular growth factors have been distinguished from nutrients and other factors essential for cell survival which will not be considered in this paper.

In type 1 and type 2 diabetes, the atherosclerotic lesions are morphologically very similar to those of nondiabetic origin. Atherosclerosis is mainly a disease of the arterial intima, where smooth muscle cells accumulate due to migration and proliferation. Vascular growth factors have been implicated in the selection process for a specific functional state or clone of smooth muscle cells, in this way initiating and facilitating migration and excessive proliferation [2–6]. Another target of vascular growth factors are the endothelial cells. In diabetic animals, early functional and morphological changes have been noted which could lead to an increased replicative turnover of endothelial cells [7] and to an increased availability of vascular growth factors to smooth muscle cells [8]. Diabetic serum from different species has been observed to stimulate increased growth of cultured fibroblasts, arterial smooth muscle and endothelial cells [9–11]. Therefore, research focused on the nature of the growth factors involved in diabetes and on their target cells in the vascular wall because the requirements for growth factors differ considerably between arterial smooth muscle and endothelial cells and some growth factors are effective exclusively in one or the other cell type.

Vascular growth factors for the arterial wall which are potentially relevant in diabetes can be related to three different groups: hormones, locally released growth factors of platelet origin, and of arterial wall cell origin (Tables 1 and 2). Growth hormone levels can increase in the plasma of both type 1 and 2 diabetics for different reasons and at different times during the day and night. There is considerable evidence implicating growth hormone in the development of diabetic microangiopathy [12]. In vitro studies have demonstrated a dose-dependent stimulation of DNA replication of arterial smooth muscle cells [13]. Therefore, increased growth hormone plasma levels might contribute to atherogenesis in diabetes, but its actual relevance still remains to be determined.

The growth hormone action has been related to the action of insulin-like growth factor (IGF) I and II. Increased plasma concentration has been described only for IGF I in selected diabetic patients with severe proliferative retinopathy [14]. Specific receptors for IGF I and II have been described in all vascular cells and IGF I and II stimulate DNA replication of endothelial and arterial smooth muscle cells and fibroblasts in vitro [15-18]. If combined with insulin, the growth effect of IGF I and II on arterial smooth muscle cells is additive [1] and regional differences in their growth effect have been observed [19]. However, the relevance of IGF I and II for the atherosclerotic development in diabetes is still unproven and requires further studies.

Hyperinsulinemia of various degrees is common in non-insulin-dependent type 2 diabetics and also occurs in insulin-treated type 2 and 1 diabetics (dosage higher than physiological need, unphysiological route of application into the peripheral circulation with continuous absorption unrelated to blood glucose concentration). There is considerable epidemiological evidence linking increased insulin levels to atherogenesis, mainly of the coronary arteries, in nondiabetic subjects (reviewed in [20]). More recently, a similar link has also been demonstrated prospectively in type 2 diabetics [21, 22]. For type 1 diabetics, such data are missing. However, insulin may also play a role in promoting other atherogenic conditions like dyslipoproteinemia.

Besides many other effects on cellular metabolism of various kinds, insulin stimulates in vitro growth of human arterial smooth muscle cells [23, 24] but not of arterial endothelial cells [18, 25]. In vitro, insulin increases growth of mesenchymal cells even further by interaction, for example, with IGF I and II and their specific receptors, platelet-derived growth factor (PDGF), fibroblasts, and epidermal growth factor (reviewed in [26]). But the relative contribution of the insulin growth effect on arterial smooth muscle cells during atherogenesis in human diabetes still remains an unresolved question.

The role of platelets as a source of growth factors for vascular cells has received widespread attention since the identification of the PDGF [27-29]. The various growth factors of platelet origin are summarized in Table 1. These growth factors are all peptides or proteins with a wide range of molecular weights. Their target cells are either endothelial cells or arterial smooth muscle cells and fibroblasts.

The best characterized growth factor of platelet origin is the PDGF (reviewed in [30]). Since PDGF is a competence factor, its overall effect on growth depends on its interaction with other factors also contained in platelets, such as endothelial growth factor (ENDO-GF) [31], transforming growth factor-β (TGF-β) [32, 33], vascular endothelial cell proliferation factor (VEPF) [34], fibroblast growth factor (FGF) [35, 36], epidermal growth factor (EGF) [37], platelet-derived endothelial cell mitogen (PDECM) [38], and the diabetic serum growth factor (DSGF) [24, 39-42]. There are also interactions between all of the growth factors of platelet origin and in addition with insulin and IGF that lead to increased in vitro growth of the target cells. But

Table 1. Vascular growth factors in diabetes mellitus

Growth factor	M_r	Target cell[a]			References
		ASMC	EC	F	
A. Hormones					
Growth hormone	21500	+	−	+	[9, 13]
IGF I	7650	+	+	+	[15–18]
IGF II	7471				[18, 20]
Insulin	6000	+	+	+	[23–26]
B. Growth factors of human platelet origin					
ENDO-GF	65000	−	+	−	[31]
PDGF	30000	+	−	+	[27–30]
TGF-β	25000	?	?	+	[32, 33]
VEPF	20000	?	+	−	[34]
FGF	16000	+	+	+	[35, 36]
EGF	6000	+	−	+	[37]
DSGF	<2000	+	?	+	[24, 39–42]
PDECM	700	−	+	−	[38]

[a] ASMC, arterial smooth muscle cell; EC, endothelial cell; F, fibroblast.

despite the fact that these factors have been studied extensively, their relevance for the atherosclerotic development in type 1 and 2 diabetics is based mainly on circumstantial evidence. As their serum or plasma concentration in the general circulation, with the exception of DSGF [24], have not been shown to be increased in diabetes, greater local availability at sites of stimulated platelet aggregation has been postulated. Platelet abnormalities, including increased aggregation and adhesion, are often found in diabetics [43, 44].

Platelets from type 1 diabetics, poorly controlled on conventional insulin therapy, released in vitro increased growth stimulating activity for arterial smooth muscle cells which returned to normal control levels after 2 months of insulin pump treatment [45]. The nature of this (these) factor(s) remained open. Platelets from poorly controlled non-insulin-dependent diabetics released in vitro increased amounts of DSGF compared to platelets from healthy subjects (Fig. 1). This is in agreement with our observation that in poorly controlled type 2 diabetics the DSGF is two to four times higher than in healthy subjects and normalized after 3–4 weeks of good metabolic control in the same diabetic patient [40].

Originally, the DSGF was observed to be increased in diabetic serum [24]. The DSGF level in plasma is only about half of that in serum from the same type 2 diabetic patient ($p < 0.01$), but still, on average, about three times higher than in normal plasma (Fig. 2). In type 2 diabetic serum, the DSGF represents about one-third of the total growth-stimulating activity and its growth potency in vitro is two to ten times higher than that of human growth hormone or insulin, added in amounts equivalent to physiological concentrations [24]. Therefore, the DSGF is a very potent growth stimulator of human vascular cells and is the first growth peptide of platelet origin that has been shown to increase in vivo in type 2 diabetes and to be regulated by the metabolic control.

In recent years, it has become evident that arterial endothelial and smooth muscle cells, fibroblasts, and monocyte/macrophages, at least in culture, release locally a

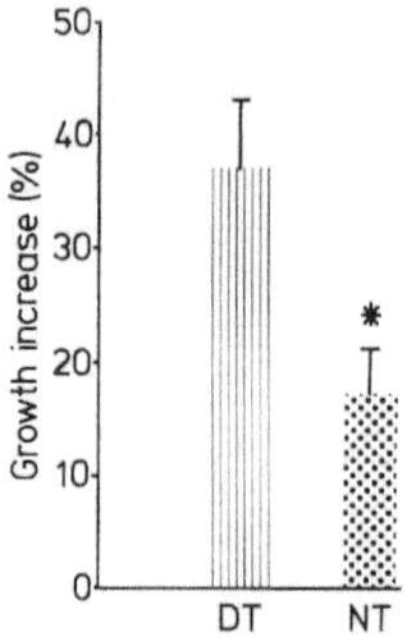

Fig. 1. Growth effect of the dialyzate fraction (mol.wt. cut off - 3500 daltons) from platelet-release products on human arterial smooth muscle cells and fibroblasts. A total of 2×10^9 platelets/per patient were isolated from plasma of three non-insulin-dependent diabetics with poor metabolic control and from three healthy subjects. The cells were grown until confluency in DMEM + 5% dialyzed diabetic serum [24] + the dialyzable platelet-release products derived from the diabetic *(DT)* and healthy subjects *(NT)*. The cell number per plate on day 5, achieved with dialyzed serum only, is set at 0% and compared to the additional growth effect of the dialyzable platelet factor(s) ($n = 3$; mean ± SD; $*p < 0.05$)

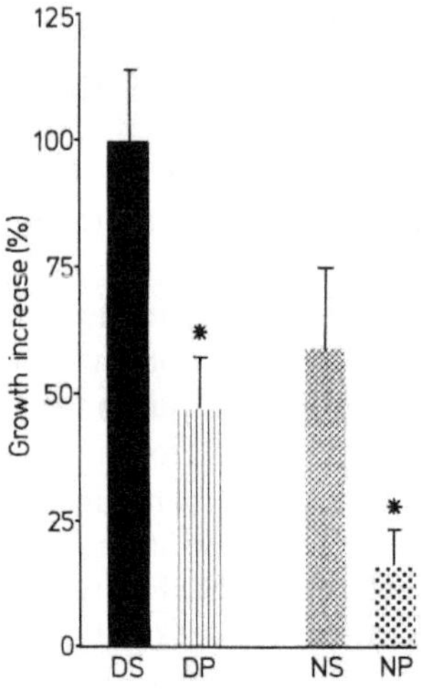

Fig. 2. Growth effect of diabetic serum growth factor [24] derived from pooled serum *(DS)* (six batches) and pooled plasma *(DP)* collected in parallel (six batches) from the same non-insulin-dependent diabetic patients with poor metabolic control on human fibroblasts and from three batches of pooled serum *(NS)* and plasma *(NP)* from healthy subjects on human arterial smooth muscle cells. The cells were grown in DMEM + 5% dialyzed diabetic or normal serum [24] + DSGF derived from equivalent amounts of the respective serum or plasma until confluency. The cell number per plate on day 5, achieved with dialyzed serum only, is set at 0% and compared to the additional growth effect of the DSGF in parallel plates (mean ± SD; $*p < 0.05$ serum vs. plasma)

Table 2. Growth factors released from vascular cells

Cell type	Growth factor	M_r	Target cells[a]			References
			ASMC	EC	F	
Endothelial cell						
EC-derived	growth factor (ECDGF)	?	+	–	+	[47, 48]
PDGF-like	growth factor	?	+	–	+	[46]
FGF-like	growth factor	?	+	+	+	[36]
Smooth muscle cell						
Smooth muscle cell-derived growth factors		?	+	–	+	[50]
PDGF-like	growth factor	?	+	–	+	[46]
IGF I-like	growth factor	?	+	?	?	[51, 52]
Fibroblast						
Fibroblast-derived growth factors		?	+	–	+	[50, 53, 54]
IGF I-like	growth factor	20500	+	?	+	[52]
Monocyte/macrophage						
Monocyte/macrophage-derived growth factors		?	+	–	+	[55, 56]
PDGF-like	growth factor	?	+	–	+	[58]
Interleukin 1		15000	–	–	+	[57]
FGF-like	growth factor	?	+	+	+	[36]
TGF-β-like	growth factor	?	?	?	+	[35]

[a] ASMC, arterial smooth muscle cell; EC, endothelial cell; F, fibroblast.

variety of growth peptides (Table 2) that could participate in an autocrine or paracrine manner in the growth regulation of the arterial wall.

Endothelial cells derived from different species and vascular regions have been shown to release PDGF-like [46], FGF-like [36], and other growth factors [47, 48] that can influence the phenotypic expression of the arterial smooth muscle cells [49] and stimulate their proliferation. Smooth muscle cells also release under various in vitro conditions at least three to four so far unidentified growth factors [50], IGF-like [51, 52] and PDGF-like growth peptides [46]. Different fibroblast-derived growth factors [50, 53, 54] for endothelial as well as arterial smooth muscle cells and also an IGF-like growth factor [52] have been described. Numerous monocyte/macrophage-derived growth factors [55, 56] including interleukin 1 [57], PDGF-like [58], FGF-like [36], and TGF-β-like [35] growth peptides have been demonstrated. Despite this growing knowledge on in vitro effects, the relevance of all these locally released factors for the growth regulation of the arterial wall in vivo is still unknown.

There is evidence in diabetics and in experimental animals with diabetes that endothelial damage or dysfunction occurs in states of poor metabolic control. These endothelial changes could alter the synthesis and release of growth factors. Circulating monocytes in type 1 diabetics with poor metabolic control have been shown to be activated [59]. The monocyte-derived macrophage can enter the arterial wall at sites of increased endothelial permeability and release some or all of the described growth factors. However, direct evidence that one or more of these alterations contribute to the acceleration of atherosclerosis in diabetic patients is still lacking.

In conclusion, there es evidence that in type 1 and type 2 diabetes, disease-related changes of vascular growth factor levels might be involved in the development of premature atherosclerosis. But their relative contribution to the proliferative response of the arterial wall cells may differ between diabetic subpopulations and still has to be determined.

Summary

There are different groups of growth factors for arterial smooth muscle and endothelial cells that are of potential relevance for atherogenesis in diabetes mellitus: hormones, locally released growth factors of platelet and of arterial wall cell origin.

The following hormones whose blood levels could increase under various conditions in diabetes have to be considered: growth hormone, insulin-like growth factor I and II, and insulin. There is circumstantial evidence that mainly insulin might contribute to premature atherogenesis in diabetes but its relative importance and mechanism of action still remains to be determined.

Human platelets contain of least eight growth peptides or proteins that all stimulate in vitro growth of arterial wall cells: platelet-derived, epidermal, fibroblast, diabetic serum, endothelial and transforming growth factors, vascular endothelial cell proliferation factor, and platelet-derived endothelial cell mitogen. In serum and plasma from type 2 diabetics only the diabetic serum growth factor has been shown to be increased, in type 1 diabetics platelets contain increased growth stimulating activity. This increased growth activity returned to normal levels in both types of diabetes after strict metabolic control. But their relative contribution to the atherogenic process is still unknown.

Arterial endothelial and smooth muscle cells, fibroblasts and monocyte/macrophages of different species release, at least in culture, a variety of growth factors that could participate in an autocrine or paracrine manner in the growth regulation of the arterial wall. Diabetes may affect the release of these factors, but direct evidence as to what degree this would contribute to atherogenesis is lacking.

In conclusion, in diabetes mellitus increased vascular growth factor levels might be involved in the development of accelerated atherosclerosis. But their relative contribution to the proliferative response of the arterial wall cells still has to be determined.

References

1. Rudermann NB, Haudenschild C (1984) Diabetes as an atherogenic factor. Progr Cardiovasc Dis 26: 373–412
2. Schwartz SM, Ross R (1984) Cellular proliferation in atherosclerosis and hypertension. Progr Cardiovasc Dis 26: 355–372
3. Benditt EP (1977) Implications of the monoclonal character of human atherosclerotic plaques. Am J Pathol 86: 693–702
4. Denes R, Lehmann R, Nienhaus R (1983) Evidence of the heterogeneity of the proliferative activity in experimental diabetes. Acta Histochem 27 [Suppl]: 259–264

5. Hauss WH, Mey J, Schulte H (1979) Effect of risk factors and anti-rheumatic drugs on the proliferation of aortic wall cells. Atherosclerosis 34: 119-143
6. Bowersox JC, Sorgente N (1985) Altered growth kinetics of dermal fibroblasts and arterial smooth muscle cells from spontaneously diabetic BB rats. Diabetes 34: 628-633
7. Grünwald J, Hesz A, Robenek H, Brücker J, Buddecke E (1985) Proliferation, morphology, and low-density lipoprotein metabolism of arterial endothelial cells cultured from normal and diabetic minipigs. Exp Mol Pathol 42: 60-70
8. Dolgov VV, Zainkina OE, Bondarenko MF, Repin VS (1982) Aortic endothelium of alloxan diabetic rabbits: a quantitative study using scanning electron microscopy. Diabetologia 22: 338-343
9. Ledet T, Fischer Dzoga K, Wissler RW (1976) Growth of rabbit aortic smooth-muscle cells cultured in media containing diabetic and hyperlipemic serum. Diabetes 25: 207-215
10. Koschinsky T, Bünting CE, Schwippert B, Gries FA (1979) Increased growth of human fibroblasts and arterial smooth muscle cells from diabetic patients related to diabetic serum factors and cell origin. Atherosclerosis 33: 245-252
11. Koh MS, Majewski BBJ, Rhodes EL (1985) Diabetic serum stimulates the proliferation of endothelial cells in culture. Diabetes Res 2: 287-289
12. Gerich JE (1984) Role of growth hormone in diabetes mellitus. N Engl J Med 310: 848-850
13. Ledet T (1977) Growth hormone anti-serum suppresses the growth effect of diabetic serum. Diabetes 26: 798-803
14. Merimee TJ, Zapf J, Froesch ER (1983) Insulin-like growth factors: studies in diabetics with and without retinopathy. N Engl J Med 309: 527-530
15. Zapf J, Schoenle E, Froesch ER (1978) Insulin-like growth factors I and II: some biological actions and receptor binding characteristics of two purified constituents of non-suppressible insulin-like activity of human serum. Eur J Biochem 87: 285-296
16. Stiles CD, Capone GT, Sher CD (1979) Dual control of cell growth by somatomedins and platelet-derived growth factor. Proc Natl Acad Sci USA 76: 1279-1283
17. Rechler MM (1979) Receptors for somatomedins and related peptides. In: Waldhäusel WK (ed) Diabetes. Excerpta Medica, Amsterdam, pp 266-271
18. King GL, Goodman AD, Buzney S, Moses A, Kahn CR (1985) Receptors and growth-promoting effects of insulin and insulin-like growth factors on cells from bovine retinal capillaries and aorta. J Clin Invest 75: 1028-1036
19. King GL (1985) Cell biology as an approach to the study of the vascular complications of diabetes. Metabolism 34 [Suppl 1]: 17-34
20. Stout RW (1985) Overview of the association between insulin and atherosclerosis. Metabolism 34 [Suppl 1]: 7-12
21. Hillson RM, Hockaday TDR, Mann JI, Newton DJ (1984) Hyperinsulinemia is associated with development of electrocardiographic abnormalities in diabetics. Diabetes Res I: 143-149
22. Standl E, Janka HU (1985) High serum insulin concentrations in relation to other cardiovascular risk factors in macrovascular disease of type 2 diabetes. Horm Metab Res [Suppl] 15: 46-51
23. Pfeifle B, Ditschuneit H (1981) Effect of insulin on the growth of cultured human arterial smooth muscle cells. Diabetologia 20: 155-158
24. Koschinsky T, Bünting CE, Rütter R, Gries FA (1985) Sera from type 2 (non-insulin-dependent) diabetic and healthy subjects contain different amounts of a very low molecular weight growth peptide for vascular cells. Diabetologia 28: 223-228
25. Taggart H, Stout RW (1980) Control of DNA synthesis in cultured vascular endothelial and smooth muscle cell. Atherosclerosis 37: 549-557
26. Straus SD (1984) Growth-stimulatory actions of insulin in vitro and in vivo. Endocrinol Rev 5: 356-369
27. Ross R, Vogel A (1978) The platelet-derived growth factor. Cell 14: 203-210
28. Antoniades HN, Scher CD, Stiles CD (1979) Purification of human platelet-derived growth factor. Proc Natl Acad Sci USA 76: 1809-1812
29. Heldin CH, Westermark B, Wasteson A (1979) Platelet-derived growth factor: purification and partial characterization. Proc Natl Acad Sci USA 76: 3722-3725
30. Ross R, Bowen-Pope DF, Raines EW (1985) Platelet-derived growth factor: its potential roles in wound healing, atherosclerosis, neoplasia, and growth and development. Ciba Found Symp 116: 98-112

31. King GL, Buchwald S (1984) Characterization and partial purification of an endothelial cell growth factor from human platelets . J Clin Invest 73: 392-396
32. Assoian RK, Komoriya A, Meyers CA, Miller DM, Sporn DB (1983) Transforming growth factor-β in human platelets. J Biol Chem 258: 7155-7160
33. Assoian RK, Grotendorst GR, Miller DM, Sporn MB (1984) Cellular transformation by coordinated action of three peptide growth factors from human platelets. Nature 309: 804-806
34. Miyazono K, Okabe T, Ishibashi S, Urabe A, Takaku F (1985) A platelet factor stimulating the proliferation of vascular endothelial cells. Exp Cell Res 159: 487-494
35. Ross R (1986) Growth factors, platelets, macrophages and atherosclerosis. In: Fidge NH, Nestel PJ (eds) Atherosclerosis VII. Elsevier, Amsterdam, pp 355-358 (International congress series 696)
36. Baird A, Esch F, Mormède P, Ueno N, Ling N, Böhlen P, Jing S-J, Wehrenberg WB, Guillemin R (1986) Molecular characterization of fibroblast growth factor: distribution and biological activities in various tissues. Hor Res 42: 143-205
37. Oka Y, Orth N (1983) Human plasma epidermal growth factor/β-urogastrone is associated with blood platelets. J Clin Invest 72: 249-259
38. Clemmons DR, William LI, Brown MT (1983) Dialyzable factor in human serum of platelet origin stimulates endothelial cell replication and growth. Proc Natl Acad Sci USA 80: 1641-1645
39. Koschinsky T, Bünting CE, Schwippert B, Gries FA (1980) Increased growth stimulation of fibroblasts from diabetics by diabetic serum factors of low molecular weight. Atherosclerosis 37: 311-317
40. Koschinsky T, Bünting CE, Schwippert B, Gries FA (1981) Regulation of diabetic serum growth factors for human vascular cells by the metabolic control of diabetes mellitus. Atherosclerosis 39: 313-319
41. Koschinsky T, Bünting CE, Rütter R, Gries FA (1983) Diabetic growth peptides of very low molecular weight for human vascular cells in serum from type 2 (non insulin-dependent) diabetic patients. Diabetologia 25: 172-173
42. Koschinsky T, Bünting CE, Rütter R, Schütze R, Gries FA (1985) Diabetic serum growth factor: a new low molecular weight growth peptide for arterial smooth muscle cells of platelet origin. Monogr Atheroscler 13: 159-163
43. Born MN (1978) Platelet function in diabetes mellitus. Diabetes 27: 342-350
44. Colwell JA, Lopes-Virella M, Halushka PV (1981) Pathogenesis of atherosclerosis in diabetes. Diabetes Care 4: 121-133
45. Hamet P, Sugimoto H, Umeda F, Lecavalier L, Franks DJ, Orth DN, Chiasson J-L (1985) Abnormalities of platelet-derived growth factors in insulin-dependent diabetes. Metabolism 34 [Suppl 1]: 25-31
46. Bowen-Pope DF, Ross R, Seifert R (1985) Locally acting growth factors for vascular cells. Circulation 72: 735-740
47. DiCorleto PE, Gajdusek CM, Schwartz SM, Ross R (1983) Biochemical properties of the endothelium-derived growth factor: comparison to other growth factors. J Cell Physiol 114: 339-345
48. Gajdusek CM (1984) Release of endothelial cell-derived growth factor (ECDGF) by heparin. J Cell Physiol 121: 13-21
49. Campbell JH, Campbell GR (1986) Endothelial cell influences on vascular smooth muscle phenotype. Annu Rev Physiol 48: 295-306
50. Stavenow L, Tejler L (1985) Growth stimulating activity from lysed cultured arterial smooth muscle cells and skin fibroblasts. Med Biol 63: 175-181
51. Clemmons DR (1985) Variables controlling the secretion of a somatomedin-like peptide by cultured porcine smooth muscle cells. Circ Res 56: 418-426
52. Clemmons DR, Van Wyk JJ (1985) Evidence for a functional role of endogenously produced somatomedinlike peptides in the regulation of DNA synthesis in cultured human fibroblasts and porcine smooth muscle cells. J Clin Invest 75: 1914-1918
53. Millis AJT, Hoyle M, Field B (1977) Human fibroblast conditioned media contains growth-promoting activities for low density cells. J Cell Physiol 93: 17-24
54. Satoh T, Kan M, Kato M, Yamane I (1986) Purification and characterization of an endothelial cell growth factor from serum-free culture medium of human diploid fibroblast cells. Biochim Biophys Acta 887: 86-93

55. Martin BM, Gimbrone MA, Unanue ER, Cotran RS (1981) Stimulation of nonlymphoid mesenchymal cell proliferation by a macrophage-derived growth factor. J Immunol 126: 1510-1515
56. Glenn KC, Ross R (1981) Human monocyte-derived growth factor(s) for mesenchymal cells: activation of secretion by endotoxin and concanavalin A. Cell 25: 603-615
57. Libby P, Wyler DJ, Janicka MW, Dinarello CA (1985) Differential effects of human interleukin-1 on growth of human fibroblasts and vascular smooth muscle cells. Arteriosclerosis 5: 186-191
58. Martinet Y, Bitterman PB, Mornex JF, Grotendorst GR, Martin GR, Crystal RG (1986) Activated human monocytes express the c-sis proto-oncogene and release a mediator showing PDGF-like activity. Nature 319: 158-160
59. Kitahara M, Eyre HJ, Lynch RE, Rallison ML, Hill HR (1980) Metabolic activity of diabetic monocytes. Diabetes 29: 251-256

Cholesterol Biosynthesis in Diabetes Mellitus

E. Andersén and K. Hellström

Introduction

Diabetes mellitus (DM) may be associated with derangements of lipid metabolism. The pattern of dyslipoproteinemia commonly encountered in noninsulin-dependent DM (NIDD) is characterized by elevated levels of VLDL-TG (very low density lipoprotein triglycerides) and subnormal concentrations of high-density lipoprotein (HDL) cholesterol. The causes of dyslipoproteinemia are multifactorial and heterogenous, and to a variable extent linked to defects in cholesterol metabolism. Thus, diabetic rats display an enhanced rate of cholesterogenesis, mainly due to high sterol production in the intestine rather than in the liver [7]. Abnormalities in line with such findings, i. e., high cholesterol production, were observed in patients with NIDD [4]. Studies in human subjects also indicate that insulin therapy, but not treatment with sulfonylurea and metformin, is able to suppress the rate of cholesterogenesis. This effect is not necessarily linked to variations in blood glucose control.

Experimental Design

The group studied comprised middle-aged patients, all regular attendants of the out-patient department. They were randomly selected from those who volunteered to participate. On the basis of the C-peptide response to i. v. glucagon they were separated into groups with IDD (insulin-dependent DM) and NIDD. Steroid balance studies were conducted in insulin-treated patients with IDD and in diet-treated patients with NIDD [4]. Patients with NIDD were also reexamined during treatment with insulin [5] and sulfonylurea [3]. Another series of sulfonylurea- and metformin-treated patients were investigated when metformin had been withdrawn [2]. Basal data are presented in Table 1.

Table 1. Basal data

Diagnosis	Therapy	No. of patients	Age (years)	Blood glucose (mmol l^{-1})	Serum cholesterol (mmol l^{-1})	Serum triglycerides (mmol l^{-1})
IDD	Insulin	6	50 ± 6	9.0 ± 0.9	4.5 ± 0.3	0.9 ± 0.1
NIDD	Diet	22	58 ± 2	10.7 ± 0.7	5.7 ± 0.1	2.2 ± 0.1
Controls	Diet	15	58 ± 2	4.5 ± 0.1	5.4 ± 0.2	1.0 ± 0.1

All patients were hospitalized during the study. The interval between two studies in the same patient was long enough to permit establishment of a new steady state. None of the patients had diseases (other than DM) known to interfere with lipoprotein or cholesterol metabolism. The diet was standardized and of a regular type. Blood glucose and lipoprotein pattern were checked repeatedly. Bile acid kinetics were studied by an isotopic technique. The sterol contents of the feces and food were determined by gas-liquid chromatography. Net steroid balance was defined as bile acid formation plus fecal excretion of cholesterol and cholesterol neutral metabolites, minus cholesterol intake.

Results

All patients were slightly to moderately hyperglycemic. As compared with controls, the diet-treated patients with NIDD had elevated levels of VLDL-TG (1.33 ± 0.11 vs 0.49 ± 0.06 mmol l^{-1}) and lower levels of HDL cholesterol (1.08 ± 0.07 vs 1.35 ± 0.07 mmol l^{-1}). The lipoprotein pattern was normal in the patients with IDD. The relative body weights averaged $98 \pm 3\%$, $93 \pm 6\%$, and $122 \pm 4\%$ in the controls and in the patients with IDD and NIDD, respectively.

The steroid balance data are summarized in Fig. 1. The mean for diet-treated patients with NIDD (3.87 ± 0.23 mmol day^{-1}) was significantly higher ($P < 0.001$) than for the controls (2.38 ± 0.20 mmol day^{-1}) and for the patients with IDD (1.59 ± 0.25 mmol day^{-1}). The high steroid balance in the patients with NIDD was mainly due to an elevated excretion of neutral steroids in the feces, while the elimination of cholesterol as bile acids remained within the upper-normal range. Upon separation of the NIDD patients by lipoprotein pattern and body weight, it appeared that the highest values (expressed per kilogram body weight) were recorded for nonobese patients. Obesity per se did not seem to be associated with an enhanced rate of cholesterogenesis.

In patients reexamined after the start of insulin therapy the blood glucose and the serum lipoprotein pattern were essentially unchanged. In diet-treated patients prescribed sulfonylurea, the fasting blood glucose dropped from 11.4 ± 1.15 to 7.4 ± 0.62 mmol l^{-1} and the serum TG level decreased slightly. Upon withdrawal of met-

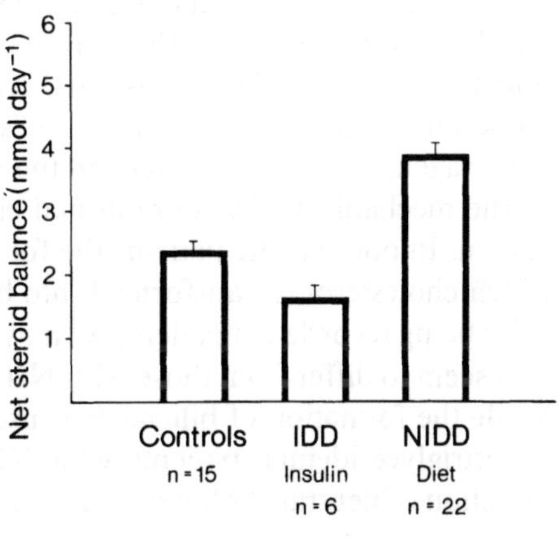

Fig. 1. Steroid balance in nondiabetic controls ($n = 15$), in insulin-treated patients with IDD ($n = 6$), and in diet-treated patients with NIDD ($n = 22$)

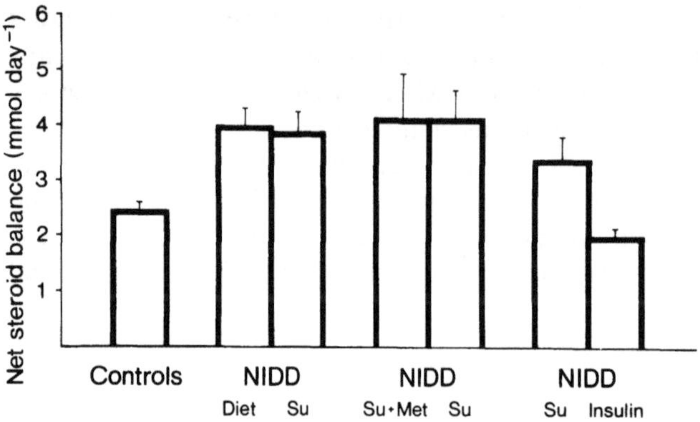

Fig. 2. Steroid balance in controls ($n=15$), in diet-treated patients before and during sulfonylurea (Su) treatment ($n=10$), in sulfonylurea-treated patients before and after withdrawal of metformin (Met; $n=6$), and in sulfonylurea-treated patients before and after sulfonylurea was replaced by insulin ($n=9$)

formin from patients also prescribed sulfonylurea, the fasting blood glucose increased by about 20%. The effect of therapy (or withdrawal of metformin) on the steroid balance is demonstrated in Fig. 2. While administration of insulin was followed by a significant reduction of the net steroid balance, this remained high and unchanged both in patients given sulfonylurea and in those given sulfonylurea and metformin.

Discussion

IDD and NIDD are different diseases. While IDD is characterized by insulin deficiency, patients with NIDD have both insulin deficiency and insulin resistance. NIDD but not IDD is commonly associated with obesity and/or dyslipoproteinemia. The hypertriglyceridemia observed is explained by overproduction and/or decreased clearance of VLDL-TG [8]. Another abnormality in NIDD demonstrated by the current studies is a highly significant rise of the net steroid balance that, in a steady state, is equivalent to the rate of cholesterol formation. A supranormal synthesis of cholesterol in diet-treated patients has also been observed by Abrams, Ginsberg and Grundy [1]. The steroid balance dropped markedly upon administration of insulin, even though insulin therapy did not normalize the blood glucose and the serum lipoproteins. In contrast, these variables were modified by the oral antidiabetic agents that had no effect on the rate of cholesterogenesis.

The mechanism of a supranormal cholesterol production in NIDD is not fully known. In nondiabetic patients the formation of VLDL-TG is related to the rate at which cholesterol is transformed into bile acids [6], the highest levels of both variables being recorded in patients with hypertriglyceridemia. Patients with such disorders seem to differ from those with NIDD in the pattern of cholesterol metabolism. While the formation of bile acids is usually increased in nondiabetic patients with hypertriglyceridemia, patients with NIDD were mainly characterized by a high excretion of neutral cholesterol products in the feces. These differences in the route of cholesterol elimination are not fully understood. They might reflect variations in the site of cholesterol production or lipoprotein degradation. In line with such a concept, diabetic rats have a high rate of cholesterol formation in the intestine, that returns to normal during insulin treatment [7].

The possible consequences of a high rate of cholesterogenesis in terms of development of macroangiopathy remain to be established. However, the recent findings of a higher incidence of macroangiopathy in NIDD than in IDD underlines the need for further studies. The lack of effects of sulfonylurea and metformin on cholesterogenesis focus interest on earlier reports of the low efficiency of such drugs in preventing the development of cardiovascular disease in diabetic patients [9].

References

1. Abrams JJ, Ginsby H, Grundy SM (1982) Metabolism of cholesterol and plasma triglycerides in non-ketotic diabetes mellitus. Diabetes 31: 903-910
2. Andersén E (1987) Cholesterol and bile acid metabolism in noninsulin-dependent diabetics - effect of discontinuation of biguanide therapy (to be published)
3. Andersén E. Hellström K (1987) Bile and kinetics and cholesterol biosynthesis in glibenclamide-treated noninsulin-dependent diabetics (to be published)
4. Andersén E, Hellström P, Hellström K (1986) Cholesterol and bile acid metabolism in middle-aged diabetics. Diabetes Metab 12: 261-267
5. Andersén E, Hellström P, Hellström K (1987) Cholesterol biosynthesis in nonketotic diabetics before and during insulin therapy. Diab Res Clin Pract (in press)
6. Angelin B, Einarsson K, Hellström K, Leijd B (1978) Bile acid kinetics in relation to endogenous triglyceride metabolism in various types of hyperlipoproteinemia. J Lipid Res 19: 1004-1016
7. Feingold KR, Wiley MH, MacRae H, Moser AH, Leah SR, Siperstein MD (1982) The effect of diabetes mellitus on sterol synthesis in the intact rat. Diabetes 31: 388-395
8. Kissebah HH, Alfarsi S, Adams PW, Wynn V (1976) Role of insulin resistance in adipose tissue and liver in the pathogenesis of endogenous hypertriglyceridaemia in man. Diabetologia 12: 563-571
9. Knatterud GL, Klimt CR, Goldner MG, Hawkins BS, Weisenfels S, Kreines K, Haddock L (1982) Effects of hypoglycaemic agents on vascular complications in patients with adult-onset diabetes, VIII. Evaluation of insulin therapy: final report. Diabetes 31, suppl 5: 1.

Effects of Diet Fat Composition on Serum Lipids and Lipoproteins in Patients with Insulin-Dependent Diabetes Mellitus*

J. Boberg, L. Abrahamsson, C. Berne, I.-B. Gustafsson, and T. Pollare

Introduction

In several countries general recommendations have been made concerning the fat content of the diet of patients with insulin-dependent diabetes mellitus (IDDM) [1-3]. A low total fat content (below 30-35 energy percent, E%), a low content of saturated fat (below 10 E%) and some increase in the content of polyunsaturated fat up to 10 E% [1] have been recommended. For patients with a high risk of future ischemic heart disease these recommendations have been urgent. Patients with IDDM constitute such a high-risk group. In addition, it has been suggested that an increased intake of polyunsaturated fat might lower the incidence of both micro- and macroangiopathy in adult-onset diabetics [4]. Recently, however, doubts have been expressed about the beneficial effects of such a diet in patients with IDDM, especially when the source of the fatty acids is fish oil, which contains mainly *n*-3 fatty acids [5].

The present study was carried out to analyze the dietary habits of a randon sample of young patients with IDDM as compared with those of a matched randomly selected reference group. It is planned that this investigation be followed by an intervention study to investigate the beneficial effects of an ideal diet given to patients with IDDM.

Materials and Methods

Subjects and Patients. The group studied comprised 101 patients with IDDM who were recruited at random from six different diabetic clinics in Sweden. The randomly recruited group was classified for age (18-35 years), size of household (one or several members), sex (males and females 1:1), and duration of disease (one-fourth less than 5 years). Excluded were patients who: had severe retinopathy; had diseases other than hypertension requiring therapy; were known to abuse alcohol or drugs; were pregnant; had continuous subcutaneous insulin infusion; did night work; and were known to have severe food allergy. The patients with IDDM were compared with 53 apparently healthy subjects randomly selected from the same geographic area as the patients and matched for age, sex, and household size. At

* Supported by grants from the Swedish Margarine Industrial Association for Nutritional-Physiology Research, the Throne-Holst Foundation and the Swedish Medical Research Council (B86-19X-07193-028).

each clinic between 12 and 24 patients and 6 and 12 controls were invited to attend for investigations. After a fasting period of at least 6 h, blood samples were drawn for measurements of blood hemoglobin, blood glucose, and serum creatinine, which were performed at the local hospital laboratory. In addition, samples were frozen and sent to Uppsala for determination of glycosylated hemoglobin, serum lipids, and lipoproteins, and of the serum lipid ester fatty acid composition. At the first visit to the clinics the blood pressure and pulse rate were recorded in a reproducible way in accordance with instructions, a form concerning the medical history was filled in, and the patients and controls were instructed how to maintain a food record by household measures for 7 days. This instruction was given by dieticians.

Laboratoy Methods. Glycosylated hemoglobin was determined as HbA_{1c} [6] in frozen samples of whole blood. Cholesterol and triglyceride concentrations in serum and in the high-density lipoprotein (HDL) fraction were determined by enzymatic methods, using Boehringer-Mannheim kits 126012 and 124087 (Munich, FRG), modified for use in a Multistat III F/LS apparatus (Instrumentation Laboratories, Lexington, USA). The HDL fraction was isolated as the supernatant of whole serum after the very low and low-density lipoproteins had been removed by precipitation with phosphotungstate/$MgCl_2$.

The fatty acid composition of plasma lipid esters was determined by extraction of plasma into chloroform to which 0.005% butylated hydroxytoluene had been added as an antioxidant. The lipid esters were separated by thin-layer chromatography and transmethylated. The fatty acid methyl esters were separated by gas-liquid chromatography as previously described [7].

Dietary Survey Method. Comprehensive oral instructions were given by specially trained dieticians attending an advanced course in dietetics at the Department of Home Economics at the University of Uppsala. In addition, written instructions were given to all patients and controls. Each dietician was responsible for about 12 patients and 6 control subjects. The study was carried out during February and March 1985 and the subjects kept a food record by household measures for 7 days [8]. All primary results were checked by the dieticians together with the patients and coded for further calculation. The data were fed into a computer for calculation of about 40 different nutrients.

Results

There was successful matching between patients and control subjects. The classification of the patient groups also meant that the samples recruited from each clinic were very similar. The clinics were distributed geographically within the southern half of Sweden.

Clinical Characteristics of the Patients. The patients were receiving between one and four doses of insulin per day (mean 2.2 ± 0.8 doses; mean total dose 46 ± 18 IU/24 h). The duration of diabetes was 12 ± 9 years (range 1-34). Mean ages for the patients and controls were 28.0 ± 5.8 and 27.5 ± 5.4 years, respectively. The blood pressure and pulse rate of the patients were 124 ± 11/76 ± 8 mmHg and 75 ± 10 min^{-1}, and those of the controls 119 ± 10/74 ± 7 mmHg and 68 ± 8 min^{-1}. None of the patients had severe nephropathy. The metabolic control was as expected in a random sample of fairly young IDDM patients (see Table 1). The mean values for serum lipid and HDL concentrations of triglycerides and cholesterol were similar in the diabetic patients and the controls (Table 2).

Fatty Acid Composition of Plasma Lipid Esters. The relative concentration of linoleic acid was significantly higher in the diabetic patients than in the controls (Table 3). The diabetic patients showed significantly lower values than the controls for the fatty acids 16:1 *n*-7 and 20:3 *n*-6. The fatty acid compositions of the plasma cholesterol esters were determined in a random subsample of the study population both before and after the food recording. No significant changes occurred in this respect during the food-recording week.

Diet Composition. The diabetic patients had a slightly lower mean energy intake than the controls. This was true both for carbohydrates and fat (Table 4). Their pro-

Table 1. Clinical characteristics of the subjects studied (mean ± SD, with range in parentheses)

	Control subjects (n=53)	Diabetic patients (n=101)
Body mass index	22.5 ± 3.0 (16–31)	22.9 ± 2.7 (14–30)
B-Hemoglobin[a] (g/l)	139 ± 15 (106–163)	146 ± 11) (115–176)
Serumcreatinine (μmol/l)	80 ± 12 (60–110)	80 ± 12 (50–142)
fB-glucose[b] (mmol/l)	4.4 ± 0.7 (2.7–6.9)	9.7 ± 5.3 (1.5–25.0)
B-Hemoglobin A_{1c} (%)	5.3 ± 0.6 (4.0–8.3)	8.4 ± 1.6 (3.7–14.3)

[a] B-Hemoglobin, Blood-Hemoglobin.
[b] fB-glucose, fasting blood glucose.

Table 2. Serum lipid and high-density liproprotein (HDL) concentrations (mean ± SD)

	Control subjects (n=53)	Diabetic patients (n=101)
S-triglyceride (mmol/l)	1.24 ± 0.78	1.27 ± 0.69
S-cholesterol (mmol/l)	4.7 ± 0.8	5.0 ± 1.2
HDL-triglyceride (mmol/l)	0.18 ± 0.06	0.19 ± 0.07
HDL-cholesterol (mmol/l)	1.2 ± 0.3	1.2 ± 0.3

Table 3. Fatty acid composition of serum phospholipids (PL) and cholesterol esters (CE) (mean ± SD)

	Control subjects		Diabetic patients	
	PL (n=53)	CE (n=9)	PL (n=101)	CE (n=26)
16:0	31.9±2.2	12.0±1.1	31.5±1.5	11.9±0.7
16:1 n-7	1.0±0.2	3.6±1.2	0.9[b]±0.2	3.0±0.9
18:0	13.9±1.5	0.9±0.2	13.8±1.1	1.1±0.2
18:1 n-9	11.8±1.3	18.1±1.4	11.9±1.3	19.1±2.4
18:2 n-6	24.6±2.3	55.9±3.3	26.3[a]±2.5	57.8±3.6
18:3 n-6	0	0.7±0.3	0	0.5±0.2
18:3 n-3	0.2±0.2	0.7±0.3	0.2±0.2	0.7±0.1
20:3 n-6	2.7±0.6	0.6±0.2	2.2[a]±0.6	0.4±0.2
20:4 n-6	7.9±1.1	6.0±1.4	7.5±1.2	4.5[b]±0.9
20:5 n-3	1.3±0.8	0.9±0.4	1.1±0.4	0.9±0.3
22:4 n-6	0	0	0	0
22:5 n-3	0.7±0.4	0	0.8±0.4	0
22:6 n-3	4.1±0.9	0.5±0.4	3.9±0.9	0.2±0.3

[a] $P<0.001$. [b] $P<0.01$.

Table 4. Body weight and diet composition of the subjects studied

	Control subjects (n=53)	Diabetic patients (n=101)
Body weight (kg)	67 ±12	66 ± 9
Energy (MJ)	10.3 ± 2.5	9.7 ± 2.8
Protein (g/day)	89 ±23	97 ±27
(E%)	15 ± 2	17 ± 3
Carbohydrate (g/day)	264 ±72	241 ±78
(E%)	44 ± 6	43 ± 6
Fat (g/day)	107 ±30	97 ±32
(E%)	39 ± 5	38 ± 5
Saturated fat (E%)	17 ± 3	16 ± 3
Mono-unsaturated fat (E%)	12 ± 2	12 ± 2
Polyunsaturated fat (E%)	5 ± 1	5 ± 1
P:S ratio	0.30± 0.10	0.31± 0.08
Cholesterol (g/day)	0.4 ± 0.1	0.4 ± 0.1
Alcohol (E%)	1.8 ± 1.8	1.6 ± 2.1

tein intake was rather higher than that of the controls. The quality of the reported fat intake was very similar in the two groups. The intake of saturated fat, 17±3 E% in the control subjects and 16±3 E% in the diabetic patients, is higher than that recommended both for the general population and, especially, for diabetic patients [1]. The recommendation for saturated fat is that it should normally not be more than 10 E%.

Relationship Between Plasma Lipids and Phospholipid Fatty Acids. In the control subjects significant negative correlations were found between the serum triglyceride (S-TG) and cholesterol concentrations and the percentage of 18:2 n-6 ($r=-0.43$

and $r = -0.36$, respectively, $P < 0.01$); no significant correlation was found in the diabetic patients ($r = -0.10$ and $r = +0.11$). For the more unsaturated fatty acids of the n-6 series (18:3 and 20:3), however, there were positive correlations. Between arachidonic acid (20:4 n-6) and the serum lipid concentrations significant negative correlations were found in the diabetic patients ($r = -0.21$, $P < 0.05$ and $r = -0.32$, $P < 0.001$ for S-TG and S-cholesterol, respectively) but not in the controls. In the diabetic patients there was also a significant negative correlation between the percentage of 22:6 n-3 and the S-cholesterol concentration ($r = -0.28$, $P < 0.01$).

Relationship Between Diet Composition and Plasma Phospholipid Fatty Acids. No significant correlations were found between the dietary intake of polyunsaturated fatty acids or the ratio of polyunsaturated to saturated fatty acids (P:S) in the diets, and the serum phospholipid content of $n = 6$ fatty acids. However, there were significant positive correlations both in the controls and in the diabetic patients between the P:S ratio and dietary intake of polyunsaturated fatty acids, on the one hand, and the serum phospholipid contents of the main n-3 fatty acids, 20:5 and 22:6, on the other.

Discussion

In the present study a random sample of young patients with IDDM was investigated concerning serum lipids and dietary habits, and was compared with a matched reference group. The diabetic patients and the controls had similar serum lipid concentrations, a finding which is in accordance with earlier reports [10] on well-controlled, insulin-treated diabetic patients.

The fatty acid compositions of serum phospholipids and cholesterol esters were also very similar in diabetic patients and controls. However, a slightly higher percentage of linoleic acid (18:2 n-6) was found in the diabetic patients, as has also been observed by Tilvis and Miettinen [11] in diabetic women and by Ewald et al. [12] in diabetic children. This probably indicates a slightly higher dietary intake of linoleic acid in the diabetic patients than in the controls [13].

Recently, De Leeuw summarized the basic aims of the diabetic diet [14]. It should provide all nutrients necessary to restore and maintain a normal nutritional status provide sufficient carbohydrates of a quality suitable to obtain the best blood glucose control possible, and apply, based on controlled studies, diet principles that could help in the prevention of long-term complications. The high-carbohydrate, high-fiber, low-fat diet that was suggested [14] seems to fulfill most of these conditions. Active fat restriction was also advised in the latest American Diabetes Association report [1]. The diabetic patients investigated in the present study had a lower energy intake and a higher protein intake than the controls. They also had an insignificantly lower intake of carbohydrates and fats as expressed in grams per day, but not when expressed in relative terms as energy percent. In addition, the quality of the fat intake was very similar, with a diet P:S ratio of 0.3. The P:S ratio of the diet and the daily intake of polyunsaturated fat were both lower than are recommended by the Swedish Nutrition Board, who consider that the P:S ratio should be about 0.5.

Using the 7-day recording, no difference in dietary fat intake was found between the patients with IDDM and the controls. However, the patients with IDDM had a higher concentration of linoleic acid in the plasma phospholipids. In the control subjects higher concentrations of linoleic acid correlated with lower serum lipid concentrations, but this was not found in the patients with IDDM. In the diabetics such negative correlations between serum lipid concentrations and polyunsaturated fatty acids in serum phospholipids were observed for arachidonic acid and also for the *n*-3 fatty acid docosahexaenoic acid (22:6 *n*-3). Positive correlations were found between P:S ratio of the dietary fat and the dietary intake of *n*-3 fatty acids, on the one hand, and the serum phospholipid contents of the fatty acids 20:5 and 22:6 *n*-3, on the other. This indicates that it might be of value to monitor the intake of fish fat by blood sample analyses during dietary treatment.

It is quite evident that the diet of the patients of the present study, who probably constitute a representative sample of patients with IDDM in Sweden, is not equivalent to the recommended diet. This is especially true for the fat intake, which is too high and includes too much saturated fat. In addition, the polyunsaturated fat should not consist of vegetable fat alone, but should also include fat of marine origin, such as fish. It would seem important that more efficient attempts be made to alter the diets of patients with IDDM. That such dietary modifications are possible has recently been demonstrated in patients with coronary heart disease [15].

References

1. American Diabetes Association (1979) Principles of nutrition and dietary recommendations for individuals with diabetes mellitus, special report. Diabetes 28: 1027–1030
2. British Diabetic Association (1982) Dietary recommendation for diabetics for the 1980's. Hum Nutr Appl Nutr 36A: 378–394
3. Huttunen JK, Aro A, Pelkonen R, Puomio M, Siltanen I, Åkerblom HK (1982) Dietary therapy in diabetes mellitus, description of a recommendation prepared by the Finnish diabetes association's committee on nutrition therapy. Acta Medica Scand 211: 469–475
4. Houtsmuller AJ, Van Hol-Ferwerda J, Zahn KJ, Heukes HE (1980) Favourable influences of linoleic acid on the progression of diabetic micro- and macroangiopathy. Nutr Metab 24 (suppl 1): 105–118
5. Illman RJ, Trimble RP, Storer GB, Topping DL, Oliver JR (1986) Time-course of changes in plasma lipids in diabetic rats fed diets high in fish or safflower oils. Atherosclerosis 59: 313–321
6. Ronquist G (1986) New Spectro-photometric method for the determination of HbA_{1c} (to be published)
7. Boberg M, Croon LB, Gustafsson I-B, Vessby B (1985) Platelet fatty acid composition in relation to fatty acid composition in plasma and to serum lipoprotein lipids in healthy subjects with special reference to the linoleic acid pathway. Clin Sci 68: 581–587
8. Marr J (1971) Individual dietary surveys; purposes and methods. World Rev Nutr Diet 13: 105–164
9. Keys A, Fidanga F, Karvonen MJ (1972) Indices of relative weight and obesity. J Chronic Dis 25: 329–343
10. Nikkilä E-A, Hormila P (1978) Serum lipids and lipoproteins in insulin-treated diabetes. Diabetes 27: 1078–1086
11. Tilvis RS, Miettinen TA (1985) Fatty acid compositions of serum lipids, erythrocytes and platelets in insulin-dependent diabetic women. J Clin Endocrinol Metab 61: 741–745

12. Ewald U, Gustafsson I-B, Tuvemo T, Vessby B (1982) Fatty acid composition of serum lipids in diabetic children and their matched healthy controls. Upsala J Med Sci 87: 111-117
13. Boberg M, Gustafsson I-B, Vessby B (1986) High content of dietary linoleic acid does not reduce platelet reactivity in patients with hyperlipoproteinaemia. Eur J Clin Invest 16: 28-34
14. De Leeuw I (1985) Diabetic diet strategy for young adults and adolescents with insulin dependent diabetes mellitus. In: Serrano-Rios M, Lefèbvre PG (eds) Diabetes. Excerpta Medica, Amsterdam, pp 810-813
15. Thuesen L, Henriksen LB, Engby B (1986) One-year experience with low fat, low cholesterol diet in patients with coronary heart disease. Am J Clin Nutr 44: 212-219

Platelets and Thrombosis

β_2-Glycoprotein-I (Apolipoprotein H): Possible Role in Platelet Activation and Coagulation

J. Nimpf and G. M. Kostner

Introduction

In 1961 Schultze et al. [1] described a new constituent of human plasma which was called β_2-mucoid. Three years later Heide et al. found a carbohydrate-rich glycoprotein in human plasma which was called β_2-glycoprotein because of its electrophoretical mobility [2]. Later, this glycoprotein was found to be identical to the previously described β_2-mucoid [3].

β_2-Glycoprotein-I (β_2-G-I) is a glycoprotein with a carbohydrate content of 16% (w/w) and a molecular mass of approximately 50 kilodaltons [4]. The normal plasma concentration of β_2-G-I ranges from 0.15–0.3 mg/ml and it is found in 94% of the European population [5, 6]. Reduced levels of the glycoprotein (0.05–0.15 mg/ml) occur in about 6% of the population; approximately 0.1% of the population seems to lack β_2-G-I totally. In the epidemiological studies cited above, no correlations between reduced plasma levels or the lack of the glycoprotein and any obvious diseases or impaired metabolic feature were found. Furthermore, the plasma concentration of β_2-G-I depends on age and sex [5].

Studies on the plasma concentrations of β_2-G-I in various diseases have revealed reduced concentrations in rheumatoid arthritis [7] and hepatic cirrhosis [8] and a two-fold increase in diabetes mellitus [5]. Contradictory results have been published in another study, where no significant differences in the concentration of the glycoprotein in rheumatoid arthritis and hepatic cirrhosis were measured in relation to healthy persons [9]. In addition, a significant reduction of β_2-G-I plasma levels occurs during pregnancy [10].

Despite these results and some other approaches discussed later, no definitive physiological or pathological function of β_2-G-I was found for a long time.

Structure of β_2-G-I

β_2-G-I is a perchloric acid-soluble protein [1] which binds with high affinity to heparin [11]. This behavior is commonly used for the preparation and purification of the glycoprotein. Finlayson et al. isolated three subfractions of β_2-G-I by ion exchange chromatography using diethylaminoethyl (DEAE-) cellulose [12]. No differences in the content of sialic acids and electrophoretic mobilities of these isoforms were detected. By isoelectric focusing Polz et al. found three immunochemically identical isoforms of the glycoprotein which differ in their isoelectric points [13]. The molecular mass of all three isoforms was determined to be 54 kilodaltons.

Amino acid analyses of the isoforms showed no significant differences in amino acid composition [14]. Similar results were found by Schousboe [15]. She isolated four isoforms of the glycoprotein by DEAE-cellulose chromatography, and found no difference in the amino acid composition, but a microheterogeneity in the sialic acid content. In our own laboratory we isolated the four main species of at least five detectable isoforms by chromatofocusing and determined the following isoelectric points: 6.1; 5.8; 5.4; and 5.2 (unpublished data). Sialic acid analysis of the isoforms did not explain definitively the microheterogeneity of the glycoprotein.

Because of the association with plasma lipoprotein fractions, β_2-G-I has also been called apolipoprotein (apo) H [16]. Studies on molecular properties indicate that β_2-G-I differs significantly from all common apolipoproteins in essential structural parameters, such as percentage of alpha-helical conformation and interaction with air-water interfaces [17]. The recent determination of the complete amino acid sequence of β_2-G-I by Lozier et al. revealed a molecular mass of 50 kilodaltons [18]. The protein consists of 326 amino acids and has attached five glucosamine-containing oligosaccharides. One of the outstanding properties is the high content of proline (10%). Thus, excluding collagen, β_2-G-I is one of the most proline-rich proteins synthesized in human or any other eukaryotic cells. Sequence homology studies have revealed the identity of the 20 amino terminal residues of β_2-G-I and a protein C-binding protein from human plasma [19]. But it has been suggested that β_2-G-I was purified instead of the protein C-binding protein and that the two proteins are not identical [18].

Involvement of β_2-G-I in the Triglyceride Metabolism

Burstein and Scholnick [20] demonstrated that chylomicrons and very low-density lipoprotein (VLDL) are precipitable with sodium dodecyl sulfate (SDS) only in the presence of a serum factor. They identified this factor as β_2-G-I by radial immunodiffusion against anti-β_2-G-I [21]. Polz et al. [14] found that β_2-G-I is a regular constituent of apo VLDL. As demonstrated later, β_2-G-I is distributed among all plasma lipoprotein fractions [22]. Approximately 17% were found in the high-density lipoprotein (HDL), 16% in the chylomicron and VLDL, and 2% in the low-density lipoprotein (LDL) fraction. The remaining part, which seems not to be associated with lipoproteins, can be isolated from the 1.21 density bottom fraction. The hydrophobic interaction of β_2-G-I with lipids was further demonstrated: (a) by the ability of the glycoprotein to bind to artificial lipid emulsions such as Intralipid [23] - in this model the dissociation constant of the binding was 10^{-8} *M*; this value is higher as is known from the binding of other apoproteins to lipids; (b) highly purified, apparently lipid-free β_2-G-I interacts with Sudan dyes and can be stained with Sudan black in electrophoresis (unpublished observation).

Nakaya et al. [16] demonstrated an in vivo activation of the lipoprotein lipase in the presence of apo CII by β_2-G-I. They suggest that a possible function of β_2-G-I might be the modulation of triglyceride metabolism in vivo. This suggestion was also supported by investigations in the rat. Rat plasma contains β_2-G-I with a similar isoform polymorphism as described in humans [24]. In a study conducted in our laboratory, rats were infused intravenously with ^{14}C-Intralipid plus β_2-G-I. Triglyceride catabolism was significantly enhanced in the group with additional β_2-G-I [25, 26]. Finally it was reported that in some types of hypertriglyceridemias there are decreased levels or a total absence of the glycoprotein [20].

Interaction of β_2-G-I with Platelets

In addition to these results concerning triglyceride metabolism, several other properties of β_2-G-I have been described. Binding to DNA [27], binding to and agglutination of mitochondria [28], binding to deoxycholate [29], and binding to platelets [30]. The common feature of this behavior seems to be an interaction of β_2-G-I with negatively charged groups on the above-mentioned substances or cells, as demonstrated by Wurm [31]. β_2-G-I binds to liposomes containing negatively charged phospholipids such as phosphatidylserine (PS) and phosphatidylinositol (PI). The binding affinities calculated from Scatchard plots were 1.8×10^{-8} *M* for PS and 1.1×10^{-8} *M* for PI.

The finding of the interaction of β_2-G-I with platelets focused our attention on the investigation of a possible biological function of this glycoprotein. We found that β_2-G-I does not bind to gel-filtered platelets, but only to platelets "washed" by centrifugation, which causes partial or total activation of these cells. On the other hand, independently of this binding, β_2-G-I inhibited the second phase of the adenosine diphosphate-(ADP-) induced platelet aggregation (Fig. 1) [32, 33]. This effect was specific for ADP and did not occur if other triggers such as thrombin, collagen,

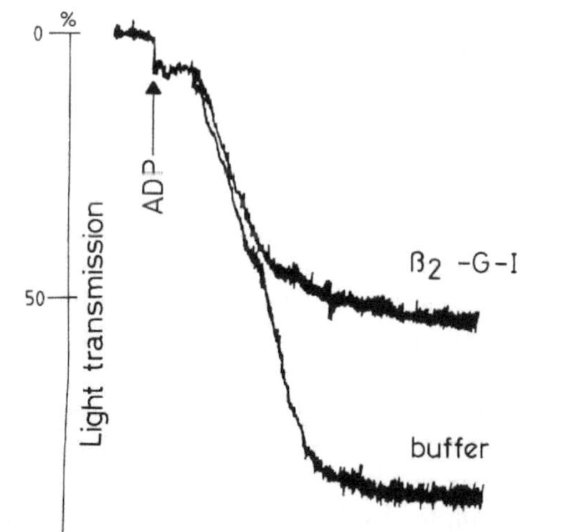

Fig. 1. Influence of β_2-G-I upon the ADP-induced aggregation of human platelets. Platelet aggregation was measured by a turbidometric method using a dual channel aggregometer. Aggregation is expressed as a percentage of light transmission of platelet-free buffer. A suspension of gel-filtered platelets was preincubated for 1 min with buffer of β_2-G-I and than stimulated by adding ADP (5 μ*M*) in the presence of fibrinogen (6 mg/ml)

platelet activating factor (PAF), or arachidonic acid were used. Measurements of the content of cyclic nucleotides during platelet activation showed no influence of the glycoprotein upon cyclic adenosine monophosphate (cAMP) levels in platelets [34]. The cGMP level, which rises during trigger-induced aggregation, was significantly enhanced during ADP and collagen aggregation in the presence of the glycoprotein. The in vitro modulation of the ADP-induced activation described is caused by a selective inhibition of the ADP-induced release reaction [35]. The concentration of the glycoprotein needed to induce these effects in vitro is in the range of 0.1-0.15 mg/ml. This is well within the physiological plasma concentration. At the moment these in vitro results cannot be related to an in vivo study where we failed to demonstrate a correlation between the concentration of β_2-G-I and platelet aggregability in young healthy persons [36]. A possible reason for this lack of correlation could be the fact that the inhibitory effect of β_2-G-I might only be relevant in some pathological states and does not become apparent in an undisturbed system.

β_2-G-I and Blood Coagulation

According to current concepts, two reactions of blood coagulation, the generation of activated factor X and thrombin, are catalyzed in vivo by activated platelets [37]. Unstimulated platelets have only minute amounts of PS in the outer monolayer of their plasma membrane [38]. In vitro activation of platelets by the combined action of thrombin and collagen leads to a drastic reorientation of phospholipids in the plasma membrane [39]. PS becomes exposed at the outer surface of the membrane, which strongly correlates with the generation of procoagulant activity of these cells [37, 40]. The prothrombinase complex is composed of activated factors V (V_a) and X (X_a), Ca^{++}, and the reoriented platelet membrane. X_a and prothrombin bind via Ca^{++} bridges to the PS of the outer surface of platelets, whereby the apparent K_m value of prothrombin is lowered to values below its physiological concentration [41]. In a similar manner X_a is produced by the tenase complex [42]. Inspired by the fact that β_2-G-I strongly interacts with negatively charged phospholipids, especially with PS, we became interested in investigating a possible interference of the glycoprotein with procoagulant activity of platelets. Indeed, in an in vitro assay β_2-G-I inhibited the production of thrombin by stimulated platelets in a concentration-dependent manner [43]. As shown in Fig. 2, stimulation of platelets with a combination of thrombin and collagen in the presence of β_2-G-I led to a similar increase of prothrombinase activity in the first 10 min as can be seen without β_2-G-I. Thereafter, prothrombinase activity decreased, reaching, after 60 min, a value of 20%-30% of the activity observed in the absence of β_2-G-I. The inhibition of the prothrombinase complex by β_2-G-I cannot be abolished by increasing the concentration of coagulation factors V_a and X_a. This suggests that the glycoprotein reduces prothrombinase binding sites rather than competing with the binding of these coagulation factors to platelets. In a model system, where activated platelets were replaced by phospholipid vesicles containing PS, the production of thrombin was inhibited in a similar manner to that shown for platelets. The time dependence of this inhibition indicates a relatively slow process and electron microscopy experiments with PS-containing vesicles and β_2-G-I demonstrated a structural alteration of the vesi-

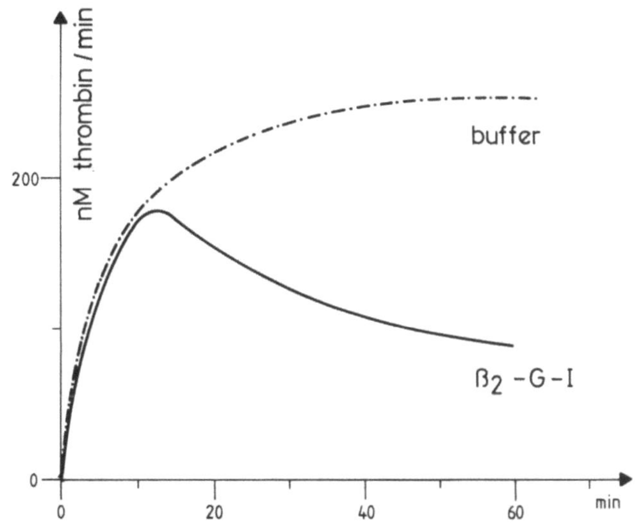

Fig. 2. Influence of formation of prothrombinase activity of platelets stimulated with collagen plus thrombin. Washed human platelets were preincubated with buffer or β_2-G-I and than activated with collagen (10 µg/ml) plus thrombin (4 n*M*) in the presence of 3 m*M* $CaCl_2$. Prothrombinase activity was measured at different times, as indicated in the *abscissa*, using a chromogenic substrate assay for thrombin. Prothrombinase activity is expressed as thrombin (n*M*) formation per 1 min

cle structure, which is strongly correlated with the inhibition of the procoagulant activity of these vesicles. It is suggested that the mechanism by which β_2-G-I alters the procoagulant activity of stimulated platelets is the same as demonstrated for vesicles, but final proof awaits further experiments. Recently Schousboe also found that β_2-G-I inhibits the activation of the contact phase system of the intrinsic pathway of blood coagulation [44]. In this step of blood coagulation, negatively charged phospholipids also play an essential role by binding Hageman factor and precallikrein.

Conclusion

β_2-G-I is an unusual apolipoprotein which might be involved in triglyceride metabolism by activating lipoprotein lipase. Despite some results in the rat it has not been clearly established that this effect also persists in humans in a physiological manner.

A more likely possibility of a physiological function is the involvement in primary and secondary hemostasis. This concept is summarized in Fig. 3.

- β_2-G-I modulates platelet aggregation by inhibiting ADP-induced irreversible aggregation and release of constituents of dense granules. This effect is possibly achieved by an increase of cGMP production during platelet activation.
- As shown by many results, β_2-G-I exerts strong interaction with negatively charged phospholipids, inhibits the prothrombinase complex and the contact activation of blood coagulation. Thus this glycoprotein is a good candidate for:

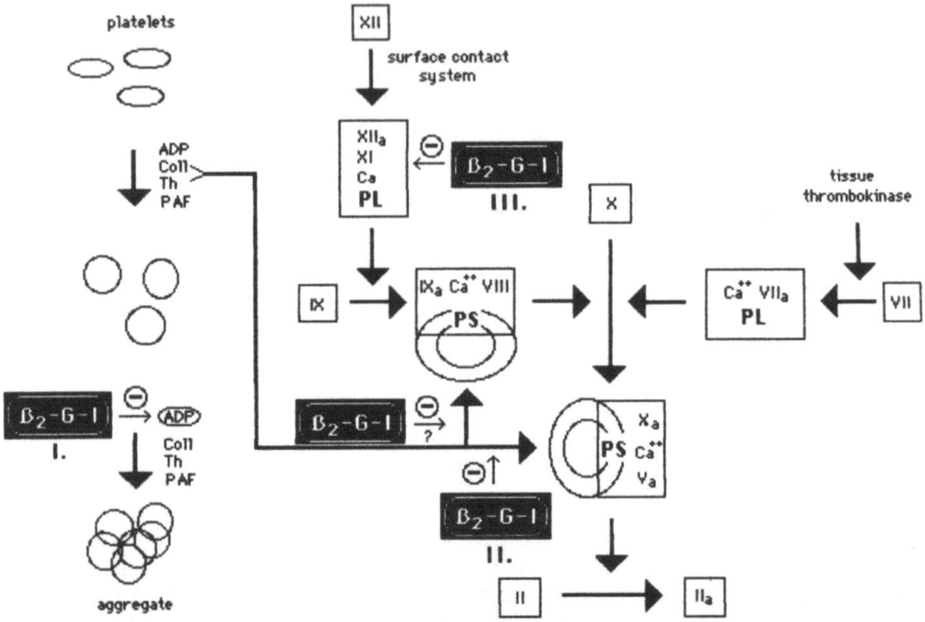

Fig. 3. Suggested interactions of β_2-G-I with primary and secondary hemostasis: *(I)* β_2-G-I inhibits the second wave of ADP-induced aggregation without influencing platelet activation triggered by collagen *(coll)*, thrombin *(Th)*, or platelet activating factor *(PAF)*; *(II)* β_2-G-I inhibits prothrombinase activity of phospholipid *(PL)* surfaces containing PS and prothrombinase activity of activated platelets; *(III)* β_2-G-I inhibits the surface contact system of blood coagulation. Blood coagulation factors are expressed in *Roman numbers (II–XII)*

(a) preventing a latent activation of coagulation by procoagulant lipid surfaces such as damaged blood cells (e.g., platelets, erythrocytes, and lymphocytes) or tissue cells; and

(b) a feedback inhibitor of prothrombinase activity of activated platelets in order to prevent a persisting stimulation of coagulation over longer periods of time.

Acknowledgement. This work was supported by a grant from the Austrian Research Foundation P5566, and the Austrian National Bank, grant No. 2663.

References

1. Schultze HE, Heide K, Haupt H (1961) Über ein bisher unbekanntes niedermolekulares β_2-Globulin des Humanserums. Naturwissenschaften 23: 719
2. Heide K, Haupt H (1964) Darstellung noch nicht therapeutisch angewandter Plasmaproteine. Behringwerke Mitt 43: 161–193
3. Schultze HE, Heremans JF (1966) Methods of plasma fractionation. Mol Biol Hum Proteins 1: 221
4. Heimburger N, Heide K, Haupt H (1964) Bausteinanalyse von Humanserumproteinen. Clin Chim Acta 10: 293–307
5. Haupt H, Heide K (1965) Isolierung und Eigenschaften eines β_2-Glykoproteins aus Humanserum. Clin Chim Acta 12: 419–424

6. Cleve H, Rittner C (1969) Further family studies on the genetic control of β_2-glycoprotein-I concentration in human serum. Humangenetik 7: 93-97
7. Kosaka S, Tohoku J (1977) β_2-Glycoprotein-I in rheumatoid arthritis. J Exp Med 122: 223-228
8. Cohnen G (1970) Immunochemical quantitation of β_2-glycoprotein-I in various diseases. J Lab Clin Med 75: 212-216
9. Chio LF, Oon CJ (1979) Changes in serum α_1, antitrypsin, α_1 acid glycoprotein and β_2-glycoprotein in patients with malignant hepatocellular carcinoma. Cancer 43: 596-604
10. Cleve H (1968) Genetic studies on the deficiency of β_2-glycoprotein-I of human serum. Humangenetik 5: 294-304
11. Polz E (1979) Isolation of a specific lipid binding protein from human serum by affinitychromatography using heparinsepharose. In: Peeters H (ed) Protides of biological fluids. Pergamon, Oxford, pp 817-820
12. Finlayson JS, Mushinski JF (1967) Separation of subfractions of human β_2-glycoprotein-I. Biochim Biophys Acta 147: 413-420
13. Polz E, Wurm H, Kostner GM (1981) Studies on the composition of the protein part of triglyceride-rich lipoproteins of human serum: isolation of polymorphic forms of β_2-glycoprotein-I. Artery 9: 305-315
14. Polz E, Kostner GM, Holasek A (1979) Studies on the protein composition of human serum very low lipoproteins: demonstration of the β_2-glycoprotein-I. Hoppe Seylers Z Physiol Chem 360: 1061-1067
15. Schousboe I (1983) Characterization of subfractions of β_2-glycoprotein-I: evidence for sialic acid microheterogeneity. Int J Biochem 15: 35-44
16. Nakaya Y, Schaefer EJ, Brewer HB (1980) Activation of human post heparin lipoprotein lipase by apolipoprotein H (β_2-glycoprotein-I). Biochem Biophys Res Commun 95: 1168-1172
17. Lee NS, Brewer HB, Osborne JC (1983) β_2-glycoprotein-I: molecular properties of an unusual apoliprotein, apolipoprotein H. J Biol Chem 258: 4765-4770
18. Lozier J, Takahashi N, Putnam FW (1984) Complete amino acid sequence of human plasma β_2-glycoprotein-I. Proc Natl Acad Sci USA 81: 3640-3644
19. Canfield WM, Kisiel W (1982) Evidence of normal function levels of activated protein C inhibition in combined factor V/VIII deficiency desease. J Clin Invest 70: 1260-1272
20. Burstein M, Scholnick HR (1972) Precipitation of chylomicrons and very low density lipoproteins from human with sodium lauryl sulfate. Life Sci 11: 177-184
21. Burstein M, Legmann P (1978) Precipitation of triglyceride-rich lipoproteins by synthetic anionic detergents. Role of β_2-glycoprotein-I. In: Peeters H (ed) Protides of biological fluids. Pergamon, Oxford, pp 407-410
22. Polz E, Kostner GM (1979) The binding of β_2-glycoprotein-I to human serum lipoproteins. FEBS Lett 102: 183-186
23. Polz E, Kostner GM (1979) Binding of β_2-glycoprotein-I to Intralipid: determination of the dissociation constant. Biochem Biophys Res Commun 90: 1305-1312
24. Polz E, Wurm H, Kostner GM (1980) Investigation on β_2-glycoprotein-I in the rat: isolation from serum and demonstration in lipoprotein density fractions. Int J Biochem 11: 265-270
25. Wurm H, Beubler E, Polz E, Kostner GM (1983) β_2-glycoprotein-I: in vitro and in vivo studies with triglyceride-rich lipoproteins. In: Crepaldi G (ed) Arteriosclerotic brain disease. Raven, New York, pp 153-158
26. Wurm H, Beubler E, Polz E, Holasek A, Kostner GM (1982) Studies on the possible function of β_2-glycoprotein-I: influence in the triglyceride metabolism in the rat. Metabolism 31: 484-486
27. Kroll J, Larsen JK, Loft H, Ezban M, Wallevik K, Faber M (1976) DNA-binding proteins in Yoshida ascites fluid. Biochim Biophys Acta 434: 490-496
28. Schousboe I (1978) Characterization of an agglutinin from human serum. Biochim Biophys Acta 543: 373-382
29. Schousboe I (1982) Addition of deoxycholate in electroimmunoassay and crossed immunofocusing for quantification of β_2-glycoprotein-I and its subfractions. J Biochem Biophys Methods 6: 105-114
30. Schousboe I (1980) Binding of β_2-glycoprotein-I to platelets: effect on adenylate cyclase activity. Thromb Res 19: 225-237
31. Wurm H (1984) β_2-glycoprotein-I (apolipoprotein-H) interaction with phospholipid vesicles. Int J Biochem 16: 511-515

32. Nimpf J, Wurm H, Kostner GM (1985) Interaction of β_2-glycoprotein-I with human blood platelets: influence upon the ADP-induced aggregation. Thromb Haemost 54: 397-401
33. Nimpf J, Wurm H, Kostner GM (1985) Wechselwirkung von β_2-glycoprotein-I (Apo-H) mit Blutplättchen. In: Proceedings of the 5th international Dresden lipid symposium, pp 239-296
34. Nimpf J, Gries A, Wurm H, Kostner GM (1985) Influence of β_2-glycoprotein-I upon the content of cAMP and cGMP in human blood platelets. Thromb Haemost 54: 824-827
35. Nimpf J, Wurm H, Kostner GM (1986) β_2-glycoprotein-I (apo-H) inhibits the release reaction of human platelets during ADP-induced aggregation. Atherosclerosis (in press)
36. Nimpf J, Nimpf M, Gries A, Pfeiffer KP, Wurm H, Kostner GM (1986) Plasma lipids, lipoproteins, and apoproteins in relation to platelet activation in normolipemic persons. Atheroma 1: 10-15
37. Rosing J, van Rijen JLML, Bevers EM, van Dieijen G, Comfurius P, Zwaal RFA (1985) The role of activated human platelets in prothrombin and factor X activation. Blood 65: 319-332
38. Chap HJ, Zwaal RFA, van Deenen LLM (1977) Action of highly purified phospolipases on blood platelets. Evidence for an asymmetric distribution of phospholipids in the surface membrane. Biochim Biophys Acta 467: 146-164
39. Bevers EM, Comfurius P, Zwaal RFA (1983) Changes in membrane phospholipid distribution during platelet activation. Biochim Biophys Acta 736: 57-66
40. Bevers EM, Comfurius P, van Rijn JLML, Hemker HC, Zwaal RFA (1982) Generation of prothrombin converting activity and the exposure of phosphatidylserine at the outer surface of platelets. Eur J Biochem 122: 429-436
41. Rosing J, Tans G, Govers-Riemslag JWP, Zwaal RFA, Hemker HC (1980) The role of phospholipids and factor V_m in the prothrombinase complex. J Biol Chem 255: 274-283
42. Van Dieijen G, Tans G, Rosing J, Hemker HC (1981) The role of phospholipid and factor VIII_m in the activation of bovine factor X. J Biol Chem 256: 3433-3442
43. Nimpf J, Bevers EM, Till U, Wurm H, Kostner GM, Zwaal RFA (1986) Prothrombinase activity of human platelets is inhibited by β_2-glycoprotein-I. Biochim Biophys Acta 884: 142-149
44. Schousboe I (1985) β_2-glycoprotein-I: a plasma inhibitor of the contact activation of the intrinsic blood coagulation pathway. Blood 66: 1086-1091

Diet, Lipoproteins and Atherosclerosis

Changes in Diet, Serum Cholesterol, and Mortality from Coronary Heart Disease in Spain

R. Carmena

Introduction

In 1953, a study conducted in Madrid by Ancel Keys et al. [1] found that men 40–49 years of age had a serum cholesterol concentration of 185 mg/dl; their total fat ingestion (mostly mono-unsaturated) accounted for less that 30% of the daily total energy intake. Coronary heart disease (CHD) was not common in Spain then, and Ancel Keys gave up his project of including Spain in the Seven Countries Study "because of lack of funds and interested local personnel." Since then, however, significant changes have occurred in the eating habits of the Spanish people, together with new social habits, such as an increase in tobacco and alcohol consumption, and socioeconomic changes. Overall, they have resulted in an increase in the rate of mortality from CHD in Spain over the past 15 years. We will briefly review some of these changes here.

Changes in the Diet

As shown by several dietary surveys conducted by Varela et al. [2, 3], the consumption of meat, eggs, milk, and milk products increased by 52% between 1961 and 1979, while the consumption of bread decreased from 108 to 71 kg per capita per annum over a similar period. For instance, in 1958, meat accounted for 17% of total food expenses, a figure equal to that of bread and cereal products in the same year. In 1981, the figure for meat rose to 29%, while that for bread and cereals fell to 10% of the total cost.

In 1965, the percent ages of daily energy intake derived from proteins, fat, and carbohydrates were 10%, 34%, and 53% respectively. A more recent survey [3] finished in 1984 gave, for the same three nutrients, figures of 13%, 40%, and 46% respectively. Fish consumption has not changed, Spain still having a higher per capita fish-consumption than any other country in Europe; consumption of olive oil, the principal vegetable oil, has also remained stable over this period.

Serum Cholesterol

In 1975, the results of a study of a group of healthy male and female hospital workers in Valencia [4], when compared with the findings of a United States study published in the same year, showed that the mean serum cholesterol levels of the Spanish workers were 15 mg/dl lower than those of the same age groups in the United States. However, it is believed, that mean serum cholesterol levels have risen consistently over the 10 years since these studies were completed. Our more recent data (1985) show that 28% of males between the ages of 40 and 59 now have a cholesterol level of 250 mg/dl or higher. By comparison, in 1975 only 22% of men between the ages of 35 and 54 had a level above 250 mg/dl. In addition, judging by comparisons of cholesterol levels measured in Manresa by Balaguer-Vintró and co-workers [5] in 1968 and again in 1978, for similar age groups, mean serum cholesterol levels have risen by 10-14 mg/dl over this period. Circumstancial evidence also comes from studies of 18-year-old draftees into the Spanish army, whose mean serum cholesterol concentration has steadily risen from 180 mg/dl in the 1950s to the present 200 mg/dl.

Thus, we can conclude that the prevalence of hypercholesterolemia has increased over the past 20 years in Spain [6].

Mortality from CHD

As we have shown, the data available, although limited, suggest that dietary habits and serum cholesterol levels may be changing in an adverse way. As might be anticipated, mortality from CHD has also increased significantly over the same period of time [7, 8].

Data collected in 1979 show that mortality from CHD has risen in both males and females aged 35-64 years [7]. Trends between 1968 and 1977 showed a significant increase in annual mortality from CHD of 6.2% for men and 4.4% for women aged 40-69 years [8]. Moreover, World Health Organization figures for rates of death from CHD for European men show that in Spain, for men aged 69-77 years, the death rate has increased by more than 52%. As a result, Spain, which had a lower CHD mortality rate in previous decades, now has a mortality approaching those of Italy, France, Belgium, and other Central European countries. It should be pointed out, however, that during the last 6 years of observation mortalities from CHD for both men and women have begun to plateau, following the steep increase to 79.2 deaths/100000 in 1975.

Conclusions

The recent increase in mortality from CHD in Spain could be explained by different factors. Undoubtedly, the existence of a wide network of National Health Institute hospitals - nonexistent 20 years ago - could have contributed to a higher awareness of the disease and to an increase in the number of deaths due to CHD recorded on death certificates. Also, changes in the percentage of correct diagnosis cannot be excluded. There are, however, reasons to believe that the increase in mortality from CHD is indeed a true phenomenon, as pointed out recently by Balaguer-Vintró and Sans [8].

Besides changes in dietary habits and serum cholesterol levels, the prevalence of other factors increasing the risk of CHD should be considered. Cigarette smoking continues to be a frequent habit among the male adult Spanish population, reaching 60% of subjects in some surveys. A continuous rise in the sales of cigarettes has occurred, the increase from 1957 to 1980 being 146% [9]. Similarly, the prevalence of hypertension in different areas of Spain has been reported to be between 11% and 13% for the 40-59-year age group [6, 10]. Recently published studies by Pardell [11] on hypertension in Spain show a higher prevalence in some areas in the north of the country, where 20% of the population was found to be hypertensive.

The future trend of mortality from CHD in Spain remains uncertain, but the changes in risk factors, presented here, are a source of concern. In fact, the present levels of several risk factors in the Spanish population are higher than the mortality figures for CHD would suggest. This is probably because the time of exposure of the population to the new, high levels of risk is still short and so a rising mortality from CHD could be expected in future years. Dietary measures being advocated to prevent this include decreasing the intake of saturated fat, increasing that of polyunsaturated fat, and maintaining levels of the most widely used mono-unsaturate, olive oil. Likewise, the importance of reducing other risk factors, such as cigarette smoking and hypertension, is being emphasized by the Spanish Society of Cardiology and other professional bodies.

References

1. Keys A, Vivanco F, Rodriguez-Minon JL, Keys MH, Castro Mendoza H (1954) Studies on the diet, body fatness and serum cholesterol in Madrid, Spain. Metabolism 3: 195-212
2. Varela G, Garcia D, Moreiras-Varela O (1971) La nutricion de los españoles. Instituto de Desarrollo Económico, Madrid
3. Varela G, Moreiras-Varela O (1985) Encuesta sobre la nutricion de los españoles, 1984. Instituto Nacional de Estadística, Madrid
4. Carmena R, Sanchis J, Gonzalez-Bayo E, Llavador J, Ascaso J (1975) Valores de lípidos y lipoproteínas séricas obtenidos en una poblacion clínicamente normal. Rev Clin Esp 138: 125-130
5. Tomas L, Bernades E, Sans S, Balaguer-Vintro I (1979) Modificacion espontánea de los factores de riesgo coronario de una poblacion laboral en un intervalo de 5 años. Rev Esp Cardiol 32: 593-600
6. World Health Organization European Collaborative Group (1980) Multifactorial trial in the prevention of coronary heart disease. I. Recruitment and initial findings. Eur Heart J 1: 73-80
7. Cortina Greus P, Segarra Castello L, Sainz Sanchez C (1982) Evolucion de la mortalidad por cardiopatía isquémica y accidentes cerebovasculares en España (1951-1977). Rev Esp Geriatría y Gerontol 17: 69-80
8. Balaguer-Vintro I, Sans S (1985) Coronary-heart disease mortality trends and related factors in Spain. Cardiology 72: 97-104
9. Servicio de Estudios de la Tabacalera (1981) I. Actualidad Tabaquera. Spanish Ministry of Economy, Madrid
10. Ruiz de la Fuente S, Cortina Greus P, Sanchez J (1983) Programa sobre deteccion y control de la hipertension en el medio laboral. I. Prevalencia. Med Clin (Barc) 80: 649-651
11. Pardell H (1984) La hipertension arterial en España. Liga Española de la lucha contra la hipertension arterial, Madrid

Modified Fat Diets and Serum Lipoproteins

P. Schwandt and P. Weisweiler

Introduction

A raised serum cholesterol level is thought to be responsible for the accelerated development of coronary artery disease [1, 2]. Changes in diet are commonly proposed to reduce the risk from atherosclerotic diseases [3, 4]. Even moderate alterations of fat saturation or fat restriction, or both, can produce significant decreases in serum cholesterol levels [5–7].

The hypcholesterolemic effect of changing dietary fat is mainly due to a decrease of low-density lipoproteins (LDL) [5–8] that are considered atherogenic [9]. This effect must be contrasted with the possibly adverse effect of polyunsaturated fat diets on the concentration of high-density lipoproteins (HDL) [10, 11] that are considered an antiatherogenic factor [12]. Some nutritional studies have shown that modified fat diets lower, furthermore, the concentration of very low-density lipoproteins (VLDL), in particular that of cholesterol-enriched VLDL [13], which are considered just as atherogenic as LDL [14].

This paper presents measurements of the concentration and composition of serum lipoproteins in normolipidemic subjects eating moderately modified fat diets. The experiments were designed to determine the major dietary factor responsible for the lowering of atherogenic serum lipoprotein levels.

Materials and Methods

Subjects

After giving their written informed consents, 22 healthy women were included. They ranged in age from 22 to 55 years (mean ± SD: 36 ± 12) and weighed from 50.5 to 69.0 kg (60.1 ± 6.0). Six women were premenopausal. The mean percentage of ideal body weight was 105% ± 11%. Serum cholesterol levels on entry to the study ranged from 145 to 275 mg/dl (mean 224 ± 44) and triglyceride levels from 38 to 174 mg/dl (mean 83 ± 35). All subjects were nuns living in a nunnery and consuming the same diet for several months. Physical activity levels were moderate and remained constant throughout the study.

Table 1. Nutrient composition of the reference and therapeutic diets and body weight

	Reference diet	Polyunsaturated diet	Low-fat, polyunsaturated diet
Calories, kcal/day	2000-2200	2000-2200	2000-2200
Protein, % of energy	12	12	12
Vegetable protein (% of protein)	35	35	35
Fag (% of energy)	42	42	32
Saturated (% of energy)	21.4	13.2	10.1
Monounsaturated (% of energy)	17.2	15.6	11.8
Polyunsaturated (% of energy)	3.4	13.2	10.1
P/S ratio	0.16	1.0	1.0
Cholesterol (mg/day)	400	400	400
Carbohydrates[a] (% of energy)	46	46	56
Dietary fiber (g/day)	21	19	25
Body weight (kg ± SD)	60.1 ± 6.0	59.8 ± 6.1	60.2 ± 6.2

[a] Monosaccharides and disaccharides contributed 21% of energy in all three diets.

Study Design

Each participant consumed a reference diet followed by two modified fat diets (Table 1). Diets were prepared by a dietitian in the nunnery kitchen. All meals were eaten in the dining room under close control. Compliance was estimated by the stability of body weight, by daily personal contact between dietitian and subjects, and by 24-h dietary recalls every week.

The three diets were fed for 6 weeks each. The reference diet [polyunsaturated/saturated (P/S) ratio 0.16, fat 42%, and carbohydrate 46% of energy, respectively] was designed to simulate the composition of the previous diet and was made up of whole foods. Saturated fat and cholesterol came from meat and sausage, poultry, fish, milk, and cheese. Compared with the reference diet the first therapeutic diet (polyunsaturated diet) differed in fat saturation (P/S ratio 1.0). Polyunsaturated fatty acids were provided by sunflower oil and diet margarine. The second therapeutic diet (low-fat, polyunsaturated diet) differed in fat saturation (P/S ratio 1.0) and in the relative proportion of fats and carbohydrates (32% and 56% of energy, respectively). This diet included less whole milk and diet margarine, but more bread and potatoes, than did the polyunsaturated diet. All diets were planned so as to be precisely isocaloric with the estimated energy intake of the participants as assessed by four 24-h dietary recalls prior to the study.

Analytical Methods

Venous blood samples were drawn with minimal hemostasis from the subjects in a sitting position. All examinations were made in the morning in the fasting state after each dietary period. Specimens were centrifuged and transported immediately to the laboratory. VLDL were isolated from serum by ultracentrifugation at 1.006 *g*/ml at 105000 *g* for 22 h at 4 °C in Beckman 40.3 rotors (Munich, FRG), and the lipoprotein fractions were recovered by tube slicing [15]. HDL in the infranate were separated from LDL by precipitation of LDL using a commercially available combination of sodium phosphotungstate and magnesium chloride, according to the method described (Boehringer kit, Mannheim, FRG). The mass of cholesterol and triglycerides in whole serum and separated lipoproteins was determined in an automated analyzer by enzymatic techniques (Boehringer kits). LDL cholesterol was calculated as the difference in the mass of cholesterol in the infranate and in HDL.

Concentrations of apolipoproteins A-I (only in serum), B, C-II, C-III, and E in serum, VLDL, and infranate were measured by endpoint immunonephelometry [16, 17]. The detergent hydroxypolyethoxydodecane (Thesit, Desitinwerke Karl Klinke, Hamburg, FRG) was added to a final concentration of 0.33 g/liter in the samples and standards. Standard curves were obtained by dilution of isolated apolipoproteins and LDL and were run simultaneously with the samples. The coefficients of variation of these assays ranged from 2% to 5%.

Because each subject served as her own control, statistical analysis ($p < 0.01$) was made using the paired Wilcoxon rank test [18] for comparisons among reference and therapeutic diets.

Results

The effects of the therapeutic diets on serum and lipoprotein lipids and apolipoproteins are shown in Tables 2 and 3. Compared with the reference diet, consumption of the polyunsaturated diet decreased the mean levels of serum cholesterol, triglycerides, and apolipoprotein B by 11.4%, 19.8%, and 9.5%, respectively. VLDL cholesterol, triglyceride, and apolipoprotein B levels fell by 33.1%, 33.9%, and 23.8%, respectively, while LDL cholesterol and apolipoprotein B (infranate) levels decreased by 13.5% and 8.8%, respectively. Mean concentration of HDL cholesterol and apolipoproteins C-II, C-III$_1$, and E were statistically unaltered by this diet.

Table 2. Response to therapeutic diets: serum and lipoprotein lipid levels

	Reference diet	Polyunsaturated diet	Low-fat, polyunsaturated diet
Cholesterol	219 ± 43	194 ± 40[a]	193 ± 28[a]
Triglycerides	80 ± 24	64 ± 18[a]	75 ± 23[b]
VLDL cholesterol	12 ± 6	8 ± 3[a]	9 ± 4[a]
VLDL triglycerides	50 ± 18	33 ± 13[a]	47 ± 13[b]
LDL cholesterol	156 ± 43	135 ± 38[a]	132 ± 33[a]
HDL cholesterol	47 ± 9	49 ± 8	48 ± 9

Results in mg/dl are mean ± SD, $n = 22$.
[a, b] $p < 0.01$ ([a] reference diet versus therapeutic diets; [b] polyunsaturated diet versus low-fat polyunsaturated diet).

Table 3. Response to therapeutic diets: serum and lipoprotein apolipoprotein levels

	Apolipoprotein levels (mean ± SD) of 22 subjects		
	Reference diet	Polyunsaturated diet	Low-fat, polyunsaturated diet
Apolipoprotein A-I	137.8 ± 10.3	133.1 ± 5.8	140.1 ± 6.5
Apolipoprotein B			
Total	105.6 ± 18.2	95.6 ± 14.6[a]	92.3 ± 11.7[a]
VLDL	12.1 ± 3.5	9.2 ± 3.8[a]	7.0 ± 2.3[a,b]
Infranate	92.9 ± 13.8	85.5 ± 12.6[a]	85.2 ± 12.1[a]
Apolipoprotein E			
Total	10.0 ± 0.9	9.8 ± 0.6	9.3 ± 0.7
VLDL	3.4 ± 0.4	3.3 ± 0.2	2.1 ± 0.3[a,b]
Infranate	6.4 ± 0.8	6.4 ± 0.7	6.9 ± 0.8
Apolipoprotein C-II			
Total	3.8 ± 0.3	3.6 ± 0.3	3.5 ± 0.3
VLDL	1.1 ± 0.2	1.0 ± 0.1	1.2 ± 0.3
Infranate	2.6 ± 0.2	2.3 ± 0.2	2.4 ± 0.3
Apolipoprotein C-III			
Total	10.9 ± 2.1	9.7 ± 2.5	9.9 ± 2.6
VLDL	3.1 ± 0.8	2.4 ± 0.5	2.6 ± 0.6
Infranate	7.6 ± 1.9	7.3 ± 2.0	7.2 ± 1.8

Results in mg/dl are mean ± SD, n = 22. [a, b] $p < 0.01$ ([a]reference diet versus therapeutic diets; [b]polyunsaturated diet versus low-fat, polyunsaturated diet).

Consumption of the low-fat, polyunsaturated diet also resulted in a decrease in the mean concentrations of serum, VLDL, and LDL cholesterol by 11.8%, 26.8%, 15.4%, respectively, and of apolipoprotein B by 12.5%, 41.6%, and 8.7%, respectively. Furthermore, the apolipoprotein E distribution in lipoproteins changed: VLDL apolipoprotein levels fell by 25.9%, while serum and VLDL triglyceride levels and the concentrations of HDL cholesterol and apolipoproteins A-I, concentrations of HDL cholesterol and apolipoproteins A-I, C-II, and C-III remained statistically unchanged. The mean cholesterol-triglyceride mass ratio within VLDL declined from 0.24 ± 0.12 to 0.19 ± 0.08 ($p < 0.01$) during this diet.

When compared to the polyunsaturated diet, the low-fat, polyunsaturated diet had reduced apolipoprotein B and E contents (−23.9% and −36.1%, respectively) in VLDL. In VLDL, the mean lipid/apolipoprotein mass ratio rose, therefore, from 3.49 ± 0.80 to 5.91 ± 1.07 ($p < 0.01$) during the low-fat, polyunsaturated diet.

Discussion

The purpose of the present work was to separate the effects of changes of dietary fat saturation from changes of the dietary fat intake in normolipidemic subjects. Substituting polyunsaturated fats for saturated fats in one characteristic feature of the modified fat diet. The first therapeutic diet was typical of a conventional polyunsaturated diet, by using a moderately increased P/S ratio of 1.0. This diet was designed to answer the question of how far serum, VLDL, and LDL cholesterol levels could be reduced and whether adverse effects on HDL could be observed during this diet. The second therapeutic diet takes account of the recommendations [19, 20] to replace part of dietary fats by complex carbohydrates. This diet was, therefore, designed to point out the additive effect of changes in the relative proportion of dietary fats and carbohydrates on serum lipoproteins.

The concentrations of both VLDL and LDL seen when the polyunsaturated diet was consumed have been associated with a reduced rate of synthesis in both classes of lipoproteins [21, 22]. Another investigation found an increased fractional catabolic rate of LDL during the polyunsaturated diet [23]. The uniform decrease in VLDL and LDL cholesterol and apolipoprotein B levels appear to be typical for polyunsaturated diets [24], while lowered HDL values after diets high in polyunsaturated fats [10] can obviously be prevented by even moderate changes in fat saturation [10].

Replacing as little as 10% of the fats with carbohydrates during the low-fat, polyunsaturated diet was followed by profound alterations in the VLDL components. It is well-known that VLDL triglyceride levels increase after diets low in total fat are consumed [25-27]; this increase has been explained by a raised hepatic synthesis and secretion of triglyceride-rich, large VLDL. The marked decrease of VLDL apolipoprotein B on the other hand, reflects a reduced production rate of LDL precursor lipoprotein particles by the liver [28]. Possible changes in the VLDL apolipoprotein B degradation during low-fat feeding have been, furthermore, assumed [29]. However, somewhat different effects on VLDL apolipoproteins C have been reported: although short-term, high-carbohydrate intake raises the levels of serum and VLDL apolipoprotein C-II and C-III [30, 31], therapeutic diets seem to have only small or no effects on the concentration and distribution of these apolipoproteins ([32] and our study).

Beside the decrease of VLDL apolipoprotein B, the decrease of apolipoprotein E is a constant finding after fat restriction [7, 13]. Opposite effects have been observed after high-cholesterol and/or saturated fat diets [33-37]. Changes in VLDL apolipoprotein composition are of interest because apolipoprotein B [38] and apolipoprotein E [38] serve as recognition markers for the cellular receptors through which some lipoproteins are taken up by cells [39]. Small VLDL are taken up more readily than the larger ones [40], a difference that may be related to differences in the conformation or surface disposition of apolipoprotein B on the VLDL particle. Beside the effects on LDL, the apparent modification of VLDL (rich in triglycerides, poor in apolipoproteins B and E) by fat restriction must be, therefore, considered in mediating possible effects of therapeutic diets on atherogenesis.

Summary

We investigated the effects of fat saturation and fat restriction on very low-, low-, and high-density lipoproteins (VLDL, LDL, and HDL). Twenty-two normolipidemic women were given a reference diet, a polyunsaturated fat diet, and a low-fat, polyunsaturated fat diet for 6 weeks each. The polyunsaturated diet decreased cholesterol and apolipoprotein B levels in VLDL (−33.1% and −23.8%) and in LDL (−13.5% and −8.8%) without affecting HDL. The low-fat, polyunsaturated fat diet resulted in a reincrease of VLDL triglycerides, but not of VLDL cholesterol. The concentration of VLDL apolipoprotein B fell further (−41.6%). VLDL apolipoprotein E also fell (−25.9%). This study indicates that a low-fat, polyunsaturated fat diet lowers VLDL and LDL without affecting HDL and alters the composition of VLDL.

References

1. Marmot MG (1979) Epidemiological basis for the prevention of coronary heart diesease. Bull WHOrg 57: 331-347
2. Stamler J (1979) Population studies. In: Levy R, Rifkind B, Dennis B, Ernst N (eds) Nutrition, lipids and coronary heart disease. Raven, New York, pp 25-88
3. Stamler J (1980) Lifestyles, major risk factors, proof and public policy. Circulation 58: 3-19
4. Lewis B (1980) Dietary prevention of ischemic heart disease - a policy for the 80's. Br Med J 281: 177-180
5. Ernst N, Bowen P, Fisher M, Schaefer EJ, Levy RI (1980) Changes in plasma lipids and lipoproteins after a modified fat diet. Lancet 2: 111-113
6. Lewis B, Katan M, Merkx I, Miller NE, Hammett F, Kay RM, Nobels A, Swan AV (1981) Towards an improved lipid-lowering diet: additive effects of changes in nutrient intake. Lancet 2: 1310-1313
7. Weisweiler P, Janetschek P, Schwandt P (1985) Influence of polyunsaturated fats and fat restriction on serum lipoproteins in humans. Metabolism 34: 83-87
8. Schaefer EJ, Levy RJ, Ernst ND, van Sant FD, Brewer HB (1981) The effects of low-cholesterol, high-polyunsaturated fat, and low-fat diets on plasma lipid and lipoprotein cholesterol levels in normal and hypercholesterolemic subjects. Am J Clin Nutr 34: 1758-1763
9. Kannel WB, Castelli WP, Gordon T (1979) Cholesterol in the prediction of atherosclerotic disease. Ann Intern Med 90: 85-91
10. Shepherd J, Packard CJ, Patsch JR, Gotto AM (1978) Effects of dietary polyunsaturated and saturated fat on the properties of high-density lipoproteins and the metabolism of apolipoprotein A-I. J Clin Invest 61: 1582-1592
11. Schwandt P, Janetschek P, Weisweiler P (1982) High-density lipoproteins unaffected by dietary fat modification. Atherosclerosis 44: 9-17
12. Castelli WP, Doyle JT, Gordon T, Hames CG, Hjortland MC, Hulley SB, Kagan A, Zukel WJ (1977) HDL cholesterol and other lipids in coronary heart disease. The cooperative lipoprotein phenotyping study. Circulation 55: 767-772
13. Weisweiler P, Drosner M, Janetschek P, Schwandt P (1983) Changes in very low- and low-density lipoproteins with dietary fat modification. Atherosclerosis 49: 325-332
14. Tatami R, Mabuchi H, Ueda K, Ueda R, Haba T, Kametani T, Ito S et al. (1981) Intermediate-density lipoprotein and cholesterol-rich very low-density lipoprotein in angiographically determined coronary artery disease. Circulation 64: 1174-1184
15. Havel RJ, Eder HA, Bragdon JH (1955) The distribution and chemical composition of ultracentrifugally separated lipoproteins in human serum. J Clin Invest 34: 1345-1353
16. Weisweiler P, Schwandt P, Friedl C (1984) Determination of human apolipoprotein A-I, B and E by laser nephelometry. J Clin Chem Clin Biochem 22: 113-118
17. Weisweiler P, Schwandt P, Friedl C (1984) Determination of human apolipoproteins C-II and C-III by laser nephelometry. Fresenius Z Anal Chem 317: 708-709
18. Geigy (1980) Wissenschaftliche Tabellen, Teilband Statistik. Ciba-Geigy, Basel, p 230
19. Grundy SM, Bilheimer D, Blackburn H, Brown WV, Kwiterowich PO, Mattson F, Schonfeld G, Weidman WH (1982) Rationale of the diet-heart statement of the American Heart Association. Circulation 65: 839 A-854 A
20. NACNE Report (1983) Proposals for nutritional guidelines for health education in Britain. Lancet 2: 835-837

21. Cortese C, Levy Y, Janus ED, Lewis B (1983) Modes of action of lipid-lowering diets in man: studies of apolipoprotein B kinetics in relation to fat consumption and dietary fatty acid composition. Eur J Clin Invest 13: 79-85
22. Nestel PJ, Connor WE, Reardon MF, Connor S, Wong S, Boston R (1984) Suppression by diets rich in fish oil of very low-density lipoprotein production in man. J Clin Invest 74: 82-89
23. Shepherd J, Packard CJ, Grundy SM, Jeshuran D, Gotto AM, Taunton OD (1980) Effects of saturated and polyunsaturated fat diets on the chemical composition and metabolism of low-density lipoproteins in man. J Lipid Res 21: 91-99
24. Vega GL, Groszek E, Wolf R, Grundy SM (1982) Influence of polyunsaturated fats on composition of plasma lipoproteins and apolipoproteins. J Lipid Res 23: 811-822
25. Quarfordt SH, Frank A, Shames DM, Berman M, Steinberg D (1970) Very low-density lipoprotein triglyceride transport in type IV hyperlipoproteinemia and the effects of carbohydrate-rich diets. J Clin Invest 49: 2281-2297
26. Schonfeld G (1970) Changes in the composition of very low-density lipoprotein during carbohydrate induction in man. J Lab Clin Med 75: 206-211
27. Ruderman NB, Jones AL, Krauss RM, Shafrir E (1974) A biochemical and morphologic study of very low-density lipoproteins in carbohydrate induced hypertriglyceridemia. J Clin Invest 50: 1355-1368
28. Melish J, Le NA, Ginsberg H, Brown WU, Steinberg D (1980) Dissociation of the rates of production of apoprotein B and triglycerides of very low-density lipoproteins during high-carbohydrate feeding in man. Am J Physiol 239: E354-362
29. Ginsberg HN, Le NA, Melish J, Steinberg D, Brown WV (1981) Effect of a high-carbohydrate diet on apoprotein B catabolism in man. Metabolism 30: 347-353
30. Falko JM, Schonfeld G, Witztum JL, Kolar JB, Salmon P (1980) Effects of short-term, high-carbohydrate, fat-free diet on plasma levels of apo C-II and apo C-III and on the apo C subspecies in human plasma lipoproteins. Metabolism 29: 654-661
31. Kashyap ML, Barnhart RL, Srivastava LS, Perisutti G, Vink P, Allen C, Hogg E, Brady D, Glueck CJ, Jackson RL (1982) Effects of dietary carbohydrate and fat on plasma lipoproteins and apolipoproteins C-II and C-III in healthy men. J Lipid Res 23: 877-886
32. Witztum JL, Schonfeld G (1978) Carbohydrate diet-induced changes in very low-density lipoprotein composition and structure. Diabetes 27: 1215-1229
33. Tan MH, Dickinson MA, Albers JJ, Havel RJ, Cheung MC, Vigne JL (1980) The effect of a high-cholesterol and saturated-fat diet on serum high-density lipoprotein cholesterol, apoprotein A-I, and apoprotein E levels in normolipidemic humans. Am J Clin Nutr 22: 2559-2665
34. Mistry P, Miller NE, Laker M, Hazzard WR, Lewis B (1981) Individual variation in the effects of dietary cholesterol on plasma lipoproteins and cellular cholesterol homeostasis in man. J Clin Invest 67: 493-502
35. Nestel P, Tada N, Billington T, Huff M, Fidge N (1982) Changes in very low-density lipoproteins with cholesterol in man. Metabolism 31: 398-405
36. Cole TG, Patsch W, Kuisk J, Gonen B, Schonfeld G (1983) Increases in dietary cholesterol and fat raise levels of apoprotein E-containing lipoproteins in the plasma of man. J Clin Endocrinol Metab 56: 1108-1115
37. Fisher EA, Blum CB, Zannis VI, Breslow JL (1983) Independent effects of dietary saturated fat and cholesterol on plasma lipids, lipoproteins, and apolipoproteins E. J Lipid Res 24: 1039-1048
38. Mahley RW (1978) Alterations in plasma lipoproteins induced by cholesterol feeding in animals including man. In: Dietschy J, Gotto AM, Outko JA (eds) Disturbances in lipid and lipoprotein metabolism. American Physiology Society, Bethesda, pp 181-197
39. Mahley RW, Hui DY, Innerarity TL, Weisgraber KH (1981) Two indipendent lipoprotein receptors on hepatic membranes of dog, swine, and man. Apo-B, E and Apo-E receptors. J Clin Invest 68: 1197-1206
40. Schonfeld G, Patsch W, Pfleger B, Witztum JL, Weidman SW (1979) Lipolysis produces changes in the immunoreactivity and cell reactivity of very low-density lipoproteins. J Clin Invest 64: 1288-1297

Essential Fatty Acids, Marine Oils, Olive Oil and Coronary Heart Disease

M. F. Oliver

Introduction

Interest in the specific effects of individual fatty acids on the pathogenesis of coronary heart disease (CHD) has been limited. There are a number of reasons for this. They include (1) the fact that the whole field of CHD has been dominated for years by cholesterol metabolism, (2) the indication from cross-cultural surveys of food habits that there are strong relationships between dietary saturated fat (as a whole) and serum cholesterol, on the one hand, and age-standardised 5-year CHD rates, on the other [1], and (3) the fact that virtually all polyunsaturated fatty acids have quite a profound effect in lowering plasma cholesterol and low-density lipoprotein (LDL) cholesterol, and this has come to be regarded as an adequate end in itself because of the presumed but unproven benefit which populations and individuals (with the exception of those with very high levels) may obtain from reduction of raised serum and LDL cholesterol.

Far less attention has been given to the effects of specific fatty acids on lipoproteins, thrombosis, membrane fluidity and function, blood pressure and other pathogenic mechanisms. The possibility that some monoenoic fatty acids may differ in their effects on serum lipoprotein concentrations compared with polyenoic fatty acids has recently re-emerged. The fact that CHD-prone populations and patients with CHD might be relatively deficient in some fatty acids, particularly linoleic acid, has only recently been considered seriously. Interest in the effects of marine oils on thrombosis is not new but has also been slow to develop.

Essential Fatty Acids

The main essential fatty acid for the maintenance of normal biology in man is linoleic acid (18: 2, n-6); it is the principal precursor of arachidonic acid (20: 4, n-6), which is itself an essential, fatty acid in some species. Linoleic acid (n-6) should be distinguished from the n-3 family of fatty acids of which α-linolenic (18: 3, n-3) is the parent and also an essential fatty acid (Fig. 1).

Over the last 10 years, we in Edinburgh have demonstrated that there is an inverse relationship between adipose linoleic acid and CHD. The Edinburgh-Stockholm Study [2] showed that healthy men in a CHD-prone population (Edinburgh) had significantly less adipose linoleic acid than comparable men aged 40 in Stockholm, where the incidence of CHD was one-third. This interpopulation difference in the concentration of adipose linoleic acid has recently been confirmed by us with the

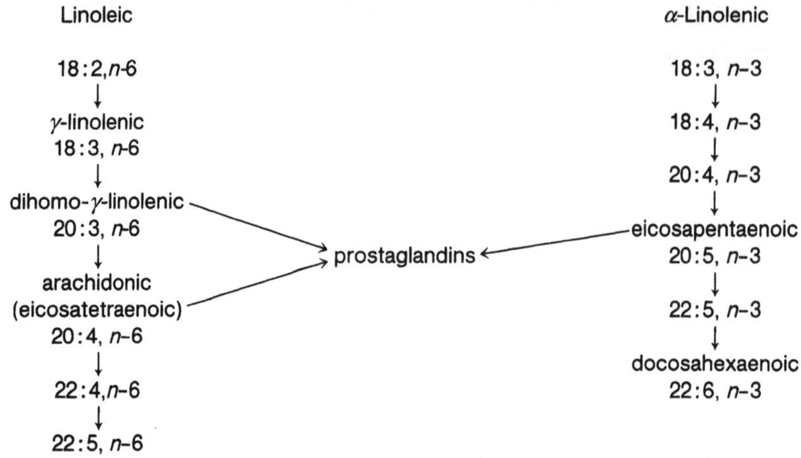

Fig. 1. Simplified metabolic pathways leading to increased unsaturation

demonstration of low adipose linoleic acid concentrations in North Karelia and Scotland, in contrast to relatively high levels in South Italy where CHD is far less common [3].

We have also demonstrated that, within a random population of 400 men in Scotland, apparently healthy individuals who were found to have occult CHD had lower adipose linoleic acid concentrations than comparable healthy men without CHD [4]. These data were obtained from 28 men who answered an angina questionnaire positively or who were found to have electrocardiographic evidence of *Q*-wave infarction. As men were unaware that they had CHD, and therefore could not have reported it to anyone, there can be no question of them having been advised to change their diet.

Thus, it has been possible to demonstrate between populations and within a population that CHD is associated with low concentrations of adipose linoleic acid. The turnover time of adipose linoleic acid is in the region of 10–12 months [5], and so the low concentrations of linoleic acid in adipose tissue found in these cross-sectional surveys reflect long-term eating habits and do not reflect last weeks' food, as it were.

Confirmation of these findings is now available from our recently completed formal case-control study [6]. This shows that there is an inverse relative risk of angina pectoris and myocardial infarction of more than 3:1 according to the proportions of adipose linoleic acid; thus, there were more than three times the number of cases in the lowest quintile of adipose linoleic acid concentration than in a large control population (Fig. 2). The data for patients with angina were obtained from those who had angina for the first time during the preceding 1 month, and in these subjects a multivariate analysis indicated that the inverse relative risk of low adipose linoleic acid concentration and CHD was independent of all other risk factors. The data from patients with myocardial infarction were obtained from those arriving without previous myocardial infarction or angina in an intensive care unit. The reason for emphasising the recent onset of symptoms is that neither the angina patients nor the

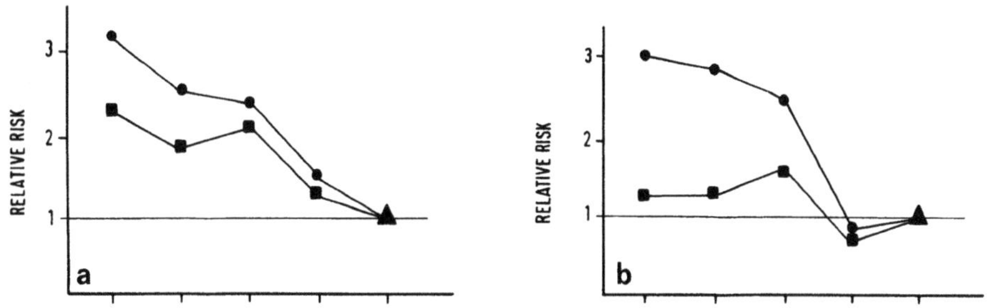

FIFTHS	1	2	3	4	5
INTERVAL (%)	<7·8	7·8-	8·8-	10·0-	≥11·5
No OF CASES	32	26	24	15	10
No OF CONTROLS	78	78	78	79	79

FIFTHS	1	2	3	4	5
INTERVAL (%)	<7·7	7·7-	8·7-	9·9-	≥11·4
No OF CASES	24	22	20	6	8
No OF CONTROLS	78	78	78	79	79

Fig. 2. The risks of ***a*** angina pectoris and ***b*** acute myocardial infarction, relative to the highest quintile of adipose linoleic acid concentration in the control population ($n = 392$). ▲, relative risk is 1.0; ●, unadjusted risk; ■, adjusted for other risk factors. (Reproduced by permission of the Lancet)

patients with myocardial infarction were aware of impending CHD and therefore we assume that the adipose linoleic acid concentrations truly reflect their long-term dietary habits. Multivariate analysis for the patients with myocardial infarctions showed that the low adipose linoleic acid content was independent of all other risk factors, with the exception of cigarette smoking.

We have now identified that cigarette smokers, independently of the presence of CHD, have lower concentrations of adipose linoleic acid than non-smokers [6]. More important, perhaps, cigarette smokers consume less linoleic acid. Why this should be is not clear, although it is possible that non-smokers are more health conscious and therefore take more edible oils. This is one of the first indications that cigarette smoking might lead to CHD by influencing food consumption adversely.

Low adipose linoleic acid concentration must result from a low dietary intake of linoleic acid and, from a 7-day prospective weighed record in 140 normal men [7], the correlation coefficient with dietary linoleic acid was + 0.58. However, it is difficult to believe that CHD-prone people select a diet low in linoleic acid months before they develop any symptoms and the possibility therefore arises that there are also major metabolic differences, either in absorption, catabolism, storage or mobilisation of fatty acids; these are under study.

Marine Oils

It has been known for many years that the very long chain polyunsaturated fatty acids which occur in fish, such as menhaden oil, have a profound effect in lowering raised serum and LDL cholesterol concentrations [8]. Such diets are poor in essential fatty acids. More recently, it has been shown that eicosapentaneoic acid (20:5, n-3) (EPA), which is present in relatively high concentrations in many fish oils, also influences plasma lipids in the same direction [9]. EPA when taken in large quantities reduces platelet count and alters platelet function and there is also prolongation of bleeding time [10].

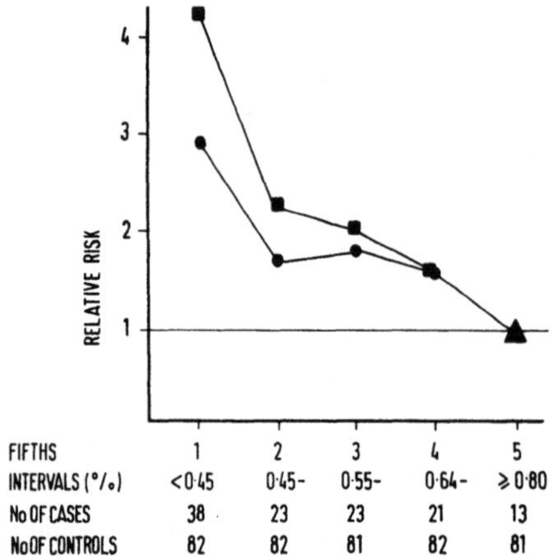

Fig. 3. The risk of angina pectoris relative to the highest quintile of platelet membrane eicosapentaenoic acid concentration in the control population ($n = 408$). ▲, relative risk is 1.0; ●, unadjusted risk; ■, adjusted for other risk factors. (Reproduced by permission of the Lancet)

Recently, some but not all studies have suggested that a relatively low weekly consumption of fish oils may be associated with less CHD [11–14]: such diets may also lower blood pressure [15]. These studies should be evaluated cautiously, because they mostly rely on dietary data collected many years ago, usually without exact dietary quantification of the amount of fish oil consumed, and they do not provide data to indicate continuity of eating habits over the intervening years. More important, a diet rich in fish oils is likely to be one low in saturated fatty acids and the putative beneficial effects may relate to this. Nevertheless, our case-control study [6] also showed that angina patients had significantly lower platelet EPA than controls and the order of magnitude of the inverse relative risk was the same as that for adipose linoleic acid (Fig. 3). It has yet to be established whether the relatively small concentrations of EPA that are available commercially in capsules will be sufficient to have any effect on the incidence of CHD, although it has been demonstrated that they are capable of altering prostanoid concentrations [16]. Appropriate large controlled trials to test this question have yet to be initiated.

Olive Oil

Monoenoic fatty acids have received little attention until recently, partly because they have been considered neutral in effect, partly because calculation of the polyunsaturated : saturated ratio does not include them, and partly because of their cost as edible oils. Olive oil is the most easily available source of monoenes and oleic acid (18:1, n-9) may have potentially beneficial effects. Cetoleic acid (22:1, n-9) may also be beneficial because of its effects on haemostasis and is found in fish and marine mammals.

Grundy [17] has clearly shown that the effects of olive oil in lowering raised serum cholesterol and LDL concentrations are as impressive, if not more so, than those of polyunsaturated edible oils such as corn oil. Moreover, a diet rich in olive oil does not reduce HDL cholesterol, while diets rich in polyunsaturated fat do. Olive oil is generally more expensive, but it may have other advantages over some of the very polyunsaturated fatty acids which have a higher proportion of *trans* fatty acids; these are metabolised as saturated fatty acids and the higher the proportion of *trans* fatty acids in edible oils the less the benefit of these oils.

Commentary

An important emerging concept of atherosclerosis and/or CHD is the likelihood that individual polyunsaturated fatty acids have specific effects on some of the mechanisms which we have come to recognise as being of crucial importance in the development of these diseases. The dominance of the cholesterol hypothesis has undoubtedly distracted attention from the effects of individual fatty acids and it is remarkable how little attention was given, even in the late 1970s, to the function of the precursor fatty acids of prostanoids and leukotrienes. Several of the long-chain polyunsaturated fatty acids are cross-inhibitory metabolically. The desaturation and chain-elongation pathways are influenced by the presence of saturated fats, alcohol and probably cigarette smoking.

It is not clear what the biological significance is of low tissue levels of the essential fatty acid linoleic acid, and it has yet to be shown whether the increased relative risk for CHD applies equally in populations with a high intake of edible oils. But the importance of the finding is emphasised further by the identification of low serum phospholipid linoleic acid concentration as a prospective marker for subsequent CHD [18]. There is evidence to suggest that, at least in the short term, linoleic acid is capable of reducing blood pressure [19]. In long-term studies, adipose α-linolenic acid (the principal n-3 essential fatty acid) has been shown to be inversely related to blood pressure [20]. Some marine oils, particularly eicosapentaneoic acid, have potentially beneficial effects on platelet function and should be regarded as being antithrombotic [21]. Other very long chain fatty acids are known to effect myocardial metabolism; for example, high concentrations of docosohexanoeic acid have been reported in patients with myocardial infarction [22] and an excess of this fatty acid has been found in the heart muscle of patients who have died from a heart attack [23].

Conclusion

Far more needs to be learned about the influences of individual long-chain mono- and polyunsaturated fatty acids on the pathogenic processes which lead to CHD. Clinical trials of the effectiveness of some fatty acids should be considered. Meanwhile, there appears to be a strong case for increasing the proportion of linoleic acid in the diet of those living in communities where the intake is low.

References

1. Keys A (1970) Coronary heart disease in seven countries. American Heart Association Monograph 29
2. Logan RL, Thomson M, Riemersma RA et al. (1978) Risk factors for ischaemic heart disease in normal men aged 40. Lancet i: 949-955
3. Riemersma RA, Wood DA, Butler S et al. (1986) Linoleic acid in adipose tissue and coronary heart disease. Br Med J 292: 1423-1427
4. Wood DA, Butler S, Riemersma RA et al. (1984) Adipose tissue and platelet fatty acids and coronary heart disease in Scottish men. Lancet 11: 117-121.
5. Van Staveren WA, Deurenberg P, Katan MB, et al. (1986) Validity of the fatty acid composition of subcutaneous fat tissue microbiopsies as an estimate of the long term average fatty acid composition of the diet of separate individuals. Am J Epidemiol 123: 455-463
6. Wood DA, Riemersma RA, Butler S et al. (1987) Linoleic and eicosapentaenoic acids in adipose tissue and platelets and risk of coronary heart disease. Lancet i: 177-183
7. Thomson M, Fulton M, Wood DA et al. (1985) A comparison of the nutrient intake of some Scotsmen with dietary recommendations. Hum Nutr Appl Nutr 39 A: 443-455
8. Ahrens EH, Insull W, Hirsch J et al. (1959) The effect on human serum-lipids of a dietary fat, highly unsaturated, but poor in essential fatty acids. Lancet i: 115
9. Phillipson BE, Rothrock DW, Connor WE et al. (1985) Reduction of plasma lipids, lipoproteins and apoproteins by dietary fish oils in patients with hypertriglyceridemia. N Engl J Med 312: 1210-1216
10. Dyerberg J, Bang HO (1979) Haemostatic function and platelet polyunsaturated fatty acids in Eskimos. Lancet i: 433-435
11. Kromhout D, Bosschieter EB, Coulander C de L (1985) The inverse relation between fish consumption and 20-year mortality from coronary heart disease. N Engl J Med 312: 1205-1209
12. Shekelle RB, Paul O, Stamler J (1985) Fish consumption and mortality from coronary heart disease. N Engl J Med 313: 820
13. Vollset SE, Heuch I, Bjelke E (1985) Fish consumption and mortality from coronary heart disease. N Engl J Med 313: 821
14. Curb JD, Reed DM (1985) Fish consumption and mortality from coronary heart disease. N Engl J Med 313: 821
15. Puska P, Iacono JM, Nissinen A et al. (1983) Controlled randomised trial of the effect of dietary fat on blood pressure. Lancet i: 1-5
16. Knapp HR, Reilly IAG, Alessandrini P et al. (1986) In vivo indexes of platelet and vascular function during fish-oil administration in patients with atherosclerosis. N Engl J Med 314: 937-942
17. Grundy SM (1986) Comparison of monounsaturated fatty acids and carbohydrates for lowering plasma cholesterol. N Engl J Med 314: 745-748
18. Miettinen TA, Naukkarinen V, Huttunen JK et al. (1982) Fatty-acid composition of serum lipids predicts myocardial infarction. Br Med J 285: 993-996
19. Heagerty AM, Ollerenshaw JD, Robertson DI et al. (1986) Influence of dietary linoleic acid on leucocyte sodium transport and blood pressure. Br Med J 293: 295-297
20. Berry EM, Hirsch J (1986) Does dietary linoleic acid influence blood pressure? Am J Clin Nutr 44: 336-340
21. Dyerberg J, Bang HO (1979) Haemostatic function and platelet polyunsaturated fatty acids in Eskimos. Lancet ii: 433-435
22. Kirkeby K, Ingvaldsen P, Bjerkedal I (1972) Fatty acid composition of serum lipids in men with myocardial infarction. Acta Med Scand 192: 513-519
23. Gudbjarnason S, Hallgrimsson J (1979) In: Hayase S, Murao S (eds) Proceedings of the VIII world congress of cardiology, Tokyo, 17-23 September 1978. Excerpta Medica, Amsterdam pp 245-247 (International Congress Series No. 470)

What Are the Alpha-Linolenic Acid Supplies to Be Recommended to the Normal Adult?

B. Jacotot

Some polyunsaturated fatty acids of the n-3 family have metabolic activities and could be useful in the prevention or treatment of ischemic diseases. The main fatty acids of this group are alpha-linolenic acid (18:3n-3), eicosapentaenoic acid (20:5n-3) and docosahexaenoic acid (22:6n-3). They are found in small amounts in most of animal tissues, but mainly in the phospholipids of brain, nerves, retina, and testis. Their structural function is important, and many studies on this subject are at present in progress. The role of the n-3 family of fatty acids, which are the source of the biosynthesis of some prostaglandins (series 3 and 4), has only recently been discovered and much remains to be studied.

Dietary Sources of the n-3 Family of Fatty Acids

Linolenic acid is provided by the intestinal hydrolysis of triglycerides or phospholipids containing this fatty acid. It is found in very small quantities in all foods of animal origin, but mainly in marine animals. Considerable amounts are also found in some vegetable oils (rapeseed oil: 7%-9% and soybean oil: 6%-8%).

Eicosapentaenoic (EPA) and docosahexaenoic (DHA) acids are provided by marine animals (fish, seals, whales). The EPA content in marine animal fats is higher than in land-living mammals. Salmon fat contains 9% EPA and 8% DHA, while human plasma phospholipids contain about 1% EPA and 4% DHA. Vegetable fats do not contain these two fatty acids.

The human body seems quite unable to synthesize alpha-linolenic acid; so this appears to be an essential fatty acid [1]. The other derivatives, EPA and DHA, can be synthesized from linolenic acid in man.

The main proof that alpha-linolenic acid is an essential fatty acid was given by Holman et al. in 1982 [2]. These authors described the case of a 6-year-old girl under total parenteral nutrition (TPN) after an extensive intestinal resection. Nutrition was provided by an emulsion enriched in linoleic acid and practically devoid of alpha-linolenic acid. After 4 to 5 months of TPN neurologic symptoms had appeared (paresthesia, difficulties in walking, pains, and visual disturbances). The analysis of the plasma phospholipid fatty acids revealed a slight deficiency in linoleic acid and a severe deficiency in linolenic acid. After substitution of the first emulsion by another preparation made with soybean oil and containing 42% linoleic acid and 6.9% alpha-linolenic acid, the symptoms disappeared. A new analysis of plasma lipids showed the correction of the linolenic acid deficiency. The author concluded that the amount of linolenate necessary to give normal values of n-3

Table 1. Daily dietary supply of linoleic and alpha-linolenic acids provided by the different diets of the Jouarre study [14] (in g/day - person - and as a percentage of the total caloric intake)

	Sunflower oil		Corn oil		Peanut oil		Olive oil		Rapeseed oil		Soybean oil	
	(g/day)	(%)	(g/day)	(%)	(g/day)	(%)	(g/day)	(%)	(g/day)	(%)	(g/day)	(%)
Linoleic acid	30	13.5	26	11.6	15	6.8	3.3	1.5	14.6	5.6	23.8	10.7
Alpha-linolenic acid	0.1	0.05	0.4	0.19	0.2	0.09	0.3	0.12	3.5	1.5	3.2	1.3

fatty acids was 0.54% of the total caloric intake. These values are close to the needs for n-3 determined in rats (0.5% of the total caloric intake) [3], but they are much less than the needs of fish (1% of the total caloric intake) [4]. The quantity determined corresponded to a daily caloric intake of 2.2 g of alpha-linolenic acid for a human subject consuming 2000 kcal/day. This is provided by 25-30 g rapeseed or soybean oil, or by 200 g butter.

In addition to this information concerning the n-3 fatty acid needs of humans, recent data has shown the interest in increasing the dietary supplies of linolenic and EPA acids. Dyerberg et al. [5] and Sinclair et al. [6] showed the unexpected effects of fatty acids on prostaglandin metabolism on the one hand, and plasma cholesterol levels on the other. The low incidence of myocardial infarction in the populations which consume significant quantities of marine animals was emphasized [7]. At the same time, several studies, experimental as well as clinical, have emphasized the interest in increasing the dietary supplies of alpha-linolenic acid and EPA, mainly to decrease platelet aggregation [8, 9] and to prevent coronary heart disease [10].

However, high levels of alpha-linolenic acid are able to induce a competition between the n-6 and n-3 families, and to inhibit the synthesis of the major derivatives of linoleic acid [11], particularly series 2 prostaglandins [12]. But it is difficult to evaluate the linoleic acid/linolenic acid ratio below which an effect on the metabolism of the n-6 family can appear.

Some answers to these various questions were provided by the study we carried out over several years in a group of Benedictine nuns in which we strictly applied special diets for long periods of time (the Jouarre study) [13, 14]. By stabilizing the daily caloric intake and, in particular, the lipid supply (30% of the total caloric intake), and by decreasing the structural fats (one-third of the dietary lipids), we could evaluate the effects on lipid metabolism and platelet aggregation of different fatty acid supplies (provided by different vegetable oils) (Table 1).

Effect on Plasma Total Cholesterol

It is known that cholesterolemia mainly depends on the saturated fat supply and increases with the rise of the dietary supply of saturated fats (and cholesterol). With the different vegetable oils we tested (Table 2) the supply of saturated fatty acids was almost the same whatever the oil considered (between 19 and 24.5 g day - person -, i.e., 8.5%-10.6% of the total caloric intake). Thus what was the effect of the unsaturated fatty acid supply, namely that of linoleic and alpha-linolenic acids? If

Table 2. Total Blood cholesterol levels observed after the different diets of the Jouarre study [14]

	Sunflower oil (g/liter) *n*	Corn oil (g/liter)	Peanut oil (g/liter)	Olive oil (g/liter)	Rapeseed oil (g/liter)	Soybean oil (g/liter)
Mean	1.93	2.20	2.10	2.10	2.01	2.19
SD	±0.36	±0.42	±0.28	±0.35	0.34	0.38
n	62	65	59	64	61	62

Table 3. Prostanoid precursor amounts in plasma phospholipids measured after the different diets of the Jouarre study [14-15] (in 10^{-3} μmol/ml of plasma)

		Sunflower oil	Corn oil	Arachide oil	Olive oil	Rapeseed oil	Soybean oil
20:3n-6	mean	16	19	39	29	26	22
	SD	± 2	± 9	± 9	±18	±15	±12
20:4n-6	mean	75	72	131	102	95	105
	SD	± 8	±32	±24	±34	±30	±28
20:5n-3	mean	6.6	3.3	10	20	16	12
	SD	± 2	± 2.5	± 2	±14	±12	± 7
22:6n-3	mean	36		73	73	63	65
	SD	±16		±26	±18	±12	±20

we compare the diet with peanut oil (15 g/day linoleic acid and 0.2 g/day alpha-linolenic acid) and the diet with olive oil (3.3 g/day linoleic acid and 0.3 g/day alpha-linolenic acid), we can observe that the mean blood cholesterol levels were identical. On the other hand, if we compare the mean blood cholesterol level in two diets providing a high and almost identical amount of linoleic acid (sunflower oil and corn oil diets), we can observe very different blood cholesterol levels (1.93 g/liter with sunflower oil and 2.19 g/liter with corn oil). Thus it is not possible to conclude that the *n*-6 polyunsaturated fatty acid supply intervenes specifically on the total blood cholesterol level.

We will now try to evaluate the real effect of alpha-linolenic acid by comparing two diets containing identical amounts of linoleic acid, but amounts or very different alpha-linolenic acid, i.e., the peanut oil diet and the rapeseed oil diet; the first provides a very low amount of alpha-linolenic acid (0.2 g/day), the second much more (3.5 g/day). The mean of serum cholesterol was lower after the rapeseed oil diet than after the peanut oil diet.

Effect on the Fatty Acid Composition of Plasma Phospholipids

The rapeseed oil diet was characterized by a linoleic acid supply close to the one which is usually recommended for the general population (10.7 g/day, i.e., 4.5% of the total caloric intake) and a high alpha-linolenic acid supply (3.5 g/day i.e., 1.5% of the total caloric intake). (Table 3, [15]). Thus the linoleic acid/linolenic acid ratio

Table 4. In vitro ADP platelet aggregation indexes observed after the different diets of the Jouarre study [15]

	Sunflower oil	Corn oil	Peanut oil	Olive oil	Rapeseed oil	Soybean oil
Mean	43.0	41.1	39.0	34.5	38.5	34.6
SD	±5.6	±5.1	±3.6	±4.3	±6.0	±6.2
n	21	22	18	22	20	19

is 3, which is much lower than that which is usually encountered. We observed that with this diet, the EPA and DHA levels in plasma phospholipids were higher than with the diets containing low amounts of alpha-linolenic acid. The same observation can be made with the soybean oil diet which also provided a high amount of 18:3*n*-3. These high *n*-3 fatty acid levels in phospholipids can be considered to be favourable for the prevention of ischemic cardiovascular disease. When examining the results obtaining with rapeseed and soybean oil diets, it now appears that di-homo-gamma-linolenic and arachidonic acids were present at a concentration which can be considered as normal (according to the results obtained by Holman in healthy subjects). So, the supply of 3.5 g alpha-linolenic acid (1.5% of the total caloric intake), with a linoleic acid/linolenic acid ratio of 3, did not induce a competition between the two main fatty acid families. That could happen if the ratio were lower, either with a markedly higher supply of alpha-linolenic acid, or with a lower supply of linoleic acid. On the other hand, it is important to note that a high supply of linoleic acid could induce a decrease in di-homo-gamma-linolenic and arachidonic acid levels: that was observed with the sunflower and corn oil diets, supplying 30 and 28.5 g/day linoleic acid, respectively, with linoleic acid/linolenic acid ratios of 300 and 65, respectively! These two diets also provided very low levels of EPA and DHA in plasma phospholipids. These data explain why platelet aggregation was higher after the sunflower and corn oil diets than after the other diets (Table 4).

In conclusion, it seems that for a diet with a low lipid supply (30% of the total caloric intake), the recommendation of the following amounts of essential fatty acids is justified:

- Linoleic acid: 5%-7% of the total caloric intake
- Alpha-linolenic acid: 0.5%-1% of the total caloric intake

In consequence, the ratio: $\frac{\text{linoleic acid}}{\text{linolenic acid}}$ should be between 5 and 10.

References

1. Holman RT (1981) Essential fatty acids in nutrition and disease. Chem Indust 17: october
2. Holman RT, Johnson SB, Hatch TF (1982) A case of human linolenic acid deficiency involving neurological abnormalities. Am J Clin Nutr 35: 617
3. Pudelkewicz C, Seufert J, Holman RT (1968) Requirements of the female rat for linoleic and linolenic acids. J Nutr 94: 138
4. Yu TC, Sinnhuber RO, Hendricks JD (1979) Reproduction and survival of rainbow trout *(Salmo gairdneri)* fed linolenic acid as the only source of essential fatty acids. Lipids 14: 572

5. Dyerberg J, Bang Ho Stoffersen, Moncada S, Vane JR (1978) Eicosapentaenoic acid and prevention of thrombosis and atherosclerosis. Lancet 2: 117
6. Sinclair HM (1980) Prevention of coronary heart disease. The role of essential fatty acids. Postgrad Med J 56: 579
7. Saynor R, Verel D, Gillott T (1984) The long-term effect of dietary supplementation with fish concentrate on serum lipids, bleeding time, platelets and angina. Atherosclerosis 50: 3
8. Jacotot B (1979) Effet de l'ingestion de l'huile de colza à basse teneur en acide érucique sur l'agrégation plaquettaire. Rev Fr des Corps Gras 26: 171
9. Hirai A, Hamazaki T, Terano T (1980) Eicosapentaenoic acid and platelet function in Japanese. Lancet 2: 1132
10. Kromhout D, Bosschieter EB, de Lezenne Coulander C (1985) The inverse relation between fish consumption and 2-year mortality from coronary heart disease. N Engl J Med 312: 1205
11. Marshall LA, Szezesniewski PV, Johnston SB (1983) Dietary alpha-linolenic acid and prostaglandin synthesis: a time course study. Am J Clin Nutr 38: 895
12. Adam O, Wolfram G, Zöllner N (1986) Effect of alpha-linolenic acid in the human diet on linoleic acid metabolism and prostaglandin biosynthesis. J Lip Res 27: 421
13. Lasserre M, Kerautret M, Navarro N, Martin C, Jacotot B (1984) Effects of several alimentary fats on serum lipids during long-term stabilized diets. Ann Nutr Metab 28: 334
14. Jacotot B, Lasserre M, Esteva O, Baudet MF, Dachet C (1985)Corps gras alimentaires et prévention des maladies vasculaires; étude chez le sujet sain. Rev Fr des Corps gras 32: 11
15. Lasserre M, Mendy F, Spielman D, Jacotot B (1985) Effects of different dietary intake of essential fatty acids on C20:3ω6 and C20:4ω6 serum levels in human adults. Lipids 20: 227

Animal and Vegetable Protein Effects in Experimental Atherosclerosis

D. Kritchevsky

The first purely nutritional experiments in atherosclerosis were carried out by Ignatowski [10, 11]. Ignatowski's hypothesis was that atherosclerosis was due to toxic products of protein digestion. Adult rabbits fed meat (up to 15 g/day) developed atherosclerosis as did weanling rabbits fed milk and egg yolk. The atherogenic effect of dietary cholesterol observed independently by Anitschkow and Chalatow [1] and Wacker and Hueck [33] turned attention to this sterol and away from other dietary factors, an oversight that persisted for half a century.

Newburgh and Squier [26] fed dried beef to rabbits and caused atherosclerosis. Diets containing 36% protein were more atherogenic than those containing 27% protein. The two diets provided 36 or 28 mg cholesterol daily, amounts insufficient to cause atherosclerosis. The atherogenic effect was attributed to protein [25]. To prove this point Clarkson and Newburgh [3] fed rabbits 25, 113, 253 or 507 mg cholesterol daily for extended periods of time. Rabbits fed 25 mg cholesterol for up to 288 days were normocholesterolemic and free of atherosclerotic lesions. Feeding of 113 mg of cholesterol for as long as 302 days produced no elevation in levels of cholesterol and only one of 19 rabbits exhibited slight atherosclerosis. Higher daily doses of cholesterol (253 or 507 mg) required long feedings to produce modest levels of atherosclerosis. The amount of cholesterol required to cause atherosclerosis was at least ten times the amount present in the beef diets.

Meeker and Kesten [22, 23] were the first investigators to compare the atherogenicity of animal and vegetable protein, using casein and soy protein in diets which provided 45%-50% protein. Their data show casein to be atherogenic even in the absence of dietary cholesterol.

The current resurgence of interest in dietary protein was stimulated by the experiments of Carroll and Hamilton [2] who fed a variety of defatted animal or plant proteins to rabbits and showed that, in general, proteins of animal origin were more cholesterolemic than those of plant origin but there was a wide range of effects within each group.

Huff et al. [9] fed rabbits mixtures of amino acids corresponding to the composition of casein or soy protein but the casein-like mixture had no effect on serum cholesterol while that resembling soy protein raised cholesterol levels by 80%. Partial enzymic hydrolyzates of casein and soy protein lowered cholesterol levels by 16% and 41%, respectively. We have examined the possibility that the ratio of lysine to arginine (L/A) present in a given protein may influence its cholesterolemic effect. The L/A ratio of most animal proteins is about 2.0 and that of plant proteins is about 1.0. Rabbits were fed semipurified diets containing casein, soy protein, casein plus arginine (to give L/A of soy protein), and soy protein plus lysine (to give L/A

Table 1. Influence of added amino acids on atherogenicity of casein or soy protein for rabbits

Regimen[a]	Rabbits (*n*)	Serum cholesterol (mg/dl)	Average atherosclerosis	
			Arch	Thoracic
C	7	174±30	2.2±0.5	1.5±0.4
S	7	77±21	1.1±0.4	0.7±0.3
CA	6	129±12	1.4±0.4	0.8±0.3
SL	6	106±29	1.6±0.4	1.1±0.2
C	8	283±28	1.1±0.3	0.8±0.3
S	11	234±20	0.5±0.2	0.4±0.1
CA	7	343±65	1.3±0.4	0.7±0.2
SL	11	242±22	0.9±0.3	0.5±0.2
C	5	377±59	1.6±0.2	0.9±0.3
S	7	117±10	0.6±0.2	0.1±0.1
CA	7	271±74	1.2±0.2	1.3±0.2
SL	8	242±43	0.5±0.2	0.7±0.1

[a] Diets contained 40% sucrose, 25% protein, 14% coconut oil, 5% mineral mix, 1% vitamin mix - fed for 8 months.
C, casein; S, soy; CA, casein + arginine; SL, soy + lysine.

of casein). The results have been reported in part [5, 6, 13, 15, 17, 19]. Table 1 details the results of those studies; it is evident that addition of arginine to casein does not affect total serum cholesterol but reduces atherosclerosis, whereas addition of lysine to soy protein is both cholesterolemic and atherogenic. To address the possibility that the observed effect might be due only to lysine, we fed rabbits three proteins (fish, casein, and whole milk) whose lysine content is similar (6.81, 6.91, and 6.61 mg/g, respectively) but whose L/A ratios were 1.44, 1.89, and 2.44. The degree of atherogenicity was fish, 1.25; casein, 1.58; whole milk, 2.08, and this correlated significantly with the L/A ratio [18].

Other amino acids have been implicated in the control of cholesterol metabolism in rabbits. Methionine has been found to be hypercholesterolemic, and glycine and alanine hypocholesterolemic [7, 12]. In rats methionine [30] and tyrosine [24] are hypercholesterolemic. Cystine and glycine have been found to be hypocholesterolemic [30] while arginine has been reported to be effective by some authors [28] but not others [29].

The mechanism underlying the animal vs. vegetable protein effect is under study. Huff and Carroll [8] found cholesterol turnover in casein-fed rabbits to be slower than that in soy-fed rabbits. We have found the turnover times of cholesterol in rabbits fed soy protein or soy protein plus lysine to be 18.4 and 33.7 days, respectively. Turnover time of cholesterol in rabbits fed casein in 36.8 days and it is not affected by addition of arginine (36.3 days), which reflects the effects on cholesterolemia. The influences of the various diets on fecal steroid excretion are detailed in Table 2.

Rats fed casein exhibit higher serum cholesterol levels than those fed soy protein or casein plus arginine. Rats fed fish protein have significantly lower serum cholesterol levels than those fed casein, milk protein or beef protein. Rats fed casein show

Table 2. Fecal steroids of rabbits fed various proteins

Protein	Feces (gm/day)	Steroids (mg/day)	
		Acidic	Neutral
Casein	5.6	9.4 ± 2.2	8.5 ± 2.6
Soy	11.7	33.0 ± 10.3	15.4 ± 4.2
Casein + arginine	5.3	12.9 ± 2.6	7.9 ± 3.0
Soy + lysine	6.7	12.1 ± 10.0	10.9 ± 0.6
Laboratory ration	20.0	31.6 ± 10.0	19.3 ± 2.9

significantly lower hepatic HMG-CoA reductase levels than do those fed soy protein or casein plus arginine [20].

Absorption of cholesterol into the thoracic duct lymph of rats fed casein proceeds faster than in those fed soy protein. The situation is reversed in rats fed casein plus arginine or soy plus lysine [31].

The serum lipoproteins or rats fed casein, soy proteins, casein plus arginine, or soy plus lysine have been analyzed [32]. Concentration of triglycerides was highest in chylomicrons of rats fed casein or soy plus lysine. Triglyceride levels in very low-density lipoprotein (VLDL) or low-density lipoprotein (LDL) were highest in rats fed soy protein or casein plus arginine. Triglyceride levels of high-density lipoprotein (HDL) were the same in all four groups. Cholesterol levels were highest in chylomicrons of rats fed casein and lowest in the soy-fed rats. Cholesterol distribution in VLDL was the same for all groups but LDL cholesterol levels were lowest in rats fed casein and highest in the soy-lysine group. HDL cholesterol levels were highest in the casein-arginine group and lowest in rats fed soy protein and lysine.

The mechanism(s) underlying the difference between casein and soy protein involve reduced clearance of cholesterol in casein-fed rabbits. Furthermore, reduced clearance of triglyceride-rich lipoproteins has been observed in casein-fed rabbits [4, 27]. Almost half the circulating triglyceride of casein-fed rats has been found in chylomicrons which is in accord with the clearance data for rabbits.

The evidence suggests that the hyperlipidemic response to casein-rich diets is due, in part, to altered kinetics of chylomicrons or of other triglyceride-rich lipoprotein fractions. These responses are also mediated by gastrointestinal hormones and insulin levels. Arginine supplementation of casein modifies these responses and addition of lysine to soy protein does so to a lesser degree. The effects of other amino acids have been studied to some extent but await elucidation.

It is important to bear in mind the role of dietary interactions as they relate to serum lipids and atherosclerosis [14]. Interactions between protein, fat, and cholesterol in pigeon atherosclerosis revealed that there was no independent variable [21]. Carroll and Hamilton [2] found that rabbits fed casein and dextrose exhibited cholesterol levels of 208 mg/dl compared to 70 mg/dl for soy-dextrose fed animals. When the dextrose was replaced by wheat starch, cholesterol levels in casein-fed rabbits were unaffected but those in rabbits fed soy protein were normalized. When the carbohydrate was potato starch, cholesterol levels of rabbits fed casein or soy protein were 48 and 52 mg/dl, respectively. The type of fiber present in the diet also affects cholesterolemia and atherosclerosis in rabbits fed casein or soy protein [16].

The role or dietary protein in atherosclerosis and, indeed, in lipid metabolism is assuming greater interest and is coming under renewed investigation. Perhaps consideration of protein will provide further insight into the development of atherosclerosis.

Acknowledgement. The author wishes to express his gratitude for their skilful assistance to the colleagues whose names are listed in the cited references. This work was supported, in part, by a Research Career Award (HL 00734) from the National Institutes of Health.

References

1. Anitschkow N, Chalatow S (1913) Über experimentelle Cholesterinsteatose und ihre Bedeutung für Entstehung einiger pathologischer Prozesse. Z Allg Pathol Anat 24: 1-9
2. Carroll KK, Hamilton RMG (1975) Effects of dietary protein and carbohydrate on plasma cholesterol levels in relation to atherosclerosis. J Food Sci 40: 18-23
3. Clarkson S, Newburgh LH (1926) The relation between atherosclerosis and ingested cholesterol in the rabbit. J Exp Med 43: 595-612
4. Cohn JS, Krimpton WG, Nestel PJ (1984) The effect of dietary casein and soy protein on cholesterol and very low density lipoprotein metabolism in the rat. Atherosclerosis 52: 219-231
5. Czarnecki SK (1982) Effects of dietary proteins on lipoprotein metabolism and atherosclerosis in rabbits. PhD dissertation, University of Pennsylvania, Philadelphia
6. Czarnecki SK, Kritchevsky D (1979) The effect of dietary proteins on lipoprotein metabolism and atherosclerosis in rabbits. J Am Oil Chem Soc 56: 388 A
7. Hermus RJJ, Dallinga-Thie GM (1979) Soya, saponins and plasma cholesterol. Lancet 1: 48
8. Huff MW, Carroll KK (1980) Effects of dietary protein on turnover, oxidation and absorption of cholesterol and on steroid excretion in rabbits. J Lipid Res 21: 546-558
9. Huff MW, Hamilton RMG, Carroll KK (1979) Plasma cholesterol levels in rabbits fed low fat, cholesterol-free semipurified diets: effects of dietary proteins, protein hydrolysates and amino acid mixtures. Atherosclerosis 28: 187-195
10. Ignatowski A (1908) Influence de la nourriture animale sur l'organisme des lapins. Arch Med Exp Anat Pathol 20: 1-20
11. Ignatowski A (1909) Über die Wirkung des tierischen Eiweisses auf die Aorta und die parynchomatosen Organe der Kaninchen. Virchows Arch Pathol Anat Physiol Klin Med 198: 248-270
12. Katan MB, Vroomen LHM, Hermus RJJ (1982) Reduction of casein-induced hypercholesterolemia and atherosclerosis in rabbits and rats by dietary glycine, arginine and alanine. Atherosclerosis 43: 381-391
13. Kritchevsky D (1979) Vegetable protein and atherosclerosis. J Am Oil Chem Soc 56: 135-146
14. Kritchevsky D (1979) Dietary interactions. In: Levy RI, Rifkind BM, Dennis BH, Ernst ND (eds) Nutrition lipids and coronary heart disease: a global view. Raven, New York, pp 229-246
15. Kritchevsky D (1980) Dietary proteins in atherosclerosis. In: Noseda G, Lewis B, Paoletti R (eds) Diet and drugs in atherosclerosis. Raven, New York, pp 9-14
16. Kritchevsky D, Tepper SA, Williams DE, Story JA (1977) Experimental atherosclerosis in rabbits fed cholesterol-free diets. 7. Interaction of animal or vegetable protein with fiber, Atherosclerosis 26: 397-403
17. Kritchevsky D, Tepper SA, Story JA (1978) Influence of soy protein and casein on atherosclerosis in rabbits. Fed Proc 37: 747
18. Kritchevsky D, Tepper SA, Czarnecki SK, Klurfeld DM (1982) Atherogenicity of animal and vegetable protein: influence of the lysine/arginine ratio. Atherosclerosis 41: 429-431

19. Kritchevsky D, Tepper SA, Czarnecki SK, Klurfeld DM, Story JA (1983) Effects of animal and vegetable protein in experimental atherosclerosis. In: Gibney MJ, Kritchevsky D (eds) Animal and vegetable proteins in lipid metabolism and atherosclerosis. Liss, New York, pp 85-100
20. Kritchevsky D, Tepper SA, Czarnecki SK, Mueller MA, Klurfeld DM, Story JA (1984) Effects of dietary protein on lipid metabolism in rats. J Washington Acad Sci 74: 1-8
21. Lofland HB, Clarkson TB, Rhyne L, Goodman HO (1966) Interrelated effects of dietary fats and protein on atherosclerosis in pigeons. J Atheroscler Res 6: 395-403
22. Meeker DR, Kesten HD (1940) Experimental atherosclerosis and high protein diets. Proc Soc Exp Biol Med 45: 543-545
23. Meeker DR, Kesten HD (1941) Effect of high protein diets on experimental atherosclerosis of rabbits. Arch Pathol 31: 147-162
24. Nagaoka S, Aoyama Y, Yoshida A (1985) Effect of tyrosine and some other amino acids on serum level of cholesterol in rats. Nutr Rep Int 31: 1137-1148
25. Newburgh LH, Clarkson S (1922) Production of arteriosclerosis in rabbits by diets rich in animal protein. JAMA 79: 1106-1108
26. Newburgh LH, Squier TL (1920) High protein diets and arteriosclerosis in rabbits: a preliminary report. Arch Int Med 26: 38-40
27. Roberts DCK, Stalmach ME, Khalil MW, Hutchinson JC, Carroll KK (1981) Effects of dietary protein on composition and turnover of apoproteins of plasma lipoprotein of rabbits. Can J Biochem 56: 642-647
28. Ryzhenkov VE, Schanygina KI, Chistyakova AM, Miroshkina VN, Parfenova NS, Kalashnikova NM (1984) Action of arginine on the lipid and lipoprotein content in blood serum of animals. Vopr Med Khim 30: 76-79
29. Sugano M, Ishiwaki N, Nagata Y, Imaizumi K (1982) Effects of arginine and lysine addition to casein and soya-bean protein on serum lipids, apolipoproteins, insulin and glucagon in rats. Br J Nutr 48: 211-221
30. Sugiyama K, Kushima Y, Muramatsu K (1985) Effects of sulfur containing amino acids and glycine on plasma cholesterol level in rats fed on a high cholesterol diet. Agric Biol Chem 49: 3455-3461
31. Vahouny GV, Chalcarz W, Satchithanandam S, Adamson I, Klurfeld DM, Kritchevsky D (1984) Effect of soy protein and casein intake on intestinal absorption and lymphatic transport of cholesterol and oleic acid. Am J Clin Nutr 40: 1156-1164
32. Vahouny GV, Adamson I, Chalcarz W, Satchithanandam S, Muesing R, Klurfeld DM, Tepper SA, Sanghvi A, Kritchevsky D (1985) Effects of casein and soy protein on hepatic and serum lipids and lipoprotein lipid distributions in the rat. Atherosclerosis 56: 127-137
33. Wacker L, Hueck W (1913) Über experimentelle Atherosklerose und Cholesterinamie. MMW 60: 2097-2100

Food Proteins and Atherosclerosis

G. Debry

Ever since the demonstration by Ignatowski in 1908 [1] of the action of animal proteins promoting the development of atherosclerosis in rabbits, the subject has been under discussion. Until the last 15 years, the relationships between proteins and atherosclerosis had been almost completely forgotten, particularly because of the success of the "lipid theory."

Nevertheless, in 1913 Anitschkow had not excluded the possible influence of dietary proteins. In 1923 Newburgh et al. [2, 3] pointed out a positive correlation in the rabbit between consumption of animal protein, blood cholesterol levels, and the intensity of atherosclerosis, in spite of an absence of dietary cholesterol: Meeker and Kestens [4, 5] obtained the same results but observed the absence of any detrimental effect of soy proteins and the protective actions of these proteins when cholesterol was added to the diet. In 1965 Howard et al. [6] confirmed these observations. Although the relationships between food proteins and atherosclerosis have undergone a recent revival of interest they are complex and still not fully understood.

The data presented here concern clinical observations, epidemiological surveys, and experimental results.

Clinical Data

In clinical situations it is always difficult to differentiate the effects of protein intake and energy intake, because of the composition of conventional foods. The influence of undernutrition on the incidence of cardiovascular disease is not well known. During periods of famine, the incidences of coronary disease and myocardial infarction decrease, but the incidences of hypertension and congestive heart failure are not modified. In kwashiorkor plasma cholesterol increases, but the duration of the illness is too short for atherosclerosis to develop, either because of death or because of recovery through nutritional rehabilitation.

Data concerning the effects of a high-protein diet are somewhat conflicting. One study found no influence of supplementing dietary protein (from 8.6% to 17% of daily energy intake) with skimmed milk in middle-aged people [7], whereas another found a moderate increase of body weight, and more often a decrease than an increase of plasma cholesterol, when milk concentrate was added to the diet of elderly people [8]. A moderate decrease of plasma proteins and cholesterol was found in young women consuming a high-protein diet (25% of daily energy intake), but no variation was observed in young men [9]. In addition, there are difficulties in discriminating between the effects of food proteins and the effects of fats when one studies the correlation between a normal diet and autopsy observations [10].

Epidemiological Data

The positive correlations between fat or animal protein consumption and mortality from and incidence of coronary heart disease are strong, probably because of the composition of foods of animal origin [11-13]. Data obtained from people on vegetarian or vegan diets are inconclusive because these diets include high quantities of dietary fibers and very few saturated fats. Thus, epidemiological and clinical data are not sufficiently convincing. For practical and ethical reasons, it is impossible to obtain in humans sufficiently clear evidence, while the extrapolation of animal experimental results to humans is always hazardous.

Experimental Data

Many animal and human experiments have demonstrated the effects of low and high dietary protein contents on plasma cholesterol and on the development of atherosclerosis, and especially the great importance of whether the food proteins are of animal or vegetable origin [4, 5].

Influence of the Protein Content of the Diet. In pigeons, a low-protein diet (10%) decreases body weight and increases plasma cholesterol and the rate of mortality is high: a high-protein diet (20% and 40%) does not increase blood cholesterol, aortal cholesterol or indices of aortic atherosclerosis [14].

In rats, protein undernutrition decreases cholesterol, triglycerides, phospholipid, total protein, and hydroxyproline levels in both the aorta and the plasma [15]. Conversely, when associated with dietary cholesterol, protein malnutrition in rats increases cholesterol and triglyceride in both the plasma and the aorta. Protein consumption can therefore modulate the effect of dietary cholesterol [16]. Generally, a low-protein diet increases plasma cholesterol in humans and animals [9, 17-30]. This increase can be explained by various metabolic changes including sulfur amino acid deficiency [17], hypertriglyceridemia [23], and hepatic synthesis of fatty acids [25, 26]. However, this effect depends on the animal species. In monkey and pig, a low-protein diet did not change the composition of aortic tissue [27, 28]. In rats receiving a low-protein diet [6.5%), the overall aorta/protein content was not modified, but the elastin content decreased, though only during the first 20 weeks of the experiment [29]. Regression of atherosclerotic lesions in the aorta of the cockerel is obtained only of the protein content of the diet is over 15%, or occasionally 10% [31].

The varying results obtained in the different experiments could be due to variations in the real daily protein intake of the animals. Unfortunately, most reports mention only the protein content of the diet, and we remain ignorant of the real quantities of protein ingested and of the status of the nitrogen balance [29].

Influence of the Nature of the Diet Proteins. In the past 10 years numerous papers have been published on the subject of the influence of the nature of dietary proteins. A high content of animal protein in the diet increases plasma cholesterol levels and favors the development of atherosclerosis, whatever the origin of the dietary proteins (milk [32, 34], fish [32, 33], egg [32]). Numerous experiments and general reviews have dealt with this particular aspect [32–42].

Among animal proteins, casein has been the most extensively investigated, often in comparison with soy protein [46–53]. Young individuals are more susceptible to hypercholestorelemia on casein-rich diets than adults [43], but the exposure of rabbits to dietary casein in early life had no detrimental effect on atherosclerotic lesions or on cholesterol and biliary acid metabolism [44]. Casein has a similar effect to saturated fats on the plasma cholesterol response to dietary cholesterol in rabbits [45]. In healthy humans, casein-rich and soy protein diets have similar effects on blood lipids [53–57], although sometimes soy protein has a slight beneficial effect on the distribution of cholesterol between the various lipoprotein fractions [56].

Conversely, in type II hyperlipoproteinemic men the substitution of soy protein for animal protein, with or without dietary cholesterol [57–64], or, most interestingly, the simple addition of soy protein to a standard low-lipid diet [61], has been found to induce a significant decrease in plasma cholesterol particularly LDL cholesterol. In type IIb hyperlipoproteinemia plasma triglycerides were also reduced. However, similar results have not been obtained by other authors [65, 66].

Thus, the effects of soy protein are different in animals and in humans. Perhaps there is a species-dependent sensivity modulated by age. Soy proteins are without effects in humans in good health and the effects differ, according to various authors, between hyperlipoproteinemic patients.

Hypotheses on the Mechanisms of Casein and Soy Protein Actions

A great number of factors have been suspected as the causes of the differing metabolic effects of soy protein and casein: the presence of phytosterols, the carbohydrate composition or low methionine and choline content of soy, the presence of saponines and the mineral content of soy, and in particular the effects of soy protein and casein on intestinal absorption, lipoprotein metabolism, and sterol excretion. Finally, immunologic hypotheses have been proposed in order to explain atherosclerotic lesions.

Digestive absorption of lipids is faster in casein-fed rats than in rats fed with soy protein [67]. Addition of arginine to the casein-rich diet and addition of lysine to the soy diet decrease and increase respectively the rates of lipid absorption [67]. The casein-rich diet decreases the rate of chylomicron clearance, increases the level of circulating insulin, and can increase or depress hepatic 7-α-hydroxylase activity [68]. The addition of arginine to the casein-rich diet and of lysine to the soy diet decrease or increase respectively the level of circulating insulin, and increase or depress respectively hepatic 7-α-hydroxylase activity [68]. It has been proposed that the specific amino acid composition of dietary proteins could explain the differing actions of vegetable and animal proteins, and that the lysine : arginine ratio may be of particular significance (casein 2.04, soy protein 0.88, on a weight basis; [69]). Histidine excess in the diet may also have an effect since it increases plasma cholesterol [70], and a negative correlation has been found in rats between the serum cholesterol level and the arginine : lysine ratio of dietary proteins [71].

Having enzymatically digested protein in the diet can lead to an effect different from that of the intact protein. The mixture of amino acids corresponding to casein and casein itself have the same effects, but the mixture of amino acids corresponding to soy protein provokes a slight increase of plasma cholesterol whereas intact soy protein diminishes it [39, 42, 72]. Deficiency or excess of sulphur amino acids increase or decrease plasma cholesterol levels respectively, and a deficiency can have an atherogenetic action in mice, rat, cocks, and monkeys: however, different experiments give conflicting results [17, 29]. Several other amino acids may also have an effect on plasma cholesterol [73, 74]. Casein and soy protein produce several effects on lipoprotein metabolism. The increase of VLDL cholesterol by a casein-rich diet is due to decreased removal and catabolism of VLDL [60, 75, 76]. According to different authors, HDL cholesterol may be unchanged [75] or increased by a soy protein diet, with an increase of lecithin-cholesterol acyl transferase [77]. In humans, casein or soy protein, when the quantities given are above minimal requirements, do not change plasma HDL and LDL cholesterol levels [78]. Nevertheless, the role of the lysine : arginine ratio as a major determinant of the cholesterolemic properties of proteins is felt by several authors to be of secondary importance, because results are not always in agreement [79], and also because one cannot neglect the possible pharmacological action of oligopeptides that have been absorbed intact [80]. The lipid-binding properties of proteins in the intestine depend upon the tertiary and quaternary structure of the proteins and cannot be produced by free amino acids [80]. Finally, the metabolic effects are not always similar with intact protein and with free amino acids [81]. The increase of blood cholesterol in casein-fed animals is due to an increase in the influx of cholesterol and bile acids from the intestine to the liver, a decrease of liver microsomal 3-hydroxymethylglutaryl coenzyme A, decreased biosynthesis of cholesterol, and a reduction of apolipoprotein B/E receptors that provokes an increase in lipoprotein concentration. The increased influx of bile acids depresses the conversion of cholesterol to bile acids and increases absorption of cholesterol [82, 83].

In soy-fed animals, the protein absorption of cholesterol is decreased, the excretion of fecal steroids is increased, the turnover of cholesterol is faster, and hepatic sterogenesis is increased [81, 84]. Some findings also support the hypothesis that the effect of casein on the enterohepatic cycle of bile acids depends on the degree of its phosphorylation [85, 86]. The phosphorylation state could also interfere with divalent cations that have an action on lipid metabolism, especially on cholesterol metabolism [87].

Finally, dietary proteins, especially animal proteins, cause an important immunological reaction [88]. Oligopeptides can be significantly absorbed through the intestine, sometimes even faster than amino acids from equivalent mixtures [89, 90], 36% of a casein hydrolysate being absorbed as peptides rather than as free amino acids [91]. Trace amounts of large polypeptides can also be absorbed through the intestine. Nevertheless, while many factors that may be involved in an immunologically provoked lesion of the arterial tissues are present, their true role in atherogenesis is not yet demonstrated [80], even if it is potentially important (41).

In conclusion, the relationships between food proteins, cholesterol metabolism, and atherosclerosis are very complex: further research is necessary to determine their real importance in human atherosclerosis.

References

1. Ignatowski A (1908) Influence de la nourriture animale sur l'organisme des lapins. Arch Med Exp Anat Pathol 20: 1-20
2. Newburgh LH, Squier TL (1920) High protein diets and atherosclerosis in rabbits. Arch Int Med 26: 38-40
3. Newburgh LH, Clarkson S (1923) The production of atherosclerosis in rabbits by feeding diet rich in meat. Arch Int Med 31: 653-676
4. Meeker DR, Keesten HD (1940) Experimental atherosclerosis and high protein diets. Proc Soc Exp Biol Med 45: 543-545
5. Meeker DR, Keesten HD (1941) Effect of high protein diets in experimental atherosclerosis of rabbits. Arch Pathol 31: 147-162
6. Howard AN, Gresham GA, Jones D, Jennings IW (1965) The prevention of rabbit atherosclerosis by soya bean meal. J Atheroscler Res 5: 330-337
7. Keys A, Anderson JT (1957) Dietary protein and the serum cholesterol in man. Am J Clin Nutr 5: 29-34
8. Albanese AA, Higgons RA, Lorenze EJ, Orto LA (1959) Effect of dietary proteins on blood cholesterol levels of adults. Geriatrics 14: 237-243
9. Bevedridge JMR, Connel WF, Robinson C (1963) Effect of the level of dietary protein with and without added cholesterol on plasma cholesterol levels in man. J Nutr 79: 289-295
10. Moore MC, Guzman MA, Schilling PE, Strong JP (1981) Dietary atherosclerosis study on deceased persons. J Am Diet Assoc 79: 668-672
11. Yudkin J (1957) Diet and coronary thrombosis: hypothesis and fact. Lancet II: 155-162
12. Connor WE, Connor SL (1972) The key role of nutritional factors in the prevention of coronary heart disease. Prev Med I: 49-83
13. Stamler JE (1979) Population studies. In: Levy RI, Rifkind BM, Dennis BM, Ernst ND (eds) Nutrition, lipids and coronary heart disease. Raven, New York, pp 25-88
14. Little JM, Angell EA (1977) Dietary protein level and experimental aortic atherosclerosis. Atherosclerosis 26: 173-179
15. Bydlowski SP, Stivaletti VLG, Douglas CR (1984) Biochemical observations on rats aortas: effect of protein refeeding after a protein depletion period. Ann Nutr Metabol 28: 85-91
16. Bydlowski SP, Stivaletti VLG, Douglas CR (1986) Biochemical observations on rat aorta: interaction of dietary protein and cholesterol. Br J Nutr 55: 295-304
17. Fillios L, Mann GV (1954) Influence of sulfur aminoacid deficiency on cholesterol metabolism. Metabolism 3: 16-26
18. Li TW, Freeman S (1946) Experimental lipaemia and hypercholesterolemia by protein depletion and by cholesterol feeding in dogs. Am J Physiol 145: 660-666
19. de Groot AP (1958) The influence of dietary protein on serum cholesterol level in rats. Voeding 19: 375-385
20. Chen LH, Liao S, Packett LV (1972) Interaction of dietary vitamin E and protein level on lipid source with serum cholesterol level in rats. J Nutr 102: 729-732
21. Leveille GA, Fischer H (1958) Plasma cholesterol in growing chicken as influenced by dietary protein and fat. Proc Soc Exp Biol Med 98: 630-632
22. Nikkila EA, Ollila O (1957) Effect of low protein diet on serum lipids and atherosclerosis of cholesterol fed chicken. Acta Pathol Microbiol Scand 40: 177-180
23. Guita PP, Tandow HD (1974) Experimental atherosclerosis in swine: effect of dietary protein and high fat. Exp Mol Pathol 20: 115-131
24. Kokatnur M, Rand NT, Kummerow FA, Scott HM (1958) Effect of dietary protein and fat on changes in serum cholesterol in mature birds. J Nutr 64: 177-184
25. Nishida T, Yenu A, Kummerow FA (1960) Effect of dietary protein on the metabolism of sodium acetate-1-C^{14} in chicks. J Nutr 71: 379-386

26. Cohen AM, Teitelbaum A (1966) Effect of different level of protein in sucrose and starch diets on lipid synthesis in the rat. Israel J Med Sci 2: 727-732
27. Deo MG, Sood SK, Ramalingaswani V (1965) Experimental protein deficiency. Pathologic features in the Rhesus Monkey. Arch Pathol 80: 14-23
28. Greer SHN, Hays AW, Speer VC, McCall JT (1966) Effect of dietary fat, protein and cholesterol on atherosclerosis in swine. J Nutr 90: 183-190
29. Laurent G (1983) Contribution à l'étude du rôle des protéines alimentaires dans l'athérogénèse. Etude chez le lapin "Fauve de Bourgogne" Oryctologus Cuniculus Dom L. Thesis, Nancy University
30. Carroll KK (1978) The role of dietary protein in hypercholesterolemia and atherosclerosis. Lipids 13: 360-365
31. Pick R, Savitri J, Katz LN, Johnson P (1965) Effect of dietary protein level on regression of cholesterol induced hypercholesterolemia and atherosclerosis of cockerels. J Atheroscler Res 5: 16-25
32. Susano M, Ishiwaki N, Nakashima K (1984) Dietary protein-dependent modification of serum cholesterol level in rats. Ann Nutr Metab 28: 192-199
33. Goulding NJ, Gibney MJ, Taylor G, Gallagher PJ (1983) Reversible hypercholesterolemia produced by cholesterol free fish meal protein diets. Atherosclerosis 49: 127-137
34. Lee HS, O'Donnell JAO, Hurt HD (1981) Influence of various dietary protein sources on plasma and liver lipids in gerbils. Fed Proc 40: 685
35. Hamilton RMG, Carroll KK (1976) Plasma cholesterol levels in rabbit fed low fat, low cholesterol diets. Effects of dietary proteins, carbohydrates and fibers from different sources. Atherosclerosis 24: 47-62
36. Hermus RJ (1975) Experimental atherosclerosis in rabbits on diet with milk, fat and different proteins. The Netherland Center of Agricultural Publishing and Documentation, Wageningen
37. Kritchevski D (1980) Dietary protein in atherosclerosis. In: Noseda G, Lewis B, Paoletti R (eds) Diet and drug in atherosclerosis. Raven, New York, pp 9-14
38. Kritchevski D, Tepper SA, Czarneski SK, Klurfeld DM, Story JA (1983) Effect of animal and vegetable protein in experimental atherosclerosis. In: Gibney HG, Kritchevski D (eds) Animal and Vegetable protein in lipid metabolism and atherosclerosis. Current topics in nutrition and disease, vol 8. Alan, Liss, New York, pp 85-100
39. Huff MW, Carroll KK (1980) Effect of dietary proteins and aminoacid mixtures on plasma cholesterol level in rabbits. J Nutr 110: 1676-1685
40. Terpstra AHM, Hermus RJJ, West CE (1983) Dietary protein and cholesterol metabolism in rabbits and rats. In: Gibney MG, Kritchevski D (eds) Animal and vegetable protein in lipid metabolism and atherosclerosis. Current topics in nutrition and disease, vol 8. Alan, Liss, New York, pp 19-49
41. Sugano M (1983) Hypocholesterolemic effect of plant protein in relation to animal protein. Mechanism of action. In: Gibney MG, Kritchevski D (eds) Animal and vegetable protein in lipid metabolism and atherosclerosis. Current topics in nutrition and disease, vol 8. Alan, Liss, New York, pp 51-84
42. Carroll KK (1981) Dietary protein and cardiovascular disease in new trends in nutrition, lipid research and cardiovascular disease. Alan, Liss, New York, pp 169-177
43. West CE, Deuring K, Ben Schutte J, Terpstra AHM (1982) The effect of age on the development of hypercholesterolemia in rabbits fed semipurified diets containing casein. J Nutr 112: 1287-1295
44. Hassan AS, Logas LL, Hackley JJ (1985) Dietary protein and atherosclerosis. Effect of exposure to dietary casein in early life on cholesterol and bile acid metabolism in the adult rabbit. Fed Proc 44: 1856
45. Beynen AC, West CE, Katan MB, Van Zutphen LFM (1986) Hyperresponsiveness of plasma cholesterol to dietary cholesterol saturated fatty acid and casein in inbred rabbits. Nutr Rep Int 33: 65-70
46. Terpstra AHM, West CE, Fennis JTCM, Schouten JA, Van der Veen A (1984) Hypocholesterolemic effect of dietary soy protein versus casein in Rhesus monkeys (Macaca Mulatta). Am J Clin Nutr 39: 1-7
47. Nagata Y, Imaizumi K, Sugano M (1980) Effects of soya-bean protein and casein on serum cholesterol levels in rats. Br J Nutr 44: 113-121

48. Terpstra AHM, Van Tintelen G, West CE (1982) The hypocholesterolemic effect of dietary soy protein in rats. J Nutr 112: 810-817
49. Lacombe C, Nibbelink M (1980) Lipoprotein modifications with changing dietary proteins in rabbits of a high fat diet. Artery 6: 280-289
50. Barth CA, Pfeuffer M, Hahn G (1984) Influence of dietary casein or soy protein on serum lipids and lipoproteins of monkeys (Macaca Fascicularis). Ann Nutr Metab 28: 137-143
51. Beynen AC, Schouten JA (1983) Influence of dietary soybean protein and casein on the level of plasma cholesterol in hamsters. Nutr Rep Int 28: 835-841
52. Terpstra AKM, van Tintelen G, West CE (1982) The hypocholesterolemic effect of dietary soy protein in rats. J Nutr 112: 810-817
53. Raheja KL, Lindscheer WG (1982) Comparative effects of soy and casein protein on plasma cholesterol concentrations. Ann Nutr Metab 26: 44-49
54. Wiebe SL, Brule VM, McDonald BE (1984) A comparison of the effect of diets containing beef protein and plant protein on blood lipids of healthy young men. Am J Clin Nutr 40: 928-989
55. Van Raaij JMA, Katan MB, Hautvast JGAJ, Hermus RJJ (1981) Effect of casein versus soy protein diets on serum cholesterol and lipoprotein in young healthy volunteers. Am J Clin Nutr 34: 1261-1271
56. Van Raaij JMA, Katan MB, West CE, Hautvast JGA (1982) Influence of diets containing casein, soy isolate and soy concentrate on serum cholesterol and lipoproteins in middle-aged volunteers. Am J Clin Nutr 35: 925-934
57. Grundy SM, Abrams JJ (1983) Comparison of action of soy protein and casein on metabolism of plasma lipoproteins and cholesterol in humans. Am J Clin Nutr 38: 245-252
58. Sirtori CR, Agradi E, Conti F, Mantero O, Gatti E (1977) Soy bean protein diet in the treatment of type II hyperlipoproteinemia. Lancet I: 275-277
59. Sirtori CR, Gatti E, Mantero E, Conti F, Agradi E, Tremoli E, Sirtori M, Fraterrigo L, Tavazzi L, Kritchevsky D (1979) Clinical experience with the soy bean protein diet in the treatment of hypercholesterolemia. Am J Clin Nutr 32: 1645-1658
60. Huff MW, Giovanetti PM, Wolfe BM (1984) Turnover of very low density lipoprotein-apoprotein B in increased by substitution of soybean protein for meat and dairy protein in the diets of hypercholesterolemic men. Am J Clin Nutr 39: 888-897
61. Verrillo A, de Teresa A, Giarrusso PC, La Rocca S (1985) Soybean protein diets in the management of type II hyperlipoproteinemia. Atherosclerosis 54: 321-331
62. Descovich GD, Ceredic C, Gaddi G (1980) Multicenter study of soybean protein diet for outpatient hypercholesterolemic patients. Lancet II: 709-712
63. Wolfe BM, Giovanetti PM, Cheng DCH, Roberts DCK, Carroll KK (1981) Hypolipidemic effect of substituting soybean protein isolate for all meat and dairy protein in the diets of hypercholesterolemic men. Nutr Rep Int 24: 1187-1197
64. Goldberg AP, Lim A, Kolar JB, Grundhauser JJ, Steinke FM, Schonfeld G (1982) Soybean protein independently lowers plasma cholesterol levels in primary hypercholesterolemia. Atherosclerosis 43: 355-368
65. Holmes WL, Rubel GB, Hood SS (1980) Comparison of the effect of dietary meat versus dietary soybean protein on plasma lipid of hyperlipidemic individuals. Atherosclerosis 36: 379-387
66. Shorey RL, Bazan B, Lo GS, Steinke FH (1981) Determinants of hypercholesterolemic response to soy and animal protein based diets. Am J Clin Nutr 34: 1769-1778
67. Vahouny GV, Chalcarz W, Satchithanandam S, Adamson I, Klurfeld DM, Kritchevsky D (1984) Effect of soy protein and casein intake on intestinal absorption and lymphatic transport of cholesterol and oleic acid. Am J Clin Nutr 40: 1156-1164
68. Vahouny GV, Adamson I, Chalcarz W, Satchithanandam S, Muesing R, Klurfeld DM, Tepper SA, Sanghvi A, Kritchevsky D (1985) Effects of casein and soy protein on hepatic and serum lipids and lipoprotein lipid distributions in the rat. Atherosclerosis 56: 127-137
69. Kritchevsky D, Tepper SA, Czarnecki SK, Klurfeld DM (1982) Atherogenicity of animal and vegetable protein. Influence of the lysine to arginine ratio. Atherosclerosis 41: 429-431
70. Aoyama Y, Yoshida A, Ashida K (1983) Changes in lipids in liver and serum of rats fed a histidine excess diet. Nutr Rep Int 28: 643-651
71. Sugano M, Ishiwaki N, Nakashima K (1984) Dietary protein-dependent modification of serum cholesterol level in rats. Ann Nutr Metab 28: 192-199
72. Huff MW, Hamilton RMG, Carroll KK (1977) Plasma cholesterol levels in rabbits fed low fat,

low cholesterol semi-purified diets. Effect of dietary proteins, protein hydrolysates and aminoacid mixtures. Atherosclerosis 28: 187-195
73. Carroll KK, Hamilton RMG (1975) Effects of dietary protein and carbohydrate on plasma cholesterol levels in relation to atherosclerosis. J Food Sci 40: 18-23
74. Carroll KK, Woodward CJM (1982) Hypocholesterolemic effects of soy protein in relation to aminoacid composition. Experimental researches. In: Lenzi S, Descovich GC (eds) Evaluation and therapy. Atherosclerosis, clinical. MTP Press, Lancaster, pp 225-230
75. Cohn JS, Kimpton WG, Nestel PJ (1984) The effect of dietary casein and soy protein on cholesterol and very low density lipoprotein metabolism in the rat. Atherosclerosis 52: 219-231
76. Scholz KE, Beynen AC, West CE (1983) Regression of casein and cholesterol induced hypercholesterolemia in rabbits. Z Ernährungswissensch 22: 85-96
77. Park MSC, Liepa GV (1982) Effects of dietary protein and aminoacids on the metabolism of cholesterol carrying lipoproteins in rats. J Nutr 112: 1892-1898
78. Sacks FM, Breslow JL, Wood PG, Kass EM (1983) Lack of an effect of dairy protein (casein) and soy protein on plasma cholesterol of strict vegetarious. J Lipid Res 24: 1012-1020
79. Gibney MJ (1983) The effect of dietary lysine to arginine ratio on cholesterol kinetics in rabbits. Atherosclerosis 47: 263-270
80. Redgrave TG (1984) Dietary proteins and atherosclerosis. Letter to the editors. Atherosclerosis 52: 349-351
81. Nagata Y, Ishiwaki N, Sugano M (1982) Studies on the mechanism of antihypercholesterolemic action of soy protein and soy protein-type aminoacid mixtures in relation to the casein counterparts in rats. J Nutr 112: 1614-1625
82. Beynen AC, van der Meer R, West CE (1986) Mechanism of casein induced hypercholesterolemia. Primary and secondary features. Letter to the editors. Atherosclerosis 60: 291-293
83. West CE, Beynen AC, Terpstra AHM, Scholz KE, Carroll KK, Woodward CJM (1983) The nature of dietary protein and serum cholesterol. Letter to the editors. Atherosclerosis 46: 253-256
84. Fumagalli R, Paoletti R, Howard AN (1978) Hypocholesterolaemic effect of soya. Life Sci 22: 947-952
85. Van der Meer R (1983) Is the hypercholesterolemic effect of dietary casein related to its phosphorylation state? Letter to the editors. Atherosclerosis 49: 339-341
86. Van der Meer R, de Vries H, West CE, de Waard H (1985) Casein induced hypercholesterolaemia in rabbits in calcium dependent Atherosclerosis 56: 139-147
87. Samman S, Roberts DCK (1984) The phosphorylation state of casein and its hypercholesterolaemic effect. The role of divalent cations. Atherosclerosis 52: 347-348
88. Gallagher PJ, Gibney MJ (1983) Immunological aspect of atherosclerosis. The role of dietary proteins. In: Gibney MG, Kritchevsky D (eds) Animal and vegetable protein in lipid metabolism and atherosclerosis. Current topics in nutrition and disease, vol 8. Alan, Liss, New York, pp 149-168
89. Silk DBA, Clark ML, Marrs TC, Addison JM, Bursten D, Matthews DM (1975) Jejunal absorption of an aminoacid mixture simulating casein and an enzymatic hydrolyzate of casein prepared for oral administration to normal adults. Br J Nutr 33: 95-100
90. Adibi SA (1971) Intestinal absorption of dipeptides in man. Relative importance of hydrolysis and intact absorption. J Clin Invest 50: 2266-2275
91. Gardner MLG (1975) Absorption of aminoacids and peptides from a complex mixture in the isolated small intestine in the rat. J Physiol 253: 233-256

Cholesterol-Lowering and High-Density Lipoprotein-Raising Properties of Lecithinated Soy Proteins in Type II Hyperlipidemic Patients

G. Noseda, C. R. Sirtori, and G. C. Descovich

Numerous dietary factors may favour an increased incidence of atherosclerosis. Among atherogenic factors in the diet, animal fat is the most widely recognized. A direct correlation has been established between saturated fatty acid and cholesterol intake, hypercolesterolemia, and the development of coronary heart disease [1]. In recent years, considerable interest has also been devoted to nutrients from vegetable sources. This interest has been particularly addressed to dietary components such as fibres, vegetable fat, and vegetable proteins. Epidemiological data show, in fact, that vegetable protein intake is negatively correlated with plasma cholesterol and coronary heart disease development [2].

The first studies on the hypocholesterolemic activity of the soybean protein diet were carried out by Sirtori about 10 years ago [3]. Textured proteins extracted from soybeans and restructured to a solid product were employed, as they were easy to convert to numerous dietary items and of acceptable taste. A group of 20 patients (plasma cholesterol being mostly in excess of 300 mg/dl) were admitted to a metabolic ward and received a diet with the complete substitution of animal with soybean proteins, but otherwise similar in the lipid and carbohydrate composition to a standard therapeutic diet. The experimental regimen was given for a period of 3 weeks and compared, in a cross-over design, with a similar diet of animal proteins. The results were clearly indicative of a 20%-22% plasma total and low-density lipoprotein (LDL) cholesterol drop with the soybean regimen in both experimental sequences. The hypothesis that a soy protein has a hypocholesterolemic action per se was demonstrated by the results of a subsequent experiment in eight type II patients in whom the addition of cholesterol, 500 mg/day, to soy protein did not modify the hypocholesterolemic response.

More recently, a multicenter study carried out in Italy and Switzerland [4] confirmed that the dietary substitution is remarkably effective, even when given to outpatients with hypercholesterolemia. The animal proteins in a low-lipid, low-cholesterol diet were substituted with a textured soybean preparation for 127 outpatients with stable type II hyperlipoproteinemia selected from eight Italian and one Swiss lipid clinics. Eight weeks of the modified diet reduced plasma cholesterol by 23% in the 67 participating male patients and by 25% in the 60 females. No significant changes in plasma triglycerides, high-density lipoprotein (HDL) cholesterol, and body weight were recorded. Better reduction in plasma cholesterol occurred in nonfamilial cases and in very young male patients.

In all clinical studies, only LDL cholesterol was decreased by textured soybean proteins, with the exception of one study in normolipidemic volunteers, where a rise in HDL cholesterol was also described [5]. Preliminary investigations have shown,

Table 1. Composition of the three experimental diets

	Traditional low-lipid Phase I–III	L-TVP 100% Phase II	L-TVP 50% Phase IV
A. Major nutrient (% of total calories) and cholesterol content			
Protein	20 (60 animal, 40 vegetable)	20 (10 animal, 90 vegetable)	20 (30 animal, 70 vegetable)
Lipid	25	25	25
Carbohydrates	55	55	55
Cholesterol (mg)	140–180	20–60	80–120
B. Fatty acid composition (%)			
16:0	17.9	17.5	17.8
18:0	8.1	7.5	7.8
18:1	27.3	26.8	27.0
18:2 (6)	44.5	46.3	44.9
18:3 (3)	0.9	1.2	1.1
20:4	0.3	0.2	0.3
Mean 18:2/18:1	1.60 (range 1.33–1.70)	1.79 (range 1.68–1.87)	1.66 (range 1.55–1.73)

L-TVP, lecithinated textured soybean protein.

however, that a preparation of textured soybean proteins containing a significant amount of lecithin may exert a promising raising effect on HDL cholesterol after only a few weeks of treatment [6]. The activity of this new lecithinated product was therefore tested within a formal protocol in a multicenter study on type II A patients, given both a complete and a partial substitution of animal proteins in their diet [7]. Plasma lipoprotein changes were evaluated in 65 type II patients undergoing sequential 4-week dietary treatment with: (a) standard low-lipid diet; (b) low-lipid diet with total replacement of animal proteins with textured soy proteins containing 6% lecithin; (c) standard low-lipid diet; (d) low-lipid diet with a 50% substitution of animal proteins with textured soy proteins containing 6% lecithin (Table 1). Total cholesterolemia was significantly reduced in both periods of lecithinated textured soy proteins: −18.6% during phase II (total replacement) and −13.2% during phase IV (partial replacement) (Fig. 1). HDL cholesterol levels tended to increase during lecithinated textured soy protein administration. However, only patients in the mid- and low tertiles for HDL cholesterolemia showed a significant increase of HDL levels during lecithinated textured soybean protein substitution (Fig. 2). The cholesterol-lowering activity of lecithinated textured soy proteins was significantly correlated to the basal cholesterolemia; the correlation in the opposite direction for HDL cholesterol (increases for patients with low starting levels) may suggest a link between the two findings. Studies on the effects of lecithin on plasma lipid-lipoprotein levels and on atherosclerosis prevention, have been controversial [8, 9]. Metabolic studies with polyunsaturated lecithin from soybeans in healthy volunteers have shown that this is secreted from the intestine within small very low-density lipoproteins (VLDL), followed by a transfer to HDL, which may contain two- to six-fold higher levels of exogenous lecithin, compared to the other lipoproteins [10]. Lecithin-modified HDL seems to have a markedly enhanced capacity for cholesterol storage [11]. If this is the case, patients with low starting HDL cholesterol levels would be more likely to benefit from this treatment.

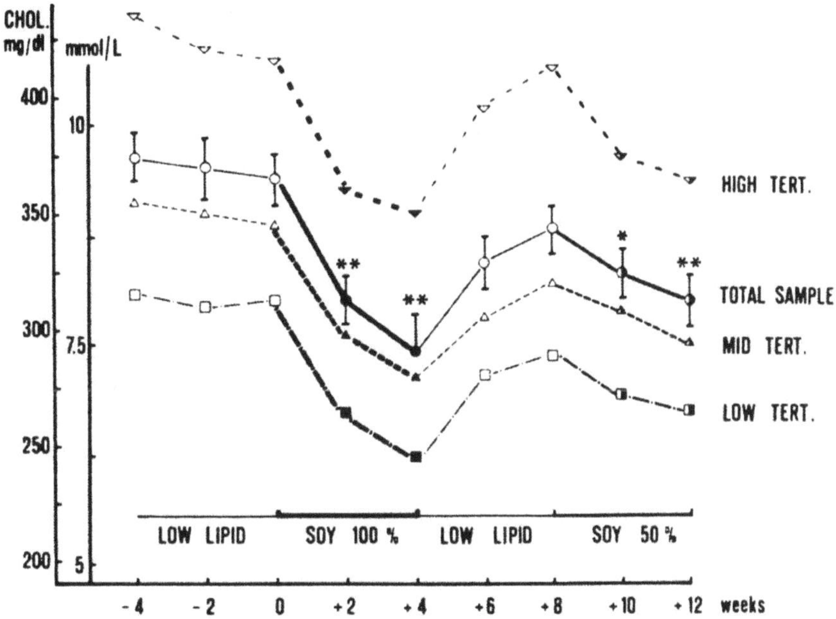

Fig. 1. Changes in plasma total cholesterol levels during the four different dietary periods in the whole patient sample ($n = 65$) and in the three tertiles with high, mid- and low cholesterolemias. Data are expressed as means ± SEM. * $p < 0.05$; ** $p < 0.01$ versus time 0

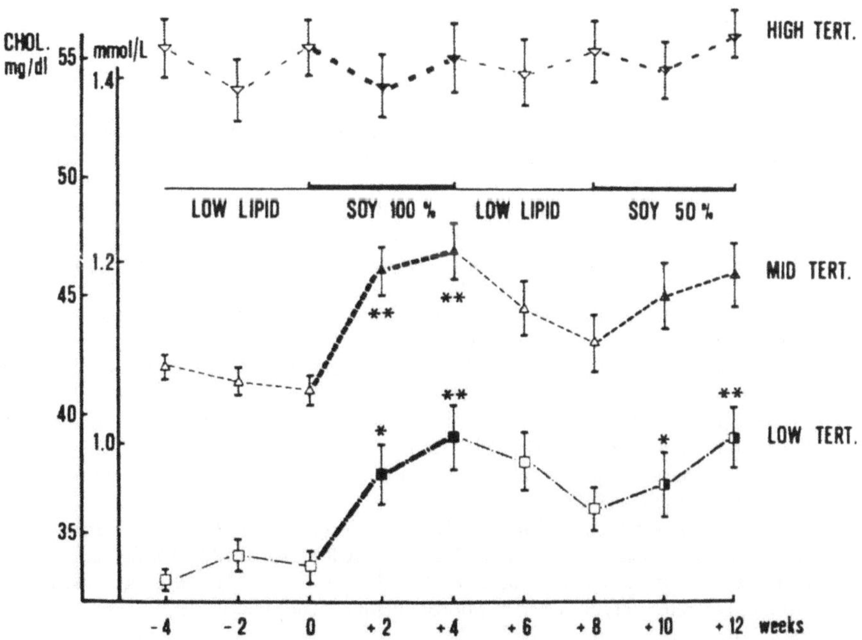

Fig. 2. Plasma HDL-C levels during each period of the study in patients divided into numerical tertiles for this parameter. The soybean regimen does not appear to modify HDL-C within the highest tertile, but significant increases are noted in both tertiles with lower HDL cholesterolemias. Mean ± SEM. * $p < 0.05$; ** $p < 0.01$ versus time 0

The demonstration that also a partial substitution of animal proteins with lecithinated textured soybean proteins, allowing a more liberal regimen, may be associated with reduced cholesterol and increased HDL, is clinically important for patients with mild forms of hypercholesterolemia.

Although a comparative evaluation of the activity of lecithin per se, without soy-proteins, was not carried out in this study, previous experience has excluded the possibility that such low levels of lecithin may significantly lower cholesterolemia and/or increase HDL [9, 12]. A possible direct link of the cholesterol-lowering properties of the lecithinated textured soyprotein diet with its high polyunsaturated/saturated ratio can also be excluded, in view of the very similar fat composition in the animal protein diet.

Although this study does not contribute to the clarification of the mechanism of action of the soybean diet, it provides further support to the growing number of observations indicating that the hypercholesterolemic condition, with a high risk of atherosclerosis development, is particularly sensitive to this regimen, especially with the addition of small quantities of lecithin.

References

1. Shekelle RB, Shryock AMC, Oglesby P, Lepper M, Stamler J, Lin S, Raynor WJ Jr (1981) Diet, serum cholesterol and death from coronary heart disease. N Engl J Med 304: 65-79
2. Carrol KK (1978) Dietary protein in relation to plasma cholesterol levels and atherosclerosis. Nutr Rev 36: 1-5
3. Sirtori CR, Agradi E, Conti F, Mantero O, Gatti E (1977) Soybean protein in the treatment of type II hyperlipoproteinaemia. Lancet I: 275-277
4. Descovich GC, Gaddi A, Mannino G, Cattin L, Senin U, Caruzzo C, Fragiacomo C, et al (1980) Multicenter study of soybean protein diet for outpatient hypercholesterolaemic patients. Lancet 2: 709-712
5. Van Raaij JMA, Katan MB, West CE, Hautoast JGAJ (1982) Influence of diets containing casein, soy isolate and soy concentrate on serum cholesterol and lipoproteins in middle-aged volunteers. Am J Clin Nutr 35: 925-934
6. Descovich GC, Mannino G, Benassi MS, Ceredi C, Cordaro CI, Dormi A, Gaddi A et al (1982) Treatment of hypercholesterolemic patients with soybean protein. In: Lenzi S, Descovich GC (eds) Atherosclerosis: clinical evaluation and therapy. MTP Press, Lancaster, pp 249-265
7. Sirtori CR, Zucchi-Dentone C, Sirtori M, Gatti E, Descovich GC, Gaddi A, Cattin L et al (1985) Cholesterol-lowering and HDL-raising properties of lecithinated soy proteins in the type II hyperlipidemic patients. Ann Nutr Metab 29: 348-357
8. Blaton V, Soeteway F, Vandanne D, Declercq B, Peeters H (1976) Effects of polyunsaturated phosphatidylcholine on human types II and IV hyperlipoproteinemias. Artery 2: 309-325
9. Greten H, Raetzer H, Stichl A, Schettler G (1980) The effect of polyunsaturated phosphatidylcholine in man. Atherosclerosis 36: 81-88
10. Zierenberg O, Grundy SM (1982) Intestinal absorption of polyenephosphatidylcholine in man. J Lipid Res 23: 1136-1142
11. Zierenberg O, Assmann G, Schmitz G, Rosseneu M (1981) Effect of polyenephosphatidylcholine and cholesterol uptake by human high density lipoprotein. Atherosclerosis 39: 527-542
12. Ter Welle HF, van Gent CM, Dekker W, Willebrands AF (1974) The effect of soya lecithin on serum lipid values in type II hyperlipoproteinemia. Acta Med Scand 195: 267-271

Prevention and Therapy

From Theory to Practice: Community-Based Studies on the Prevention of Coronary Heart Disease

P. Puska

The Nature and Need for Community-Based Studies

Since the Second World War cardiovascular diseases (CVD), and especially coronary heard disease (CHD), have become the leading public health problem in most of the industrialised world. CHD rates have increased not only among old people, but an alarming increase has also taken place among the middle-aged population. This has led to the fact that in many countries every second premature death is due to CVD. Thus it is obvious that any major new improvement in public health, especially with regard to prevention of premature mortality and disability, is greatly dependent on our ability to prevent the modern epidemic of heart disease and related chronic health problems.

The medical and epidemiological research on the aetiology of CHD has drawn the attention to the likely causal role of certain risk factors, especially elevated serum (low-density lipoprotein - LDL) cholesterol and blood pressure levels and smoking. Classical trials to prove the causality have met with problems of feasibility and study design. The community-based studies have substantial potential in introducing general lifestyle and risk factor changes in large numbers of people (since the risk factor is closely related with the general way of life and other features of the community). Thus a well-evaluated community-based study can add to our knowledge of the role of the risk factors. Furthermore, the community study examines how the existing service structure and community resources can be used and assesses the overall feasibility and consequences of such an intervention.

The central aim in the community study is to influence the risk factor levels of the whole population of the community through a comprehensive intervention using the available community structures and the naturally occurring interactions. From an *epidemiological point of view* the strength of this population approach is that it will be more effective in reducing the community disease rates than a restricted, even intensive, intervention among only high-risk people. This is because the bulk of the disease cases in the community do not come from the relatively small proportion people with clearly high-risk factor levels but from the large majority of the population that has only moderated elevation but usually in several risk factors.

From a *behavioural and social point of view,* the potential of the community approach lies in the fact that the risk-related behaviours are deeply embedded in the ways of life, in the social and even physical environments of the community. Thus it is only possible to influence permanently the health-related lifestyles in large numbers of people if the determinants of such lifestyles can be changed and thus a general social process of change introduced in the community.

Public health decisions on risk factor reduction and CHD prevention must be based on general information about the overall expected favourable and harmful consequences of such an activity. Community studies investigate several questions relevant to prevention and community health in a real-life situation. Thus these studies, besides assessing risk factors and disease changes, yield information on the feasibility of the programme and turn up other positive findings such as reduced disability payments, fewer reported general health complaints and emotional problems, and popular satisfaction with the action in progress.

Thus the question of the causal relationship between the risk factors and CHD is only one of several aspects that the community-based study deals with. In principle, this hypothesis should be approached by a classical randomised design. A classical trial with random allocation or individuals into experimental and control groups has, however, several major limitations. An individual clinical type of intervention on risk factors deals with people outside their natural living conditions; it is expensive and the results may be difficult to apply nationwide. A community-based approach that tests the effects of a comprehensive package in natural conditions overcomes these problems to a great extent. It uses more "real-life" intervention with the existing service structure and community participation and takes advantage of natural interactions of several varibles in the community. It may reduce costs significantly and obviate ethical problems which might otherwise exist.

A community-based study is thus only partially designed to study the possible causal relation between risk factors and disease. Nevertheless, because of the limitations of randomised trials and the advantages of community programmes, these may give considerable information about the role of conventional risk factors. Community programmes have other important roles as well. They demonstrate our ability to modify levels of risk factors and influence lifestyle in the population to the extent of improving the health of the people. They test the feasibility of such programmes using existing health services and other resources. Furthermore, they serve as demonstration and training models.

The North Karelia Project as an Example of the Community-Based Approach

Heart disease has not affected all industrialised countries to the same extent. In the 1960s mortality statistics showed that the highest CHD mortality rates were observed in Finland, and especially among its male population. These differences between countries were confirmed at the beginning of the 1970s in a register study coordinated by the World Health Organization (WHO) [1]. Similar studies showed that there were also some regional differences within Finland, so that the highest rates were observed in Eastern Finland and especially in the county of North Karelia [2].

The North Karelia Project was launched in 1972 as a response to the difficult problem of heart disease in North Karelia. Since this problem was by no means much smaller in other parts of Finland and in many other countries, the project was also to be a "pilot" or "demonstration" programme for wider application. In addition, since the prevention and control of CVD involved many unsolved scientific questions, careful scientific evaluative research was linked into the programme.

Both the background of the project and the nature of the problem naturally lead in the planning phase to the adoption of the community approach as the main strategy for the prevention of CHD.

The major question of the evaluation were naturally whether it was possible to influence the risk factor levels in the population and, if so, whether such changes led to respective changes in CHD rates. For this evaluation a quasi-experimental study design was used. Changes in the North Karelian population were compared with respective changes in a reference area that was chosen to be as similar to North Karelia as possible.

The assessment of the effect of the intervention on health behaviour and risk factors was based on repeated independent surveys of large representative population samples in North Karelia and in a matched reference area at the outset (spring 1972), at the end of the first 5-year period (spring 1977), and at the end of 10 years (spring 1982). The net reduction in North Karelia (the reduction in North Karelia minus the reduction in the reference area) was considered to be the programme effect. This estimate is a conservative one, because it is likely that the project also influenced the development in the reference area and nationally. Independent random sample surveys were used to assess the magnitude of changes in the whole population, since follow-up of a cohort would not have been able to distinguish intervention effect from evaluation effect. Strictly standardised and similar questionnaires were used on large samples in both areas for the three surveys. The participation rates were also high.

Disease rates in North Karelia were monitored by special myocardial infarction and stroke registers that operated in the whole North Karelia according to WHO criteria. Mortality and disability pension development in the two areas, as well as in the whole country, were assessed using national register data.

The results of the original 5-year period of the project (1972-77) have been published in a number of publications and in a monograph published by WHO [3]. After the encouraging results of the first 5 years it was decided to continue with the programme and with the follow-up of the risk factor and disease changes in the area. This was considered to be of great importance in order to learn about the long-term consequences of this type of activity. At the same time the project has been increasingly associated with the national application of the results - which is in accordance with the original aims but which at the same time reduces the availability of reference areas for evaluation.

Results of the North Karelia Project

Overall the reductions in risk factor levels observed in North Karelia during the 10 years of the programme were substantial: for men there was a 36% reduction in smoking, 11% in mean serum cholesterol concentration and 5% in mean diastolic blood pressure. The changes in biological risk factors (serum cholesterol and blood pressure) were much smaller than in smoking, which is to be expected. These changes in risk factors may be considered small for an individual but they represent mean changes for the whole population and should thus have an important effect on population disease rates. The changes in biological risk factors among women

Table 1. Relative net reductions (% ± 95% confidence interval) in the risk factor means in men and women aged 30-59 years in North Karelia (i.e. adjusted for changes in the reference area) in 1972-1977 and 1972-1982 based on cross-sectional surveys of random population samples in 1972, 1977 and 1982

Risk factor	Net reduction (%)			
	Men		Women	
	1972-1977	1972-1982	1972-1977	1972-1982
Daily smoking	14 ± 10[b]	28 ± 11[c]	8 ± 27	14 ± 38
Serum cholesterol	4 ± 1[c]	3 ± 2[c]	1 ± 2	1 ± 2
Systolic BP	3 ± 1[c]	3 ± 1[c]	5 ± 1[c]	5 ± 1[c]
Diastolic BP	3 ±	1 ± 1[a]	4 ± 1[c]	2 ± 1[c]

[a] $p<0.05$. [b] $p<0.01$. [c] $p<0.001$. BP, blood pressure.

were similar to those among men, but the results for smoking were bound to differ because of the lower initial smoking rates among women.

Risk factor levels were also clearly reduced in the reference area, as had been observed during the first 5-year period. At that time, however, the reduction had been greater in North Karelia among men for all risk factors and among women for blood pressure. During continued follow-up the net difference in favour of North Karelia further increased for smoking, remained the same for serum cholesterol concentration and systolic blood pressure, and lessened for diastolic blood pressure. Thus the results in 1982 were further evidence of the effects of the intervention programme in North Karelia. During the 10-year period 1972-1982 the following net changes (i.e. adjusted for changes in the reference area) took place for the risk factor means of the population aged 30-59 in North Karelia (Table 1): −28% for smoking ($p<0.001$), −3% for serum cholesterol ($p<0.001$) and −3% for systolic BP ($p<0.001$) [4].

The analysis of the available mortality data concerning the period from 1969 to 1979 [5] showed that the CHD mortality among the middle-aged male population in North Karelia decreased 24% (nationally 12%, $p<0.05$). Most of this decrease in North Karelia took place after 1973. During this period (i.e. 1974-1979) the reduction in CHD mortality was 22% in North Karelia, 12% in the reference area and 11% in the rest of the country (Table 2). CHD mortality also declined among women in North Karelia more than in the rest of the country but because of much smaller absolute numbers there is much more uncertainty about the significance of the results among women. A similar, although less marked pattern was also observed for cardiovascular mortality and all-cause mortality of the middle-aged population.

A continued follow-up of the CHD mortality trends up to 1982 showed that the decrease in North Karelia continued. Over the 10 years of the project the reduction in age-adjusted CHD mortality of the middle-aged male population was approximately 30%. This reduction was reflected in reduced total premature mortality. At the same time the respective reduction of CHD mortality in the rest of Finland was approximately 20%.

The comprehensive evaluation has given other evidence to support the conclu-

Table 2. Decline in age-standardised coronary heart disease mortality based on average annual regression in North Karelia, the reference area, and in Finland (less North Karelia) 1974-1979 (± % confidence intervals)

	Annual decline during 1974-1979 (%)	
	Men	Women
North Karelia	3.7 ± 1.5	2.2 ± 3.4
Reference area	1.9 ± 2.3	1.8 ± 1.4
Finland less North Karelia	1.7 ± 2.2[a]	1.2 ± 2.4

[a] Difference from North Karelia in relation to random variation $p < 0.05$.

sion that the intervention resulted in a positive effect on cardiovascular and other health problems. A net reduction among both men and women was observed in the self-reported prevalence of angina pectoris, diagnosed and/or treated by a doctor. The findings indicative a positive effect on cardiovascular disability pension rates which were based both on pension statistics and on survey data [3].

The previous evaluation showed that, as a whole, no negative psychosocial consequences of the intervention could be observed - either in the total population or in the high-risk groups. The programme was much more associated with an improvement in self-reported subjective health and perceived risk of heart disease among the North Karelian population. And a significant difference in favour of North Karelia was observed in these changes when compared with the reference area [6].

Throughout the 10-year period the feasibility of the programme was good. This was the case inspite of the fact that - at least in the early years - the health service resources were scarce and the society norms were rather traditional and likely to resist changes in lifestyle. Local health services and local health personnel co-operated well and thus formed a firm backbone for the action. The local population participated eagerly in the activities and over the years various community organisations contributed in many ways to the aims of the project in the area. Because the project aims were integrated into the existing health services and broad community participation was a key feature, the overall costs of the programme were modest. Additionally, obvious savings occurred, for instance in reduced disability payments [3].

Discussion and Conclusions

Influencing people's health-related behaviour and risk factors is obviously not an easy task. Even though the health hazards of for example smoking are well-known, many activities to fight smoking have met with limited success. We consider the results and experience presented here as an encouraging indication that, at least under favourable conditions, a comprehensive, determined and well-planned activity can indeed leat to substantial favourable changes.

It is obviously difficult to state the reason for this favourable effect in North Karelia and whether and how it could be accomplished elsewhere. A community programme like this ultimately tests whether a specific programme (designed so that it can be applied on a larger scale) is feasible and effective under given conditions. The impact of various community conditions and of different components of the project on successes and failures can be evaluated only to a limited extent.

The experience and results so far support the initial hypothesis that a well-conceived comprehensive community-based programme can have a positive impact on lifestyles and cardiovascular risk factors of a whole population and that such a development is associated with reduced cardiovascular mortality rates. These results thus give further support to the currently widely accepted risk factor theory. Furthermore, they demonstrate the potential of a community-based approach in changing the risk factors and give practical experience in organising such activities within health services and other community settings.

The programme in North Karelia continues to support further the so far favourable development. This is also considered important for national and international demonstration and training purposes. At the same time it is important to monitor further the risk factor and disease trends in order to assess fully the long-term impact of these activities. Furthermore, the scope of the programme has been extended to consider related major non-communicable diseases in an integrated way and to emphasise also the promotion of "positive" health. The project also continues the application of its experience nationwide, through the national health service system, through several mass-media channels, by the preparation of health education and other materials, etc.

Active collaboration with WHO and other agencies has helped to apply the approach used in North Karelia elsewhere. During the last few years several community-based studies and programmes have been launched in Europe and the United States. This development is of great importance, since it will show whether the results obtained in North Karelia can also be achieved elsewhere and it will tell us more about the value of different intervention approaches in different cultural settings.

References

1. World Health Organization (1976) Myocardial infarction community registers. WHO, Copenhagen (Public Health in Europe 5)
2. Pohjola S, Siltanen P, Romo M, et al (1980) Sydäninfarktin esiintyvyys ja ennuste Soumesa vuonna 1973. Helsingin, Turun, Tampereen ja Pohjois-Karjalan rekistereiden vertailua. Duodecim 96: 18-31
3. Puska P, Tuomilehto J, Salonen J, et al (1981) The North Karelia project: evaluation of a comprehensive community programme for control of cardiovascular diseases in North Karelia, Finland 1972-77. WHO, Copenhagen
4. Puska P, Salonen J, Nissinen A, et al (1983) Change in risk factors for coronary heart disease during 10 years of a community intervention programme (North Karelia project). Br Med J 287: 1840-1844
5. Salonen J, Puska P, Kottke T, Tuomilehto J, Nissinen A (1983) Decline in mortality from coronary heart disease in Finland from 1969 to 1979. Br Med J 286: 1857-1860
6. Kottke T, Puska P, Salonen JT, Tuomilehto J, Nissinen A (1984) Changes in perceived heart disease risk and health during a community-based heart disease prevention programme. The North Karelia project. Am J Public Health 74: 1404-1405

Regression of Atherosclerosis in Man

A. G. Olsson

Introduction

Methods to determine whether regression of atherosclerosis is possible in man must be indirect. Two principal methods used to demonstrate regression can be discussed: patho-anatomical studies on autopsy material, and visualisation of atheroma in vivo by other means.

Patho-Anatomical Evidence of Atherosclerosis Regression in Man

The first research to conclude that regression might be possible in man was presented by Aschoff in 1924. Of observations made during World War I he stated [1]: "With the increasing duration of war the atheromatous spots on the aorta was observed less frequently." Malinow has elegantly reviewed current evidence from post-mortem studies that atheroma regression may occur [2]. Based on observations at autopsy of atheroma in cancer and noncancer patients [3], he noted that cancer patients had a level of atherosclerosis corresponding to that of noncancer patients 16 years younger. As it is improbable that the cancer had influenced the arterial process over that many years, it was inferred that regression of already existing atherosclerosis had occurred during the shorter course of the malignant disease. This analysis by Malinow may provide statistical anatomical evidence of the occurrence of atherosclerosis regression in humans. Although the findings are consistent with the hypothesis that processes occurring during the terminal stages of cancer are associated with the arrest of progression or regression of atherosclerosis in humans, the limitations of post-mortem studies make these conclusions tentative.

Evidence of Atherosclerosis Regression in Living Man

The most precise method to study atherosclerotic change in man is by standardized serial arteriographies. By this method the effect of decreasing atherogenic serum lipoprotein concentrations on the rate of change of atheromatosis can be studied [4]. These studies of atherosclerosis development have been called regression studies, and have examined coronary (CAD) and femoral artery disease (FAD).

Assessment of Atherosclerosis and Atherosclerosis Change

In studies on the development of angiographically defined atherosclerosis, a crucial point is the reproducibility of the method. We [5] and others [6] have pointed out the considerable intra- and interindividual error in visual estimation of atherosclerosis. Therefore, improvements to the methodology of atheroma estimation have been necessary. These have been made by essentially two approaches, consensus evaluation by expert panels [7], and computer-assisted techniques [8, 9]. Data on variations between methods have been presented for both CAD [8] and FAD [9]. Here, I will consider studies on atheroma estimation in the coronary and in the femoral arteries, using both visual (expert panel) and computer methods. At present results of intervention studies with all these methods are not available.

Coronary Atherosclerosis

Hamsten et al. recently pointed out the relative importance of accurate measurement of the extent and severity of coronary atheromatosis in contrast to the number and severity of coronary stenoses [10]. They found highly significant relations between low-density lipoprotein (LDL) cholesterol and apolipoprotein B concentrations on one hand and the severity of CAD on the other. However, no relation was seen between the lipoprotein and apoprotein concentrations and the degree of stenosis. Consequently, in a study of regression of coronary atherosclerosis by lowering of serum lipid levels, the use of CAD severity as the endpoint is more likely to show any effects of treatment than using figures for stenosis. It should be pointed out that the method of Hamsten et al. for arteriographically determining CAD has so far not been validated using autopsy data. However, the work illustrates the importance of careful definition of endpoints in regression studies.

Visual Estimation of CAD

In a nonrandomized, controlled prospective study [11], Nikkilä et al. studied 28 patients with hyperlipidaemia and CAD. Coronary arteriograms were performed 7 years apart in the treatment group and 5 years apart in the control groups. Changes were extrapolated to 7 years in the latter group. Treatment consisted of diet and clofibrate, in some cases combined with nicotinic acid. CAD was estimated visually, luminal narrowing being the endpoint used.

In nine of the 28 treated patients the lesions did not progress (32%), while in only one did they not progress in the control group (8%). Those patients having plasma cholesterol above normal during the study showed a higher mean proportional increase of CAD. Those with low levels of high-density lipoprotein (HDL) cholesterol showed a higher number of segments with lesions that progressed. It could be concluded that the average angiographic progression was least in patients with the lowest cholesterol, triglyceride, and very low density lipoprotein (VLDL) plus LDL cholesterol concentrations during treatment, and in those with the highest HDL cholesterol levels.

The NHLBI study [7] examined whether lowering the plasma concentration of cholesterol by diet and cholestyramine therapy reduced the development of CAD. The study was double blind, and placebo controlled. Patients with type II hyperlipoproteinemia were randomly assigned to a low-cholesterol, low-fat diet plus active drug or placebo. CAD was assessed by coronary angiography at entry and after 5 years of therapy. An elaborate system for visual evaluation of films was set up, with three independent review panels.

59 patients were allocated to cholestyramine therapy (24 g daily) and 57 to placebo. "Definite" or "probable" progression of CAD, as determined by the review panel, was found in 32% of the cholestyramine-treated group and in 49% of the placebo group ($P<0.05$, one-tailed test). If the same definitions were applied to those with lesions producing more than 50% stenosis, the corresponding figures were 12% and 33% respectively ($P<0.05$). For other parameters studied, e.g., regression, new lesions showed favorable results in the cholestyramine-treated group.

The authors concluded that, although the results could not be considered definite, the evidence provided by the investigation suggested that lowering of cholesterol produced by diet and cholestyramine therapy inhibits the progression of CAD.

In a companion article [12], the effects of lowering plasma cholesterol, regardless of assigned treatment group, were analyzed. A significant inverse relationship was found between progression and the combination of an increase in HDL cholesterol and a decrease in LDL cholesterol. Changes in the ratio of HDL cholesterol to total and LDL cholesterol were the best predictors of changes in occurrence CAD. The authors concluded that "these observations are supportive of a redefined lipid hypothesis, i.e. that increasing concentrations of HDL cholesterol and decreasing concentrations of total cholesterol or LDL cholesterol will delay progression of CAD."

The NHLBI study has subsequently been subjected to analysis of the effects of cholestyramine on the incidence of coronary heart disease (CHD) and mortality [13]. So far very few data have been published on the relation between atheroma change and prognosis. Thus, Kramer et al. [14] reported that patients with CAD progression, measured as an increase in coronary obstruction of 20% or more, or as a change from less than total to total obstruction, were more likely to have new myocardial infarctions than those who did not have progression. In this part of the NHLBI study, 72 placebo and the 71 cholestyramine-treated patients were compared with regard to deaths, nonfatal myocardial infarctions, worsening angina, and at least one cardiac event. The evaluation of events was done blind. The cholestyramine-treated group had significantly fewer events than the placebo group ($P<0.05$). When CAD progression status was combined with the clinical endpoints, the beneficial effects of cholestyramine became uniformly significant.

Visual and Computer Estimation of Coronary Atherosclerosis

Arntzenius et al. [15] recently published the results of a study of the effect of dietary intervention on CAD progression. The study was uncontrolled but the results are nevertheless highly interesting. Thirty-nine patients were investigated by coronary arteriography over a period of 2 years.

Change in lesion size, mainly growth, was estimated both visually and by computerized image analysis. The severity of coronary obstruction was expressed as the minimum diameter in millimeters at the site of obstruction. The estimate therefore does not reflect the amount of coronary atheromatosis. Treatment consisted of a vegetarian diet in which the ratio of polyunsaturated to saturated fatty acids was at least 2:1 and dietary cholesterol was less than 100 mg per day. This resulted in a significant decrease in total cholesterol and in the ratio of total to HDL cholesterol. Both visual and computer-assisted assessment showed progression in 21 of the 39 patients but no lesion growth in 18 patients. The latter group had significantly lower total cholesterol and total to HDL cholesterol ratio, and higher HDL cholesterol, both at baseline and during the 2 years of intervention. Computer-measured lesion growth correlated positively with the mean values for the total to HDL cholesterol ratio ($n=19$), both for those with high initial total to HDL cholesterol ratio and a good response to diet ("high-low") ($n=19$), and for those with a high initial ratio and poor reduction with treatment ("high-high") ($n=11$). The CAD of the "high-high" patients showed considerable and significant progression, while no progression was seen in either "low" group or the "high-low" group. The authors concluded that "coronary lesion growth was strongly related to the total/HDL cholesterol." The results are interesting as they are the first to show that dietary change might influence the development of CAD in man. The study is also remarkable in that changes were observed after a relatively short interval of study, 2 years.

Computer-Assisted Image Reconstruction

Brown et al. [9] used coronary cine-frames to reconstruct images of diseased arterial segments. The image borders defined by subjective interpretation were digitized. Computer programs were constructed to account for distortions. Percentage diameter and area reduction in the stenoses were computed, as were lesion length, estimated atheroma mass stenosis, Reynolds number, flow resistance, and peak initial shear stress. In a careful methodological study this method was used to determine the natural history of CAD in 47 patients with clinical CHD on two occasions 18 months apart. True change was defined as 3 standard deviations of a short term difference distribution, and was found to correspond to 10.2% stenosis with 99.5% confidence. The study showed that 12% of all lesions progressed and that 4% regressed over the 18 months. More severe lesions were more likely to regress. Of these, 23% were due to thrombolytic recanalization of the atheroma mass or occluding thrombus, and 77% were due to reduction of atheroma mass. Abnormal serum lipids made progression more likely ($P<0.03$).

Brown's technique is at present being used in a number of interventions studies.

Femoral Atherosclerosis

Use of FAD as an endpoint following treatment of serum lipid levels has been made by Blankenhorn et al. [16], Duffield et al. [17], and ourselves [18], all in controlled studies.

The technique of computer estimation of FAD was developed by Blankenhorn et al. [16]. In a series of methodological publications they demonstrated that computer-estimated atherosclerosis (CEA) of the femoral artery correlated with the amount of cholesterol in the femoral lesion [19]. Average atheroma growth rate in a population of hyperlipidemics was 2% per year [8]. In a pilot intervention study those who decreased their serum cholesterol concentration by 15%, showed a reduction of CEA of 0.62% per month [4].

From the data obtained by Blankenhorn it can be calculated that, if an endpoint was tested only once in a trial, if an alpha error of 0.05 was chosen, and if 120 subjects were included in both test and control groups, there would be a greater than 97% chance of detecting an effect of therapy of 2% change per year after 3 years. Thus by careful calculations sample sizes and trial costs can be defined before an intervention study of femoral atherosclerosis development. Blankenhorn et al. are using their technology in their cholesterol lowering atherosclerosis study (CLAS) [16], which comprises 80 patients in treatment and control groups. The endpoint is the rate of change of atherosclerosis, as determined from selective femoral angiograms. Selection criteria have been that subjects should have had coronary bypass surgery, be nonsmokers, and have total plasma cholesterol between 185 and 350 mg/ 100 ml. The treatment group receives dietary advice and niacin, and the control group receives dietary advice. The interval between angiograms is 2 years. Progress reports have been published.

In a study using computer estimation of FAD we made calculations to see what could be achieved by increasing the number of observations of femoral atheroma, basing the figures of Blankenhorn's data (I. Holme, personal communication). We were interested to determine what increase of discriminatory power could be achieved if double angiograms were performed yearly instead of 2-yearly in a 36 month study ($n=8$). To be conservative we estimated the rate of change of CEA as -0.4% per month if the serum cholesterol decrease was 15% (-0.62% in Blankenhorn's study). If cholesterol-related atheroma change does not alter with time we will find an 8% decrease of CEA with a 10% decrease of cholesterol. When two estimations are made, a 0.05 significance level chosen, and 100 subjects used in treatment and control groups, these adjusted data give a power of $1-\alpha=0.53$ ($1-\alpha=0.98$ not adjusted). If the number of observations is increased to eight the power increases to $1-\alpha=0.94$.

Duffield et al. [17] investigated patients with symptoms of FAD (intermittent claudication). Twenty-four patients were randomly assigned to serum lipid lowering treatment (diet plus nicotinic acid, cholestyramine or clofibrate) or to "usual care." Peripheral atherosclerosis was estimated by arteriography and computer estimation of "edge irregularity." Visual estimation was performed before the study and after a mean period of 19 months. This indicated that the number of arterial segments showing progression decreased significantly by 60%. The edge irregularity index derived from computerized analysis showed a significant 2.5-fold increase in the usual-care group compared with the treatment group. A positive and significant correlation was found between LDL cholesterol and change in irregularity index when the treatment and usual care groups were pooled.

In our own study, asymtomatic patients (mean age at entry 53 years, range 35-65) with types II A ($n=21$), II B ($n=18$), and IV ($n=24$) hyperlipoproteinaemia were included [18]. After 6 months on a moderate diet patients were arteriographed and randomly allocated to the treatment group ($n = 31$) or control group ($n = 32$). The treatment group received a combination of nicotinic acid in doses increasing successively to 1 g four times daily, and 0.2 g fenofibrate twice daily. Patients in the control group received, twice daily, two placebo tablets identical to the fenofibrate tablets.

After 12 months a second femoral arteriography was performed.

When the study was finished visual estimation of all angiograms was done. Three radiologists independently scored atherosclerosis on four segments of the femoral artery (upper and lower segments of the superior and inferior parts, respectively) from 0 to 5 with increasing severity. Consensus evaluation between the radiologists was required. The sum of the scores was divided by the number of segments judged, and change of atheroma size was estimated in pairs of femoral arteriograms and in a random order with regard to group. For each segment, regression, progression, and no change were given the values −1, +1 and 0 respectively. The sum of the segment change scores was divided by the number of segments scored. Change of atherosclerosis score (0–5) was set to −2 or +2 as this always indicated a large change in atheroma size.

The distribution of visually estimated atherosclerosis did not differ between the two groups. Sixteen patients were excluded from the study, the reasons being (numbers in treatment/control groups) no visible atherosclerosis (8/6), or unwillingness to continue one year's treatment (1/1). One patient developed allergic symptoms to the contrast medium at the first arteriography. No significant differences of age, smoking, systolic and diastolic blood pressure, and serum lipoprotein concentrations were seen between treatment and control groups after 6 months.

The serum lipoprotein concentrations after 12 months in patients who completed 1 year of treatment are given in Table 1. Changes in femoral atheroma were seen in 11 of the 47 patients (Table 2). With Fisher's exact test, Mann-Whitney test and Stu-

Table 1. Mean serum lipoprotein concentration after 12 months' drug treatment (mmol/l) chol, cholesterol; TG, triglycerides; significance test, Wilcoxon

Group	*n*	Total		VLDL		LDL		HDL	
		Chol	TG	Chol	TG	Chol	TG	Chol	TG
Treatment	22	6.03	1.35	0.40	0.74	3.92	0.43	1.68	0.13
P		<0.001	<0.001	<0.001	<0.001	<0.001	NS	NS	<0.001
Control	25	8.41	2.97	1.32	2.12	5.64	0.47	1.42	0.19

Table 2. Number of subjects with regression and progression in treatment and control groups, respectively

Group	Regression	Progression	All
Treatment	2	1	3
Control	1	7	8
All	3	8	11

dent's t-test, *P* values for one-tailed tests were 0.15, 0.14 and 0.09 respectively. Thus the effects on atheroma development were not statistically significant in this small group of patients. The mean concentrations of VLDL and HDL triglyceride decreased significantly more in those whose atheroma regressed ($n=3$), and HDL cholesterol increased significantly more than in those whose atheroma progressed ($n=8$).

Correlation analysis showed that significant correlations existed between regression and decrease in HDL triglyceride ($r=-0.78$) (Fig. 1), and between regression and decrease in total cholesterol ($r=-0.58$). Correlations of borderline significance were seen between regression and decrease in LDL ($r=-0.49$) and HDL cholesterol ($r=0.48$). Multiple-regression analysis demonstrated that 94% of the variability in femoral atheroma ($R^2=0.94$) could be explained by the changes in HDL triglyceride ($P<0.01$), total triglyceride ($P<0.001$) and VLDL triglyceride ($P<0.001$).

Thus, lowering serum lipid for 1 year was found to have no significant effect on femoral atheroma development when compared with placebo-treated controls in this small sample of asymptomatic men with hyperlipidemia. Change in atheroma size was seen in only one-quarter of the patients, and because of the small sample size, the probability of type 2 error is high.

However, subgroup analysis showed interesting relations between change of change and effects on serum lipoproteins. The decrease in HDL triglyceride was highly significantly related to regression, but the triglyceride content of other lipoprotein fractions was shown to be of importance by multiple-regression analysis. These findings are in agreement with the results of Blankenhorn et al. [4]. They reported, in an uncontrolled study of 25 patients followed for a similar length of time (13 months), a high correlation between serum triglyceride concentration and percentage change of CEA per month in subjects with type IV hyperlipoproteinemia. No significant correlates were found in type II hyperlipoproteinemia. It thus

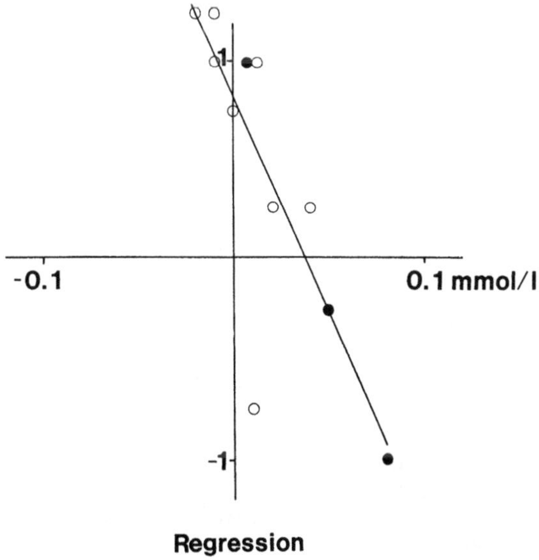

Fig. 1. Relation between change of HDL triglyceride concentration and visual estimation of change in femoral atherosclerosis. ●, Treatment group; ○, control group; $r=-0.78$

seems that the serum triglyceride, but not serum cholesterol, concentration has a bearing on atheroma changes that occur in 1 year. It is possible that this reflects a selection phenomen in the sense that triglyceride-rich atheroma more readily changes size when triglyceride is lowered than does tissue cholesterol on lowering of cholesterol.

References

1. Aschoff L (1924) Atherosclerosis. In: Lectures in pathology (delivered in the United States, 1924). Hoeber, New York
2. Malinow MR (1984) Regression of atherosclerosis in humans: anatomical evidence from post mortem studies. In Malinow MR, Blaton VH (eds) Regression of atherosclerotic lesions: experimental studies and observations in humans. Plenum, New York, pp 329-337 (Life Sciences, vol 79)
3. Wanscher O, Clemmesen J, Neilson A (1951) Negative correlation between atherosclerosis and carcinoma. Br J Cancer 5: 172
4. Blankenhorn DH, Brooks SH, Selzer RH, Barndt R (1978) The rate of atherosclerosis change during treatment of hyperlipoproteinemia. Circulation 57: 355
5. Olsson AG, Erikson U, Helmius G, Hemmingsson A, Ruhn G (1984) Regression of femoral atherosclerosis in humans: methodological and clinical problems associated with studies on femoral atherosclerosis development as assessed by angiograms. In Malinow MR, Blaton VH (eds) Regression of atherosclerotic lesions: experimental studies and observations in humans. Plenum, New York, p 311 (Life Sciences, vol 79)
6. De Rouen TA, Murray JA, Owen W (1977) Variability in the analysis of coronary arteriograms. Circulation 55: 324
7. Brensike JF, Levy RI, Kelsey SF et al (1984) Effects of therapy with cholestyramine on progression of coronary arteriosclerosis: results of the NHLBI type II coronary intervention study. Circulation 69: 313
8. Blankenhorn DH, Brooks SH (1981) Angiographic trial of lipid-lowering therapy. Arteriosclerosis 1: 242
9. Brown BG, Bolson EL, Dodge HT (1982) Arteriographic assessment of coronary atherosclerosis: review of current methods, their limitations, and clinical applications. Arteriosclerosis 2: 2
10. Hamsten A, Walldius G, Szamosi A et al (1986) Relationship of angiographically defined coronary artery disease to serum lipoproteins and apolipoproteins in young survivors of myocardial infarction. In: Hamsten A, Studies on Myocardial Infarction at Young Age, thesis, Karolinska Institute
11. Nikkilä EA, Viikinkoski P, Valle M, Frick MH (1984) Prevention of progression of coronary artherosclerosis by treatment of hyperlipidaemia: a seven year prospective angiographic study. Br Med J 289: 220
12. Levy RI, Brensike JF, Epstein SE et al (1984) The influence of changes in lipid values induced by cholestyramine and diet on progression of coronary artery disease: results of the NHLBI type II coronary intervention study. Circulation 69: 325
13. Detre KM, Kelsey SF, Levy RI (1985) Effects of cholestyramine on incidence of morbidity and mortality: NHLBI type II coronary intervention study. Council on Arteriosclerosis, American Society for the study of arteriosclerosis, Washington, DC, November 1985. Arteriosclerosis 5: 512a
14. Kramer JR, Matsuda Y, Mulligan DO (1981) Progression of coronary atherosclerosis. Circulation 63: 519
15. Arntzenius AC, Kromhout D, Barth J et al (1985) Diet, lipoproteins, and the progression of coronary atherosclerosis. N Engl J Med 312: 805
16. Blankenhorn DH (1984) Progress report on a lipid-lowering trial in men with coronary bypass surgery. In: Carlson LA, Olsson AG (eds) Treatment of hyperlipoproteinemia. Raven, New York, p 211

17. Duffield RGM, Miller NE, Brunt JNH et al (1983) Treatment of hyperlipidaemia retards progression of symptomatic femoral atherosclerosis: a randomised controlled trial. Lancet II: 639
18. Olsson AG, Erikson U, Helmius G et al (1986) The effect of pronounced serum lipid lowering for one year on the development of femoral atherosclerosis in asymptomatic hyperlipoproteinemia. In: Fidge NH, Nestel PJ (eds) atherosclerosis VII. Excerpta Medica
19. Crawford DW, Brooks SH, Selzer RH et al (1977) Computer densitometry for angiographic assessment of arterial cholesterol content and gross pathology in human atherosclerosis. J Lab Clin Med 89: 378

Plasma Exchange and Its Development in the Treatment of Familial Hypercholesterolemia

M. Mancini, A. Postiglione, and A. Gnasso

Introduction

The treatment of patients with homozygous familial hypercholesterolemia (FH) is a difficult and daunting clinical problem. Diet and drugs have little influence on the hypercholesterolemia of these patients; combinations of cholestyramine and nicotinic acid [1], compactin [2] and probucol [3] have also been tried but all have failed to provide adequate and satisfactory control of the disease. More recently mevinolin, a specific HMG-CoA reductase inhibitor, has produced good results in the treatment of heterozygous FH [4], but data on the homozygous form are still lacking.

The severity of the disease needs a strong and tireless adequate treatment. Therefore various nonpharmacological alternatives have been tried. Among the surgical possibilities, partial ileal bypass has proved to be useful in the treatment of the milder cases of heterozygous FH but ineffective in most homozygotes [5]. Portacaval shunt has yielded clinical benefit in approximately two-thirds of the operated patients, while serum cholesterol levels have remained unchanged and complications such as infertility, increased platelet aggregation and shunt closure have occurred in the remainder [6, 7].

Periodic plasma exchange (PE) in FH patients was first described by Thompson et al. [8]. PE is a procedure whereby blood is removed continously from the patients and red cells separated and returned to the donor after resuspension in plasma protein fraction (PPF), fresh-frozen plasma, or 5% albumin in physiological saline. Using the former solution, up to 4 liters plasma can be exchanged and plasma cholesterol concentration markedly lowered. As anticoagulant heparin is used for continuous flow cell separators and acid citrate dextrose (ACD) for discontinuous flow machines.

The usefulness of PE for the treatment of homozygous FH has been subsequently confirmed and reported by many others. The youngest patient treated by this procedure has been a 4-year-old FH homozygote [9]; in most instances, PE has been well-tolerated without any serious side-effect and with clinical benefit. Thompson reported that PE with up to 4 liters of PPF at 1-2 weekly intervals, combined with 3-5 g daily oral nicotinic acid, is a safe and reliable means of reducing the average level of serum total cholesterol by roughly 50% in homozygous FH on a long-term basis [10-13]. This reported efficacy of nicotinic acid to slow down the expected post-exchange rebound of plasma cholesterol has not been confirmed by Keller et al., who used beta-pyridylcarbinol or cholestyramine [14].

Biological Effects of PE

Changes in Lipids and Lipoproteins

After each procedure of PE there is a rapid decrease in serum cholesterol concentration constantly followed by a slower rebound. The magnitude of the immediate decrease (about 40%-70%) is determined by the volume of plasma exchanged and the patient's blood volume. The best control of hypercholesterolemia is undoubtedly achieved by weekly rather than biweekly PE. Figure 1 shows the decrease and the post-exchange rebound of the cholesterol mojety of various plasma lipoproteins

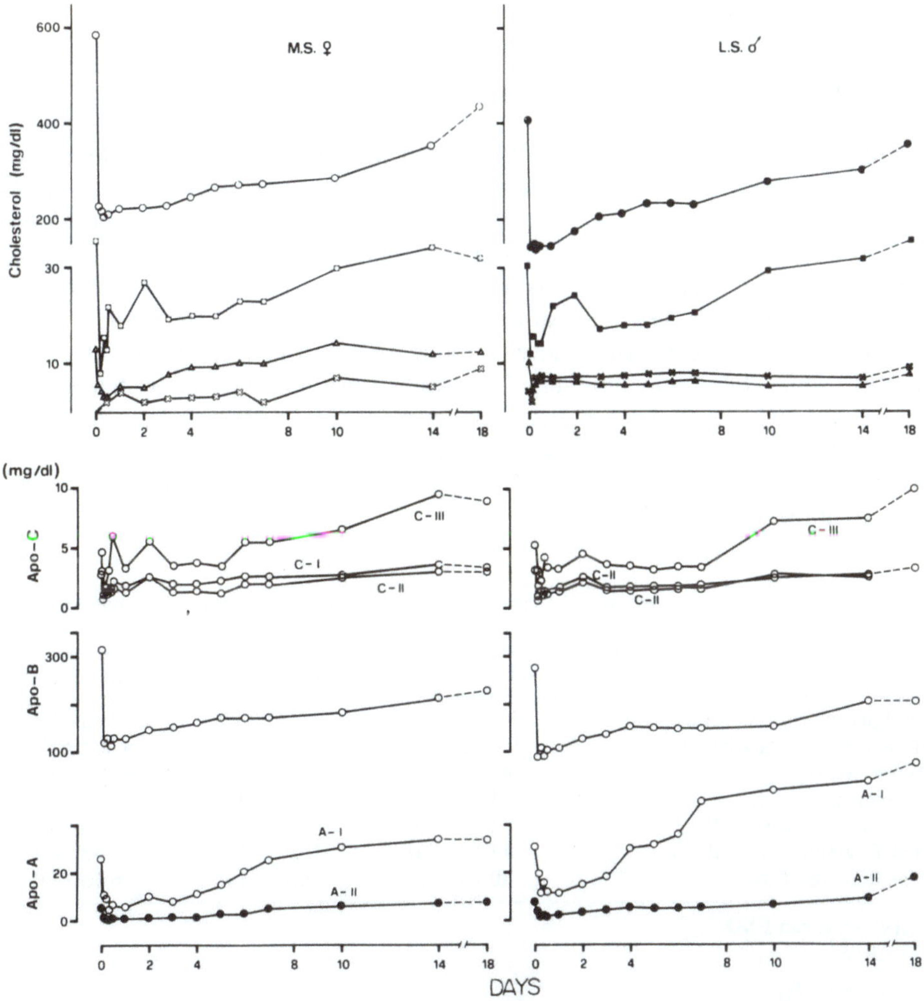

Fig. 1. Effect of PE on LDL (○ ●), HDL (□ ■), IDL (⊠ ✖), VLDL (△ ▲) cholesterol *(upper panel)* and on major plasma apolipoprotein concentrations *(lower panel)* in two homozygous FH patients

(upper panel) and of major plasma apolipoproteins (lower panel) in two homozygous FH patients. Plasma total cholesterol concentration decrease is mainly due to a reduction of low-density lipoprotein (LDL) and, to a certain extent, to the removal of high-density lipoprotein (HDL). The latter more rapidly returns to the pre-exchange level than the LDL fraction; transfer of cholesterol from the extra- to the intravascular pool after PE has been shown by radioisotopic studies. In a patient who had been given ^{14}C-cholesterol before PE, changes in the plasma cholesterol specific activity were produced, indicating that tissue cholesterol is selectively taken up by HDL during the 1th week after PE [11]. The lower panel in Fig. 1 shows that apolipoprotein B is greatly reduced after PE and progressively increases during the subsequent days. All plasma apolipoprotein C (C I, C II, C III) returned to the previous level within a short time, as did plasma apolipoprotein A I, the main constituent of HDL, whose concentration was even higher than baseline values 8-10 days after PE.

Hemodynamic and Hemorheological Effects

By reducing plasma concentration of fibrinogen and LDL, PE decreases blood and plasma viscosity by 20%-80% at low shear rate [15] and improves the erythrocyte filtration rate [16]. These positive hemorheological effects improve arterial blood flow, as shown in Table 1, where a lower limb reactive hyperemia test after PE is reported for five FH patients. As expected, plasma cholesterol, significantly reduced during the 1st week of treatment, was then found at an intermediate value as compared to the pretreatment level. Resting arterial flow was slightly increased after PE, while at the same time significant improvement in the reactive hyperemia test occurred with an increase in peak flow over the calf by about 25%. A dissociation between plasma cholesterol levels and flow rates is evident: despite a marked rise in plasma cholesterol during the 2nd week, the hemodynamic effects are not reduced at the same time [17].

Table 1. Reactive hyperemia test over the calf after plasma exchange in familial hypercholesterolemia

	Baseline	Week 1	Week 2
Total plasma cholesterol (mg/dl)	662.8 ± 107.6	478.9 ± 97.2[a]	582.9 ± 72.9
Plasma triglyceride (mg/dl)	164.6 ± 65.1	151.4 ± 59.8	149.6 ± 65.1
Packed red cell (%)	42 ± 6	41 ± 6	42 ± 6
Fibrinogen (mg/dl)	324 ± 36	300 ± 29	310 ± 41
Rest flow ($ml/min^{-1}/dl^{-1}$)	2.1 ± 0.6	2.6 ± 0.5	2.9 ± 0.5[a]
Peak flow ($ml/min^{-1}/dl^{-1}$)	13.3 ± 0.6	16.7 ± 1.3[a]	15.4 ± 0.9[a]
Peak flow/rest flow	10.1 ± 3.8	6.1 ± 1.0	6.1 ± 1.0

Values are mean ± SD.
[a] $P < 0.05$.

Effects on Hemostasis and Circulating Platelets

Platelets from FH patients aggregate in response to significantly lower concentrations of aggregating agents, such as adenosine diphosphate (ADP), collagen, arachidonic acid (AA), thrombin, than platelets from normal controls (Table 2) [18]. PE causes a short-lived reduction in the platelet counts and in coagulation factors, not giving rise to any clinical manifestation. Brook et al. [19] have also demonstrated a post-exchange decrease of in vitro platelet hyperreactivity to various aggregating agents in homozygous FH. Circulating platelets from these patients, when observed by electron microscopy, show an increased number of cell wall irregularities as compared to normocholesterolemic subjects. The extent of these abnormalities, very likely related to plasma cholesterol concentration, was markedly reduced after PE [20].

PE Developments

PE has some limitations: it lacks selectivity and specificity and its efficacy is limited for the increasing dilution of plasma cholesterol. The exchange fluids are very expensive and, furthermore, a very important disadvantage is the unwanted loss of non-atherogenic HDL as well as other precious plasma components, including albumin and immunoglobulins. It is therefore of great interest that a selective removal of LDL (LDL apheresis) has been tried in patients with FH by the following new methods:

- Heparin agarose beads [21, 22]
- Anti-LDL antibody agarose gel [23-26]
- LDL precipitation by heparin at low pH [27]
- Double membrane filtration [28]
- LDL adsorption by dextran sulphate cellulose [28, 29]

The LDL antibody and the dextran sulphate adsorption seem at present the most reliable and effective procedures. Experience with dextran sulphate cellulose columns was first described in Japan. Unpublished observations in eight FH heterozy-

Table 2. The AC 50 of platelet aggregating agents on platelet suspensions from controls and FH subjects

Aggregating agent	Controls ($n=10$)	FH patients ($n=9$)
ADP (μM)	2.15 ± 0.38	0.50 ± 0.11 [a]
Collagen (μg/ml)	0.46 ± 0.09	0.11 ± 0.02 [a]
AA (μM)	11.10 ± 1.14	2.83 ± 0.46 [a]
Thrombin (milliunits/ml)	11.06 ± 1.22	3.77 ± 0.61 [a]
U-46619 (μg/ml)	0.46 ± 0.11	0.53 ± 0.14

AC 50 is defined as the lowest concentration of an aggregating agent that causes a 50% light transmittance within 3 min.
Values are mean ± SD.
[a] $P < 0.01$.

Table 3. Comparison of selective LDL adsorption plasmapheresis procedures

	Heparin agarose	Anti-LDL antibody agarose	Dextran sulphate cellulose
Plasma separator	No	Centrifuge	Hollow fiber filter
Extracorporeal volume (ml)	400-700	500	500
Additional infusion (ml)	No	300-500	No
Operation	Intermittent	Continuous (2 columns)	Continuous (1 column)
Removal specificity	LDL, VLDL	LDL, VLDL	LDL, VLDL
Capacity of gel (g chol/l gel)	19	5	19
LDL cholesterol removal (g)	1.3-5.2	5.6	5.5-7.5
Time (h)	-	3	2

gous patients, undergoing LDL apheresis at biweekly intervals, have shown a 43%-68% decrease of total serum cholesterol, while HDL cholesterol reduction was limited at only 0%-28%. No adverse reactions, such as severe anemia or complement activation, have been noted in these studies [30]. A comparison of these selective removals of LDL is given in Table 3 [29]. Dextran sulphate cellulose columns have several advantages compared to the original PE. Columns are autoclavable and disposable, while anti-LDL antibody agarose needs a prolonged and accurate maintainance.

Conclusions

PE is currently the most effective method of controlling hypercholesterolemia in homozygous FH patients and has proved to be safe over periods of more than 5 years. In one homozygous FH patient, continuously treated by our group by PE at biweekly intervals for 5 years, cutaneous xanthomas as well as signs and symptoms of myocardial ischemia have totally disappeared. Various other patients treated by PE by Thompson [13] have lived longer than their homozygous siblings, who died at an earlier age without receiving this form of treatment. Obvious difficulties deriving for the periodicity of PE may be very likely minimized by the new developments in this technique. The effectiveness and the safety of this therapeutical approach, which has already been proven to reduce the progression of atherosclerosis, is of undoubted clinical interest.

References

1. Moutafis CD, Myant NB, Mancini M, Oriente P (1971) Cholestyramine and nicotinic acid in the treatment of familial hyperbetalipoproteinemia in homozygous form. Atherosclerosis 14: 247
2. Yamamoto A, Sudo H, Endo A (1980) Therapeutic effects of ML-236 B in primary hypercholesterolemia. Atherosclerosis 35: 259
3. Baker SG, Joffe BI, Mendelsohn D, Seftel MC (1982) Treatment of homozygous familial hypercholesterolemia with probucol. S Afr Med J 62: 7

4. Grundy SM, Bilheimer DW (1984) Influence of inhibition of 3-hydroxy-3-methylglutaryl CoA reductase by mevinolin in familial hypercholesterolemia heterozygotes: effect on cholesterol balance. Proc Natl Acad Sci USA 81: 2538
5. Miettinen TA (1980) Comparison of cholestyramine, ileal by-pass and portacaval shunt in the treatment of familial hypercholesterolemia. In: Gotto AM, Smith LC, Allen B (eds) Atherosclerosis V. Springer, Berlin Heidelberg New York, p 470
6. Stein EA, Glueck CJ (1980) Homozygous familial hypercholesterolemia, treatment of portacaval shunt. In: Gotto AM, Smith LC, Allen B (eds) Atherosclerosis V. Springer, Berlin Heidelberg New York, p 474
7. Forman MB, Baker GG, Mieny CJ, Joffe B, Sandler MP, Mendelsohn D, Seftel HC (1982) Treatment of homozygous familial hypercholesterolemia with portacaval shunt. Atherosclerosis 41: 349
8. Thompson GR, Lowenthal R, Myant NB (1975) Plasma exchange in the management of familial hypercholesterolemia. Lancet 1: 1208
9. Witztum JL, William JC, Ostlund R, Sherman L, Siccard G, Schonfeld G (1980) Successful plasmapheresis in a four year old child with homozygous familial hypercholesterolemia. J Pediatr 97: 615
10. Thompson GR (1979) Management of familial hypercholesterolemia and new approaches to the treatment of atherosclerosis. In: Paoletti R, Gotto AM (eds) Atherosclerosis Review, vol 5. Raven, New York, p 67
11. Thompson GR (1981) Plasma exchange for hypercholesterolemia. Lancet 1: 1246
12. Thompson GR (1981) Long-term plasma exchange in severe familial hypercholesterolemia. In: NIH (ed) Proceedings of the workshop on therapeutic plasma pheresis. NIH, Washington, p 1665
13. Thompson GR (1983) Plasma exchange and affinity chromatographic therapy for hyperlipoproteinemia: a review. Apheresis Bull 1: 26
14. Keller C, Hailer S, Demant T, Wolfram G, Zöllner N (1985) Effect of plasma exchange with and without concomitant drug treatment on lipids and lipoproteins in patients with familial hypercholesterolemia confirmed by tissue culture. Atherosclerosis 57: 225
15. Kilpatrick D, Fleming J, Clyne C, Thompson GR (1979) Reduction of blood viscosity following plasma exchange. Atherosclerosis 32: 301
16. Postiglione A, Soricelli A, Lamenza F, Scarpato N, Montefusco S (1982) Plasma exchange for the treatment of cerebrovascular disease in familial hypercholesterolemia. J Chronic Dis Ther Res 6: 213
17. Rubba P, Postiglione A, Scarpato N, Iannuzzi A, Mancini M (1985) Improved reactive hyperemia test after plasma exchange in familial hypercholesterolemia. Atherosclerosis 56: 237
18. Di Minno G, Silver MJ, Cerbone AM, Rainone A, Postiglione A, Mancini M (1986) Increased fibrinogen binding to platelets from patients with familial hypercholesterolemia. Arteriosclerosis 6: 203
19. Brook GI, Winterstein G, Aviram M (1983) Platelet function and lipoprotein levels after plasma exchange in patients with familial hypercholesterolemia. Clin Sci 64: 637
20. Weber G, Bianciardi G, Toti P, Scarpato N, Postiglione A, Mancini M (1984) Ultrastructural features of circulating platelets from hypercholesterolemic (type II a) patients submitted to plasma exchange. A freeze etching study. In: Carlson LA, Olsson AG (eds) Treatment of hyperlipoproteinemia. Raven, New York, p 143
21. Lupien PJ, Moorjani S, Awad J (1976) A new approach to the management of familial hypercholesterolemia: removal of plasma cholesterol based on the principle of affinity chromatography. Lancet 1: 1261
22. Lupien PJ, Moorjani S, Gagne C, Brun LD, Lou M, Dagenais G (1982) Long term treatment of two familial hypercholesterolemic heterozygote patients with batch affinity chromatography (BAC). Artery 10: 288
23. Stoffel W, Demant T (1981) Selective removal of apolipoprotein B-containing lipoproteins from blood plasma. Proc Natl Acad Sci USA 78: 611
24. Stoffel W, Borberg H, Greve V (1981) Application of specific extracorporeal removal of low density lipoprotein in familial hyperlipoproteinemia. Lancet 2: 1005
25. Stoffel W, Bode C (1984) Selective removal of low density lipoproteins. In: Pineda AA (ed) Selective plasma component removal. Mount Kisco, New York, p 1

26. Tauchert M, Stoffel W, Bode C (1982) LDL-apheresis in patients with hypercholesterolemia type II a (Abstr). Circulation 68: III-290
27. Fuchs C, Windisch M, Wieland H (1983) Selective continuous extracorporeal elimination of low density lipoproteins from plasma by precipitation with heparin without cations (Abstr). Proc Annu Meet Am Soc Artif Intern Organs 12: 82
28. Yokoyama S, Kikkawa T, Hayashi R (1983) Plasmapheresis therapy of hypercholesterolemias. In: Nose Y, Malchesky PS, Smith JW (eds) Plasmapheresis: New trends in therapeutic applications. ISAO, Cleveland, p 231
29. Yokoyama S, Hayashi R, Kikkawa T (1984) Specific sorbent of apolipoprotein B-containing lipoproteins for plasmapheresis: characterization and experimental use in hypercholesterolemic rabbits. Arteriosclerosis 4: 276
30. Sakai K, Mabuchi H (1985) Plasma exchange therapy for homozygous familial hypercholesterolemia with a dextran sulfuric acid cellulose column (KNA-01). 17th General Assembly of the Japan Society of the Study of Arteriosclerosis, Sendai

The HELP System: A Novel Technique for the Extracorporeal Treatment of Familial Hypercholesterolemia

V. W. Armstrong and D. Seidel

Introduction

Extracorporeal plasma therapy has now been used for several years in the treatment of severe hypercholesterolemia. An improved survival has been reported for five subjects with homozygous familial hypercholesterolemia (FH) who had been on regular plasmapheresis for a mean of 8 years, as compared with their untreated siblings [1]. The benefit of plasmapheresis for the treatment of heterozygous FH is less clear. Symptomatic improvement has been reported in three out of four individuals who were treated every 1-2 weeks, and in one individual whose cholesterol levels could be normalized there was also angiographic evidence of improvement [2, 3]. Other authors [4], however, came to the conclusion that plasmapheresis offered no further advantages over normal diet and drug therapy, although in this study treatment was performed only once every 4 weeks. It is important to realize in this respect that the nature of plasma exchange therapy is such that an effective lowering of plasma cholesterol concentration can only be achieved if therapy is performed on a frequent and regular basis.

Since conventional plasma exchange requires replacement of the patient's own plasma with a donor plasma, or more usually a plasma protein fraction, complications can arise due to the introduction of foreign protein and the transmission of infectious diseases. In order to circumvent such problems, specific procedures have been developed for the selective elimination of low-density lipoprotein (LDL), allowing return of the patient's own plasma. These include binding of LDL to heparin-agarose [5], anti-LDL-sepharose [6], and immobilized dextran sulfate [7], as well as cascade filtration [7, 8] and thermofiltration [9].

We have developed a further procedure [10, 11] for the elimination of not only LDL from plasma but also fibrinogen, that is based on their precipitation at acid pH in the presence of heparin. This procedure has been named HELP, *H*eparin *E*xtracorporeal *L*DL *P*recipitation, and is the subject of this article.

Heparin-Induced Precipitation of Plasma Lipoproteins and Proteins

It has long been known that lipoproteins can be precipitated by polyanions at neutral pH with divalent metal ions. However, the different lipoprotein classes also demonstrate a pH-dependent precipitation with heparin in the absence of divalent cations [12]. The actual pH at which a particular lipoprotein can be precipitated depends upon several factors including the ionic strength of the medium, the pres-

Table 1. In vitro precipitation of plasma proteins from K^+/EDTA plasma with 0.2 *M* acetate buffer containing 150 IU heparin/ml

Protein	pH of acetate buffer[a] at which maximum precipitation occurs	Protein precipitated (%)
Total protein	4.0–4.6	17
Apolipoprotein B	4.6–4.85	86
Apolipoprotein A I	4.6	6
Fibrinogen	4.2–5.0	88
Plasminogen	4.4	80
Complement C 4	5.0	82
Complement C 3	4.6	60
Antithrombin III	4.4	25
Albumin	<4.0	5
IgG	4.8	2

[a] Plasma was mixed with an equal volume of a 0.2 *M* acetate buffer adjusted to the appropriate pH.

ence or absence of other plasma proteins, and the heparin concentration. However, of the three major lipoprotein classes, high density (HDL), very low density (VLDL) and low density (LDL), the latter are precipitated at a higher pH range than the other two. A selective procedure could, therefore, be developed for the measurement of LDL cholesterol in serum or plasma by precipitation of LDL with heparin at a pH of 5.12 [13].

In addition to LDL, a limited number of plasma proteins are also precipitated by heparin at low pH. The results for some representative proteins from our in vitro investigations are summarized in Table 1. Approximately 17% of total plasma protein could be precipitated using buffers in the pH range of 4.0–4.6. The final pH range of the buffer-plasma mixture was then 4.28–4.83. Typical heparin-binding proteins such as apolipoprotein B (apo B), fibrinogen, plasminogen, and the complement factors C 3 and C 4 could all be precipitated from plasma with heparin at acidic pH. However, other proteins such as apo A I, albumin, and IgG that do not bind heparin were hardly precipitated under these conditions. A prerequisite for the effective precipitation of proteins from plasma at acidic pH would therefore appear to be their ability to form complexes with heparin at physiological pH. An exception is antithrombin (AT) III. Only 25% of this protein could be precipitated in vitro under the above conditions. A possible explanation for this limited precipitation may be the fact that AT III binds preferentially to low molecular weight heparins, whereas high molecular weight heparins are more effective in the precipitation of plasma lipoproteins and proteins (V. W. Armstrong, D. Noll and D. Seidel, unpublished observations).

The HELP System

On the basis of our in vitro studies, an extracorporeal procedure for the continuous elimination of LDL with heparin at acidic pH was developed in collaboration with

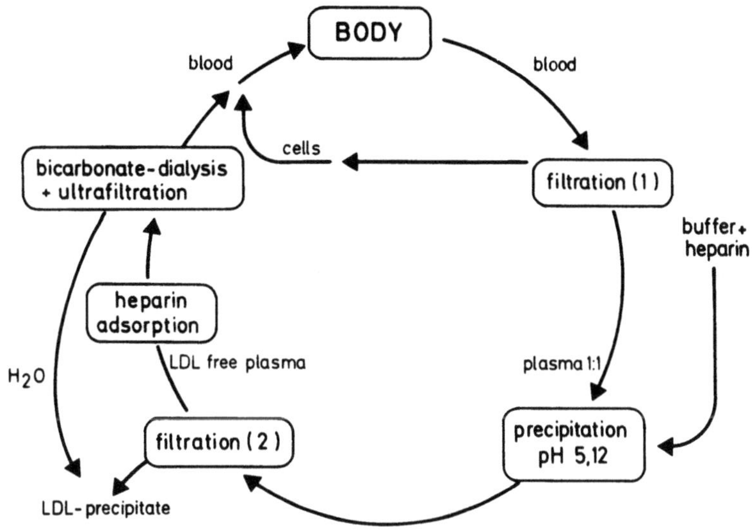

Fig. 1. Flow chart for the HELP procedure

the firm of B. Braun (Melsungen, FRG). The flow scheme is illustrated in Fig. 1. In the first step, plasma is obtained by filtration of whole blood through a 0.2-μm filter (filter 1). This is then mixed continuously with a 0.3 *M* acetate buffer of pH 4.85 containing 100 IU heparin/ml. The flow rates of plasma and buffer are normally identical and range from 20 to 30 ml/min. Precipitation occurs in a small mixing chamber at a pH of around 5.12 and the suspension is continuously recirculated through a 0.4-μm polycarbonate filter (filter 2), from which an LDL-free, clear filtrate is obtained. Approximately 50% of the heparin required for the precipitation is removed with the precipitate while the remainder is adsorbed by passage of the plasma through an anion-exchange filter. At a pH of 5.12 the polyanionic heparin is still highly negatively charged on account of its strongly acidic sulfate groups, while plasma proteins will be positively charged at this pH and therefore not retained by the filter. Table 2 shows the data from an in vitro experiment illustrating the function and effectiveness of the heparin adsorber.

After the heparin adsorption the buffer-plasma mixture is subject to bicarbonate dialysis and ultrafiltration. In this step excess fluid is removed, physiological pH is

Table 2. In vitro removal of heparin by an anion-exchange filter

	Heparin concentration (IU/ml)	Protein concentration (g/l)	Cholesterol concentration (mg/dl)
Before 0.4-μm filter	50	29.1	71.3
After 0.4-μm filter	27	26.8	24.3
After anion-exchange filter	0	26.8	22.4

4 l plasma was mixed with 4 l 0.3 *M* acetate (pH 4.85) containing 100 IU heparin/ml and the mixture was filtered through a 0.4-μm polycarbonate filter and an anion-exchange filter.

restored, and the acetate levels in the plasma are reduced by over 90% [10]. Finally, the plasma is mixed with the blood cells from filter 1 before being returned to the patient.

The filters and tubing required for treatment are all sterile, disposable systems that are intended for single use only. The total extracorporeal volume of the system amounts to approximately 1100 ml, of which half is plasma and the other half acetate buffer during treatment. Before beginning each treatment the filters are washed and primed with an isotonic salt solution. In order to treat a homozygous child, the buffer-to-plasma ratio is altered to 3:1, thereby reducing the total amount of plasma in the extracorporeal system. The plasma flow in this case is around 10 ml/min and the buffer heparin concentration can be lowered from 100 to 50 IU/ml.

Clinical Experience with the HELP System

Specificity and Efficiency. The aim of any elimination procedure must be to achieve complete elimination of LDL in a single passage through the extracorporeal circuit. If this is the case, then plasma LDL levels would be reduced from 100% to 37% of their original value if the volume of plasma treated is equivalent to the total plasma volume of the patient. The LDL cholesterol concentration at the end of treatment can then be predicted [11, 14] from the exponential equation

$$C_E = C_0 \exp \frac{(-\mathrm{PE})}{(\mathrm{PV})},$$

where C_E is the LDL cholesterol concentration at the end of treatment, C_0 is the LDL cholesterol concentration at the start of treatment, PE is the volume of plasma treated, and PV is the plasma volume of the patient. Therefore, knowing the actual LDL cholesterol concentration at the end of treatment (and the plasma volume of the patient) the efficiency of the elimination can be calculated not only for LDL cholesterol, but also for other plasma lipoproteins and proteins whose concentrations in plasma can be measured. The data obtained from a total of 20 treatments with the HELP procedure are presented in Table 3. LDL cholesterol, fibrinogen and

Table 3. Efficiency of the elimination of various plasma lipoproteins and proteins by HELP as derived from 20 different HELP procedures

Protein/lipoprotein	Elimination (%)
LDL cholesterol	102
Fibrinogen	97
Complement C4	97
Plasminogen	84
C1 inhibitor	82
C3 complement	59
AT III	44
Total protein	22
HDL cholesterol, albumin, IgG, IgA, IgM, transferrin, ferritin	<18

Table 4. Mean concentrations of LDL cholesterol, fibrinogen, and plasminogen during therapy as compared with the values before therapy

Patient	No. of HELP treatments	Duration of therapy (weeks)	LDL cholesterol (mg/dl)				Fibrinogen (mg/dl)				Plasminogen (mg/dl)			
			Before therapy	$\overline{AP}$	$\overline{EP}$	$\frac{(\overline{AP}+\overline{EP})}{2}$	Before therapy	$\overline{AP}$	$\overline{EP}$	$\frac{(\overline{AP}+\overline{EP})}{2}$	Before therapy	$\overline{AP}$	$\overline{EP}$	$\frac{(\overline{AP}+\overline{EP})}{2}$
E.S.	48	56	323	212	73	143	395	263	109	186	11.4	11.0	4.8	7.9
H.E.	39	50	365	266	107	187	410	281	137	209	14.6	14.1	7.4	10.8
R.K.	30	41	252	155	80	118	360	277	156	217	10.2	10.0	6.0	8.0
C.G.	20	23	240	152	44	98	260	201	88	145	9.2	9.2	4.2	6.7
J.C.	31	26	796	407	181	294	375	318	163	241	11.8	10.3	5.9	8.1

$\overline{AP}$, mean value at the beginning of each HELP procedure.
$\overline{EP}$, mean value at the end of each HELP procedure.

complement C4 were all virtually totally eliminated from the plasma in a single pass through the extracorporeal system. Plasminogen and C1 esterase inhibitor were also precipitated to a large extent. In agreement with our in vitro observations, complement C3 was only partially eliminated by the HELP procedure as was ATIII; the concentrations of the latter at the end of each treatment averaged approximately 75% of the original value. A small loss of total plasma protein was observed due to precipitation of the above proteins as well as unspecific losses. Of the other proteins and lipoproteins that were measured, only minor unspecific elimination occurred.

Long-Term Treatment. A total of 158 HELP procedures have now been performed in five patients, four adults (two male, two female) with heterozygous FH and one young girl with homozygous FH. The duration of therapy has ranged from 23 to 56 weeks and the average frequency is once every 9 days (Table 4). Cholesterol levels could not be normalized in these patients by diet and drug therapy alone. Treatment by HELP, however, has further reduced their LDL cholesterol levels. In two of the patients (R. K., C. G.) concentrations now remain continually within the normal range. Even in the other two patients (E. S., H. E.) pretreatment LDL cholesterol levels have been lowered by over 30% compared with the levels before HELP therapy.

In addition to LDL cholesterol, fibrinogen levels have also been reduced by HELP therapy, pretreatment levels being 15%–33% lower than the concentrations measured before beginning the therapy. This is of particular interest since fibrinogen levels are often elevated in hypercholesterolemia [15], and fibrinogen and its degradation products are implicated in the atherosclerotic process [16, 17]. Pretreatment plasminogen levels, however, were unaltered by HELP therapy, even though this protein was also effectively eliminated by the HELP procedure.

No ill-effects have yet been observed due to the coprecipitation of other plasma proteins. Overall treatment tolerance and compliance have been good and no major complications have been observed.

Conclusion

Treatment of severe hypercholesterolemia by the HELP procedure provides a safe alternative to conventional plasmapheresis. It displays the same efficiency as the latter and has the added advantage that the patient is not exposed to foreign proteins, thus avoiding immunological problems. The potential of this cholesterol-lowering therapy will depend upon its ability to cause regression of atherosclerotic plaques. Although sporadic observations have been reported in the literature, there are as yet no large-scale studies that have been directed towards this problem. Future work must therefore involve multicenter investigations to ascertain the therapeutic effectiveness of this therapy.

Acknowledgements. The development of the HELP procedure could only have been accomplished by the involvement of a large number of persons from various disciplines. We are particularly grateful in Dr. T. Eisenhauer from the Department of

Nephrology, University Clinic, Göttingen, whose experience in extracorporeal therapy has proved invaluable. We would also like to thank Dr. K. Nebendahl, director of the Department for Animal Studies at the University Clinic, Göttingen, for his assistance in the numerous animal experiments that were necessary before the first clinical application of the HELP procedure.

References

1. Thompson GR, Miller JP, Breslow JL (1985) Improved survival of patients with homozygous familial hypercholesterolaemia treated with plasma exchange. Br Med Journal 291: 1671-1673
2. Thompson GR, Myant NB, Kilpatrick P, Oakley CM, Raphael MJ, Steiner RE (1980) Assessment of long-term plasma exchange for familial hypercholesterolaemia. Br Heart J 43: 680-688
3. Thompson GR (1981) Plasma exchange for hypercholesterolaemia. Lancet I: 1246-1248
4. Simons LA, Gibson JC, Isbister JP, Biggs JC (1978) The effects of plasma exchange on cholesterol metabolism. Atherosclerosis 31: 195-204
5. Lupien PJ, Moojani S, Award J (1976) A new approach to the management of familial hypercholesterolaemia: removal of plasma cholesterol based on the principle of affinity chromatography. Lancet I: 1261-1265
6. Stoffel W, Demant T (1981) Selective removal of apolipoprotein B-containing serum lipoproteins from blood plasma. Proc Natl Acad Sci USA 78: 611-615
7. Yokoyama S, Hayashi R, Satani M, Yamamoto A (1985) Selective removal of low density lipoproteins by plasmapheresis in familial hypercholesterolemia. Arteriosclerosis 5: 613-621
8. von Bayer H, Schwerdlfeger R, Schwartzkopf W, Schrig R, Kochinke F, Marx M, Schutten D (1983) Selective removal of low density lipoproteins (LDL) by plasmapheresis combined with selective plasma-protein ultracentrifugation (SPU). Plasma Ther Transfus Technol 4: 447-458
9. Nose Y, Usani M, Malchesky PS, Emura M, Horiuchi T, Sakamoto H, Smith JW (1985) Clinical thermofiltration: initial application. Artif Organs 9: 425-427
10. Armstrong VW, Windisch M, Wieland H, Fuchs C, Rieger J, Köstering H, Nebendahl K, Scheler F, Seidel D (1983) Selective continuous extracorporal elimination of low-density lipoproteins with heparin at acidic pH. Trans Am Soc Artif Intern Organs 29: 323-327
11. Eisenhauer T, Armstrong VW, Wieland H, Fuchs C, Scheler F, Seidel D (1987) Selective removal of low density lipoproteins (LDL) by precipitation at low pH: first clinical application of the HELP-system. Klin Wochenschr 65 (in press)
12. Burstein M, Scholnick HR (1974) On the precipitation of serum lipoproteins by heparin. Nouv Rev Fr Hematol 14: 131-136
13. Wieland H, Seidel D (1983) A simple specific method for precipitation of low density lipoproteins. J Lipid Res 24: 904-909
14. Thompson GR (1980) Plasma exchange for hypercholesterolaemia: a therapeutic mode and investigative mode. Plasma Ther 1: 5-15
15. Wilhelmsen L, Svärdsudd K, Korsan-Bengtsen K, Larsson B, Welin L, Tibblin G (1984) Fibrinogen as a risk factor for stroke and myocardial infarction. N Engl J Med 311: 501-505
16. Watanabe K, Tanaka K (1983) Influence of fibrin fibrinogen and fibrinogen degradiation products on cultured endothelial cells. Atherosclerosis 48: 57-70
17. Smith EB (1985) Fibrinogen, fibrin and fibrin degradation products in relation to atherosclerosis. In Fidge NH, Nestel PJ (eds) Atherosclerosis VII. Excerpta Medica, pp 459-462

Plasma Exchange for Severe Forms of Familial Hypercholesterolemia: 10 Years' (23 Patient Years') Experience

N. Zöllner, C. Keller, and G. Wolfram

Early coronary atherosclerosis and myocardial infarction are the most disabling complications of untreated familial hypercholesterolemia (FHC) determining the prognosis of these patients. The results of the American LRC study [1] showed that the manifestation and complications of ischemic heart disease due to hypercholesterolemia can be delayed by normalization of serum cholesterol.

In a small group of FHC patients hypercholesterolemia cannot be normalized by conventional lipid-lowering drug treatment. This group consists of the rare homozygous patients with FHC who lack functional low-density lipoprotein (LDL) receptors and of a few young heterozygous FHC patients with very high total and LDL cholesterol. These patients need special attention and intensive cholesterol-lowering treatment because they develop coronary heart disease at a very young age. Plasmapheresis and related procedures seem to be the best treatment for them.

Since the development of a centrifuge allowing the continuous separation of plasma and blood cells, plasmapheresis has become the treatment of choice for severe FHC, first inaugurated by Thompson et al. in 1975 [2].

Our own experience with plasmapheresis for FHC has been gained over the past 10 years by treating three homozygous and three heterozygous patients from half a year to six years continuously. The longest continuous treatment has been conducted in a receptor-defective homozygous male who is now 41 years old. Further details concerning the patients are given in Tables 1 and 2.

Most of the time we have used conventional plasmapheresis with human albumin solution as substitute for the patient's plasma rich in LDL cholesterol.

Plasma exchange (PE) was performed with an IBM cell separator 2997 as a continuous exchange of 2.5 liters patient's plasma within 90–120 min. The centrifuge was primed with isotonic sodium chloride solution containing 1 unit per milliliter heparin and operated at 405 × *g*. Immediately before PE the patient was anticoagulated with a bolus injection of 5000 units heparin. Anticoagulation during the PE was maintained with heparin (1 unit/ml i. v. fluid). Platelet aggregation as well as complement activation were suppressed by acid citrate dextrose A (ACD-A) solution (USA Pharmacopoea) at a ratio 20:1. The blood returning to the patient was warmed up by means of a blood warmer to 37 °C. Potassium and calcium were substituted during PE according to the patient's serum electrolytes before PE. Usually 20 mmol potassium and 10 ml calcium gluconate solution (10%) were sufficient to maintain homeostasis.

With this procedure it was possible to lower cholesterol and all lipoprotein and apolipoprotein fractions acutely by 50% to 60%. The rebound of all moieties after the end of PE is fast and continuous. Within 2 weeks the initial concentrations of

Table 1. Summary of data before plasma exchange (PE). Highest known values before any treatment are listed in the first line of information for each patient; the values before the first PE are without drug treatment for 4 weeks or longer (patients 1–3, 6), or for a few days (patients 4, 5)

Patient	Sex	Age (years)	Tissue culture[a]	Year of first treatment	Plasma lipids and lipoproteins (mg/dl)				
					Total choles-terol	LDL choles-terol	HDL choles-terol	Triglyc-erides	Year of highest known value
Homozygotes									
1[c]	Female	12	Negative	1985	957	852	28	284	1981
					849	727	26	185	
2[b]	Male	24	Negative	1976	1060	–	–	–	1968
				1983	629	595	46	132	
3[c]	Male	41	Defective	1980	795	–	–	124	1972
					600	492	23	184	
Heterozygotes									
4[c]	Male	14	Defective	1986	771	724	33	75	1985
					588	546	26	82	
5[b]	Male	21	Defective	1982	680	–	–	140	1976
					512	464	33	170	
6[b]	Male	30	Defective	1983	508	439	46	122	1982
					462	366	43	213	

[a] Tissue culture of skin fibroblasts to assess LDL receptor function [6].
[b] Weekly treatment.
[c] Treatment every 2 weeks.

Table 2. Summary of cardiovascular data before PE

Patient	Cardiovascular findings
Homozygotes	
1	Angina pectoris for half a year
	Supravalvular aortic stenosis, gradient 20 mm
	Right coronary artery: 75% stenosis at the origin
2	Angina pectoris since the age of 12 years
	Ischemia during exercise ECG at the age of 10 years
	Clinically aortic stenosis and insufficiency, mild
	Massively thickened aortic and mitral valves (echocardiography)
3	Ventricular arrhythmia
	Supravalvular aortic stenosis, gradient 20 mm Hg, aortic insufficiency grade I to II, diffuse atherosclerotic changes of the coronary arteries, right coronary artery: one 50% stenosis, left coronary artery: several stenoses, max. 50%
Heterozygotes	
4	No cardiac symptoms
	Valvular aortic stenosis, gradient small, aortic leaflet calcified
	Coronary arteries normal
5	Angina pectoris since the age of 12 years
	Supravalvular stenosis, gradient 40 mm Hg, left ventricular hypertrophy
	Right coronary artery: 90% stenosis at the origin, left coronary artery: 30% stenosis of the main stem
6	Angina pectoris since the age of 25 years
	Right coronary artery: two 50% stenoses of the mid-portion, ramus interventricularis anterior of the left coronary artery: 90% stenosis of the mid-portion

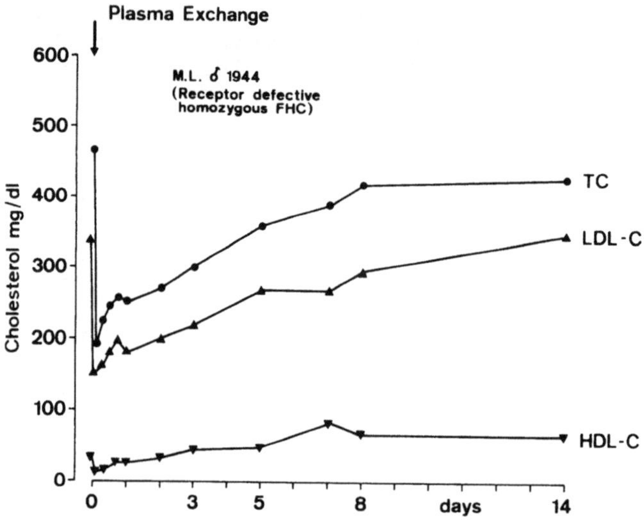

Fig. 1. Typical rebound curve of total *(TC)*, low-density lipoprotein *(LDL-C)*, and high-density lipoprotein *(HDL-C)* cholesterol following plasma exchange within 2 weeks (patient 3)

cholesterol and lipoproteins are nearly reached. The fastest increase is observed during the first week (Fig. 1). Changing the therapeutic interval from one treatment every 2 weeks to one treatment every week leads to additional lowering of cholesterol (Fig. 2) [4].

Lipid-lowering drug therapy in addition to PE does not diminish the rebound of cholesterol and lipoproteins following PE. Though Thompson et al. [3] found that nicotinic acid had an additional cholesterol-lowering effect in their patients, we did not observe the same in our patients. However, the rebound of apolipoprotein B seemed to slow down in our patients when they took either beta-pyridylcarbinol or cholestyramine (Fig. 2) [4].

The removal of lipids and lipoproteins in relation to pre-exchange concentration was about the same for all moieties. The post-exchange rebound of apolipoprotein B was faster than of LDL and total cholesterol. The apolipoproteins A I and A II increased faster than apolipoprotein B but more slowly than high-density lipoprotein (HDL) cholesterol.

The rapid drainage of cholesterol and lipoproteins by PE resulted in a comparable decrease of these moieties in all patients. The subsequent rise was also comparable even though the patients treated were receptor-defective and receptor-negative homozygous patients as shown by skin fibroblast cultures in our own laboratory, and three heterozygous patients [5].

We did not observe severe untoward effects of PE. The amount of albumin infused did not lead to persistent dysproteinemia [6] and 46% of the immunoglobulins were removed with an exchange volume of 2.5 liters [7]. It has been reported [8] that the specific antibody activity is rapidly restored after partial PE with albumin, most likely due to stimulated resynthesis of antibodies following the removal. Even though the patients being treated weekly have subnormal concentrations of immunoglobulins at the end of PE not returning to normal concentrations within one

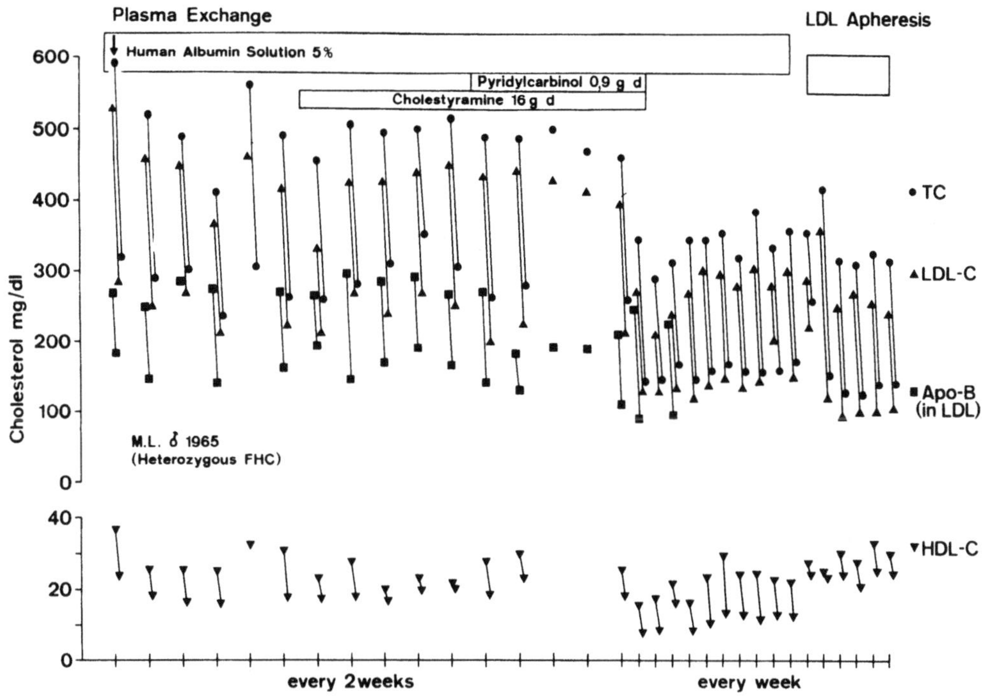

Fig. 2. Comparison of the effects of PE every 2 weeks, of PE every 2 weeks accompanied by drug treatment (cholestyramine 16 g/day; cholestyramine 16 g/day plus pyridylcarbinol 0.9 g/day), of PE every week, and LDL-immuneabsorption (LDL-apherese) every week (patient 3)

week, they have not been prone to infections. We have not observed any bleeding disorder following PE.

Months after starting PE, tuberous xanthoma start to become smaller or disappear. After an interruption of the treatment for at least 3 months tuberous xanthoma started to reappear again or to increase in size. Tendinous xanthoma take much longer to become smaller. Serial measurements of Achilles tendon thickness by xero radiography showed that PE performed every 2 weeks led to a measurable decrease of tendon thickness which became more pronounced as the treatment was carried on. In one of our patients we observed a decrease of 10–12 mm on both feet after 3 years of treatment [9].

The most important aspect of any effective cholesterol-lowering treatment is regression of atherosclerotic vascular lesions, especially in the coronary arteries. One of our patients had a second coronary angiography after 1 year of regular PE every 2 weeks. There was no obvious change in the vascular stenoses after this short period of time. Most likely 1 year is too short to induce regression recognizable by angiography. However, following 3 years of PE every 2 weeks we could demonstrate that aortic valvular stenosis of mild degree (transvalvular gradient 20 mm Hg) had disappeared. This had been suspected before recatherization because the bright reflections in the aortic root observed by echocardiography and indicating calcification of the area had diminished notably during the treatment period. Angiography revealed that the calcification of the aortic cusp rims had become less and coronary stenoses had not increased [10]. Thompson et al. [11] reported recently that the survival of his patients treated by PE continuously since 1975 has been longer than for their homozygous siblings not being treated.

Plasmapheresis is an expensive procedure due to the high price of the albumin solution in addition to the costly equipment for the centrifuge, not even considering the cost for personnel involved in the treatment. The costs of replacement fluid became lower by the development of immuneabsorption of apolipoprotein B-containing lipoproteins by a polyclonal LDL antibody produced in sheep by immunization with human LDL, inaugurated by Stoffel and Demant [12]. Borberg et al. [13] could lower LDL cholesterol by about 70% compared to initial concentration using this procedure and did not observe adverse effects. Our own experience with this method of LDL elimination is limited. One patient being treated with LDL immuneabsorption every week for the past 3 months has not reached a better interim cholesterol concentration than with weekly PE. However, immunoglobulin levels have increased and returned to low normal values since the change of the therapeutic mode.

Another way of preserving the patient's own serum proteins except for LDL cholesterol is to apply various forms of filtration as in use for treatment of autoimmune diseases. Schwerdtfeger et al. [14] have described a variation of cascade filtration which seems to be applicable in connection with a hemodialysis unit. The results he obtained seem to be acceptable except that albumin substitution was necessary in small amounts when cascade filtration was used at weekly intervals.

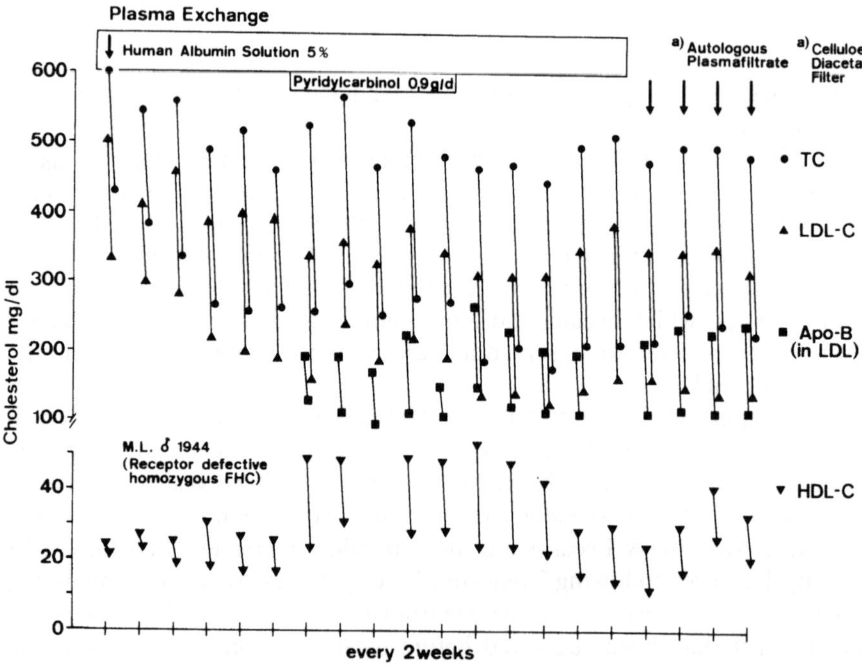

Fig. 3. Comparison of the effects of PE every 2 weeks, of PE every 2 weeks accompanied by treatment with pyridylcarbinol 0.9 g/day or PE with filtrated autologous plasma as substitution solution (patient 3)

We have tried to filter the LDL-rich plasma after the patient has finished PE to gain an autologous plasma as substitution solution for the next PE [15]. Using a filter (manufactured by Dideco) with a pore size of 0.002 μm and a surface of 0.8 m^2 it is possible to produce a plasma containing less than 20 mg/dl LDL cholesterol and about 50% of the initial concentration of albumin and immunoglobulins. As the same exchange volume of 2.5 liters is used and reinfused, the cholesterol-lowering effect of this modified PE is comparable to the conventional PE (Fig. 3). It has to be evaluated whether the patient is able to compensate for the protein loss over a longer period of time. So far, no adverse effects have been observed when applying this exchange solution every 2 weeks.

The results of long-term plasmapheresis in the treatment of FHC have shown that it is a safe procedure, well tolerated by the patient once he has got mentally used to being treated by a method processing a large extracorporeal volume of plasma in a rather short period of time. PE is promising in the respect of ameliorating the prognosis of young patients threatened by early myocardial infarction or sudden cardiac death, as could be shown during the past few years in several centers applying this treatment.

Acknowledgement. These studies have been supported by grants from the Deutsche Forschungsgesellschaft.

References

1. Lipid Research Clinics Program (1984) The Lipid Research Clinics Coronary Primary Prevention Trials results. JAMA 251: 351-364, 365-374
2. Thompson GR, Lowenthal R, Myant MB (1975) Plasma exchange in the management of homozygous familial hypercholesterolemia. Lancet 1: 1208
3. Thompson GR, Myant NB, Kilpatrick D, Oakly CM, Raffael MH, Steiner RE (1980) Assessment of long-term plasma exchange for familial hypercholesterolemia. Br Heart J 43: 680
4. Keller C, Hailer S, Demant T, Wolfram G, Zöllner N (1985) Effect of plasma exchange with and without concomitant drug treatment on lipids and lipoproteins in patients with familial hypercholesterolemia confirmed by tissue culture. Atherosclerosis 57: 225
5. Lundsgaard-Hansen P (1977) Intensive plasmapheresis as a risk factor for arteriosclerotic cardiovascular disease. Vox Sang 33: 1
6. Spengel FA, Harders-Spengel KM, Keller CF, Wieczorek A, Wolfram G, Zöllner N (1982) Use of fibroblast culture to diagnose and phenotype familial hypercholesterolemia. Ann Nutr Metab 26: 240
7. Buffaloe GW, Heineken FG (1983) Plasma volume nomograms for the use in therapeutic plasma exchange. Transfusion 23: 355
8. Orlin JB, Berkman EM (1980) Partial plasma exchange using albumin replacement - removal and recovery of normal plasma constituents. Blood 56: 1055
9. Seidl O, Keller C, Berger H, Wolfram G, Zöllner N (1983) Xeroradiographic determination of Achilles tendon thickness in familial hypercholesterolemia confirmed by tissue cultures. Atherosclerosis 46: 163
10. Keller C, Schmitz H, Theisen K, Zöllner N (1986) Regression of valvular aortic stenosis due to homozygous familial hypercholesterolemia following plasmapheresis. Klin Wochenschr 64: 338
11. Thompson GR, Miller JP, Breslow JL (1985) Improved survival of patients with homozygous familial hypercholesterolemia treated with plasma exchange. Br Med J 291: 1671
12. Stoffel W, Demant T (1981) Selective removal of apolipoprotein B-containing serum lipoproteins from blood plasma. Proc North Acad Sci USA 78: 611

13. Borberg H, Bode C, Mattele L, Oette K, Tauchert M, Stoffel W (1983) LDL-apheresis in hypercholesterolemic patients - technical and clinical aspects. In: Lysaght MJ, Gurland HJ (eds) Plasma separation and plasma fractionation. Karger, Basel, pp 266
14. Schwerdtfeger F, von Baeyer H, Schwartzkopff W, Weiss R, Kochinke F (1984) Long-term results of selective plasmapheretic treatment of familial hypercholesterolemia (FH). Ann Med Interne (Paris) 135: A53
15. Demant T, Gruss M, Keller C (1985) LDL elimination by a combination of plasma separation and plasma filtration in familial hypercholesterolemia. ASFA, 7th Annual Apheresis Symposium, Chicago

MIX
Papier aus verantwortungsvollen Quellen
Paper from responsible sources
FSC® C105338

FSC
www.fsc.org

If you have any concerns about our products,
you can contact us on
ProductSafety@springernature.com

In case Publisher is established outside the EU,
the EU authorized representative is:
Springer Nature Customer Service Center GmbH
Europaplatz 3, 69115 Heidelberg, Germany

Printed by Libri Plureos GmbH
in Hamburg, Germany